This b
self

2

The Art and Soul of Midwifery

Creativity in practice, education and research

For Elsevier:
Commissioning Editor: Mary Seager
Development Editor: Rebecca Nelemans
Project Manager: Elouise Ball
Designer: Stewart Larking

The Art and Soul
of Midwifery

Creativity in practice, education and research

Edited by

Lorna Davies

RN RM PGCEA BSc(Hons) MA

Senior Lecturer in Midwifery, Christchurch Polytechnic
Institute of Technology, New Zealand.

Foreword by Elizabeth Davis

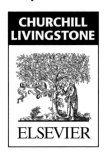

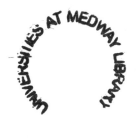

Edinburgh London New York Oxford Philadelphia St Louis Sydney Toronto 2006

CHURCHILL
LIVINGSTONE
ELSEVIER

ISBN 10: 0 443 10192 2
ISBN 13: 978 0443 101922

British Library Cataloguing in Publication Data
A catalogue record for this book is available from the British Library

Library of Congress Cataloging in Publication Data
A catalog record for this book is available from the Library of Congress

Notice
Knowledge and best practice in this field are constantly changing. As new research and experience broaden our knowledge, changes in practice, treatment and drug therapy may become necessary or appropriate. Readers are advised to check the most current information provided (i) on procedures featured or (ii) by the manufacturer of each product to be administered, to verify the recommended dose or formula, the method and duration of administration, and contraindications. It is the responsibility of the practitioner, relying on their own experience and knowledge of the patient, to make diagnoses, to determine dosages and the best treatment for each individual patient, and to take all appropriate safety precautions. To the fullest extent of the law, neither the publisher nor the editor assumes any liability for any injury and/or damage.

The Publisher

ELSEVIER
your source for books, journals and multimedia in the health sciences
www.elsevierhealth.com

The Publisher's policy is to use paper manufactured from sustainable forests

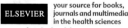

Working together to grow libraries in developing countries
www.elsevier.com | www.bookaid.org | www.sabre.org
ELSEVIER   BOOK AID International   Sabre Foundation

Printed in China

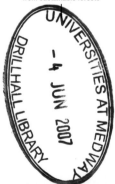

CONTENTS

Contributors vii
Foreword xi
Acknowledgements xiii

CHAPTER ONE
Introduction
Lorna Davies
Page 1

CHAPTER TWO
The Last Taboo:
Representations of Childbearing in Art Form
Lorna Davies
Page 9

CHAPTER THREE
Birth Art as a Timeless Avenue to a Soulful Birth
Pam England
Page 31

CHAPTER FOUR
The Delivery of Art in a Maternity Hospital
Mary Grehan
Page 49

CHAPTER FIVE
Weaving the Fabric of Life:
Women, Birth and Craft
Sara Wickham
Page 63

CHAPTER SIX
Poetry and childbirth:
'A light by which we may see'. From technician to midwife
Tricia Anderson
Page 75

CHAPTER SEVEN
How Do They See Us? Portrayals of Childbirth and the Role of the Midwife in Literature
Terri Coates
Page 95

CHAPTER EIGHT
Blue Moons and Wise Hands:
Birth Knowledge and Stories of Mindful Midwifery
Nessa McHugh
Page 111

CHAPTER NINE
Looking at Ourselves:
Using Theatre to Examine Structures Around Birth
Kirsten Baker
Page 127

CHAPTER TEN
The Rhythm of Life:
Music and Childbirth
Janice Marsh-Prelesnik & Lorna Davies
Page 139

CHAPTER ELEVEN
Dancing Birth:
Choreography and Improvisation
Carol Bartle
Page 157

CHAPTER TWELVE
A Soulful Journey:
Creativity and Midwife Educators
Janice Bass
Page 167

CHAPTER THIRTEEN
Feeling the Fear and Doing it Regardless!
Lorna Davies & Sara Wickham
Page 191

CHAPTER FOURTEEN
Creativity, Spirituality and Birth
Jenny Hall
Page 217

Index 235

CONTRIBUTORS

Tricia Anderson MSc BA(Hons) PGDip(THE) RM

Independent Midwife and Midwife Researcher, Bournemouth University, Bournemouth, UK.

Tricia Anderson completed her first degree in English and Music at York University prior to becoming a midwife, where her dissertation was on modern feminist poetry. She worked in both hospital and community settings prior to becoming an independent midwife. She was Course Leader for the MA Advanced Midwifery Practice at Bournemouth University as well as the Editor of the *MIDIRS Midwifery Digest* and *The Practising Midwife* and Co-Editor of *The Informed Choice Initiative*. She is widely published, teaches both nationally and internationally, and is currently a research midwife at Bournemouth University.

Kirsten Baker BA RM

Midwife, Director of Progress Theatre and Midwifery Lecturer, University of the West of England, Bristol, UK.

Kirsten Baker was seduced by the smell of greasepaint at an early age and studied English and Drama at the University of Exeter in the late 1970s. Using drama as an exploratory tool formed the basis of Kirsten's work for the next decade. Working with health professionals as a simulated patient seemed to offer rich learning potential as the layers of interaction were unfurled – for the health professionals, and for the actors too. Kirsten's interest in healthcare grew and following the birth of her first child in 1985, she decided to become a midwife. She now combines drama and midwifery and in 1999 founded Progress Theatre, a midwifery theatre group. She is currently teaching at the University of the West of England.

Carol Bartle PGDip ChAd MHea/Sc RN RM

Midwife and lactation consultant, Otago, New Zealand.

Carol Bartle has a nursing, midwifery and lactation consultant background. She has just completed a Masters thesis which explores mothers' experiences of breastfeeding in a neonatal intensive care environment. Carol works as a midwife in a primary maternity facility, as a lactation consultant in a neonatal intensive care unit and she teaches developmentally supportive breastfeeding and the politics of breastfeeding around New Zealand. Current interests include the controversies in the use of donor breastmilk in neonatal intensive care and the impact of separating mothers and babies in these environments. Carol is a member of the La Leche League New Zealand Board of Consultants and a founding member of the recently formed Infant Feeding Association of New Zealand (IFANZ), an Asia-Pacific branch of the global organisation IBFAN. Carol trained as a midwife in England but now lives happily in Christchurch, New Zealand, and she has two very grown-up children, Oliver and Louise.

Janice Bass MA BA(Hons) PGCEA ADM RM

Independent midwife and Director of 'Soul Midwifery', Christchurch, New Zealand.

Janice Bass is a midwife/educator with 23 years' experience of supporting women and families as they prepare for birth and parenthood. Her experience of being 'with woman and baby' has increasingly led her to explore the spiritual dimensions of birth, particularly the merging of soul with body consciousness and how birth practices honour and support this process. Completion of a Masters dissertation in 2003 inspired the development of an approach to midwifery practice that incorporates a soulful educative model. In her search for the authentic at a personal and professional level, she migrated with her partner and three children from the UK to New Zealand in 2004. She settled in Christchurch and is fortunate to live on a farm/homestead close to the Torlesse Mountain Range, with ski fields, forests, lakes and the beautiful Waimakariri River. Currently Janice works as an independent home birth midwife supporting parents who choose gentle birthing, and as Director for the Sacred Birthing Foundation in New Zealand.

Terri Coates MSc RN RM ADM DipEd

Independent midwifery lecturer and writer, Salisbury, UK.

Terri Coates currently works as a freelance midwifery lecturer and author. She has practised as a midwife since 1982 and has been a midwifery lecturer since 1991. She started researching literary images of midwives during the long commute to Surrey whilst studying for her MSc. She wrote an article for the *RCM Journal* entitled 'Impressions of the midwife in literature' in 1988. That article led to her contribution to this book and to a collaboration with Jennifer Worth who recorded her professional memoirs in *Call the Midwife*.

Lorna Davies RN RM PGCEA BSc(Hons) MA

Lecturer in Midwifery, Christchurch Polytechnic and Institute of Technology, New Zealand.

Lorna Davies is a qualified midwife who has worked in midwifery education for the last 11 years. She has written and published many articles in midwifery journals and authored and co-authored chapters in several midwifery textbooks. She has been interested in the issue of the arts in relation to childbirth for many years and *The Art and Soul of Midwifery* is the realization of her dream to publish a text which celebrates the value of the arts in promoting a holistic model for midwifery. She is married to Tom and has three children. She currently lives in the Canterbury region of New Zealand where she works as a Senior Lecturer in Midwifery at Christchurch Polytechnic Institute of Technology, and is an independent midwife.

Pam England RM MA

International teacher, New Mexico, USA.

Pam England was a nurse-midwife for 20 years; she also earned a Masters in psychology and counselling. After the birth of her first son (1982), she realized the chasm between what was being taught in typical childbirth classes and what women need to know to give birth in our complex and diverse birth system. Since then she has devoted her life to creating a more dynamic, matriarchal model of childbirth education. Pam is the author of *Birthing From Within, The Keepsake Journal* and numerous articles, as well as being an international teacher. Pam lives in Albuquerque, New Mexico, and is the mother of two sons, Sky and Luc.

Mary Grehan ANCAD Dip(Arts Admin)

Arts manager, curator and artist, Ireland.

Mary Grehan is an arts manager, curator and artist. In 2005, she completed a study entitled 'Mind Where You Look' which compares a public gallery and an acute hospital as sites for viewing art. She is an arts coordinator of the Waterford Healing Arts Trust, Ireland's largest and longest running hospital-based arts programme. Mary was the first Arts Manager of the National Maternity Hospital, Dublin during their centenary year in 1994. She was Director of Tallaght Community Arts Centre, Dublin (1995–2000), and curator of inSite, a programme of community-based public art in Oxford, UK (2001). Mary was the first manager of the Midland Arts Resource Centre in Mullingar, Ireland (1991), and coordinated a pilot craftworkers-in-schools scheme for the Crafts Council of Ireland (1990). She has travelled widely and lived and worked in Japan (1991–93).

Jennifer Hall RN RM ADM MSc PGDip(HE)

Senior Midwifery Lecturer, University of the West of England, Bristol, UK.

Jennifer Hall is Clinical Editor of *The Practising Midwife* and author of *Midwifery Mind and Spirit: emerging issues of care.* She has a particular interest in spirituality and its connection to pregnancy and birth. She encourages the use of art to explore spiritual aspects and has commenced an EdD looking at the use of art to facilitate qualified midwives in understanding spirituality.

Janice Marsh-Prelesnik

Midwife, massage therapist, herbalist, Director of Creative and Birthing Arts, Michigan, USA.

Janice Marsh-Prelesnik has worked as a midwife, massage therapist and herbalist since 1981. As music was her first love, she often is heard singing to mothers and babies and enjoying the rhythms of life in her organic herb gardens and while preparing herbs for her herbal line, Granny Janny Herbs. Janice recently authored the book *The Roots of Natural Mothering: Through the Seasons of Pregnancy, Journey of Birth, and Motherbaby Moon Time.* She can be reached at www.creativebirthingarts.com.

Nessa McHugh RM RGN BA(Hons) MA PGDE

Midwifery Lecturer, Napier University, Edinburgh, UK.

Nessa McHugh has been a midwife for over 10 years and is currently a midwifery lecturer at Napier University. Occasionally she publishes a piece on whatever she happens to be interested in at the time. She has always found the stories of women and midwives deeply fascinating because they reveal so much about the culture of birth and there is so much to learn when you listen to other people's experiences. Nessa lives in Scotland with her husband, Tony, and their two children.

Sara Wickham RM MA BA (Hons) PGCERT

Independent midwifery Lecturer and Consultant.

Sara Wickham is a midwife, lecturer, researcher and author who discovered the joys of craft at an early age and has rarely been seen without a knitting or sewing project about her person since. She is the Editor of the Midwifery: Best Practice series, has written a number of midwifery books and articles and is the webmistress of www.withwoman.co.uk. She is currently attempting to find space in between knitting projects in which she can write her PhD thesis.

FOREWORD

I have had the pleasure of teaching with several of the contributors to this book for many years. They are all distinguished in the field, recognized as both visionaries and pragmatists with a concern for the integrity of the mother-baby unit at the forefront.

This book clearly springs from this concern: that women are losing the power and transformational aspects of childbirth through medicalisation, that babies and families bear the consequences, and that midwives have somehow become complicit. The situation in the United States is different from that in Europe in that midwifery was virtually eradicated by medicine and is only now reestablishing itself as an autonomous profession. This has given us the distinct advantage of forging our institutions of education and regulation to reflect current values on the principles and ethics of holism.

What we have discovered in this process is that our practice, our philosophy, our very approach to our work reflects a paradigm diametrically opposed to the medical model. For example, medicine sees the "patient" under the jurisdiction of the doctor; holistic midwifery sees the "client" responsible for making her own informed decisions. Medicine sees the body as a machine in need of testing and tinkering; holistic midwifery sees the body as blended with mind and spirit so that optimal health is always a matter of integration. Where medicine teaches "clinical detachment," holistic midwifery teaches involvement, relationship. And where medicine would deny the existence of fear in practice, holistic midwifery acknowledges it and gives guidelines for its incorporation in the work.

Birth is the teacher in all of this. In birthing naturally, a woman will often encounter fear greater than any she has ever known. Emotions of self-doubt arise, along with fears of losing control, of death, of splitting apart—and what does the wise midwife advise? "Let go, just go right into your fear, surrender to the process—let yourself open, open like a flower..." In any life-threatening situation fear comes naturally, but if we panic and tighten-up in response, we lose our place and waste precious moments being disconnected from what we need to do. So the mandate springs from the work: we must teach midwives to face their fears, to know themselves, to be prepared, to do their work in the same state of integration that they encourage in their clients. Perhaps the simplest way of saying it: if we want midwives to be truly "with woman," we must educate them to be true to themselves. Thus students must be midwifed into the work—not terrorized and separated from the power of their own instinctual knowing (as birthing women today so often are).

And here is where this wonderfully potent and timely book comes in. This book holds the keys!! Keys to educating midwives to empower themselves and the women they serve. Keys to bringing back the power and mystery of childbirth. Keys to restoring the primacy of family. Keys to a healthy society.

To lend a bit more context to this goal: there was a time when midwifery meant care from womb to tomb, when midwives were the primary caregivers for women not only day-to-day but at life's great passages—the Blood Mysteries of menarche, birth, and menopause. We call these physiologic milestones Blood

Mysteries because they are borne on the body, and mysteriously usher women quite quickly and dramatically to a new phase of life. Historically, midwives have been the honored wise women that facilitate these transitions.

Whether you are an aspiring midwife or already practicing, consider what it would take for you to assume this role. What would you need to know and do to feel prepared? And what sort of tools would you want to have at the ready to assist women in making these crossings consciously and joyously? This is the true work of midwifery, our heritage which was devastated by the Inquisition, otherwise known as the "Holocaust of Women" when as many as six million lost their lives for believing in the beauty of the body and the healing power of nature. Society has trivialized our work ever since, and medicine has exacerbated this by limiting our scope of practice to births only, often without the ability to do prenatal care or provide continuity of care, and in some cases "only with a doctor in the room." In losing midwifery, we have not only lost the work, we have lost our identity as women healers and community leaders.

Bringing the mystery back to our Blood Mysteries will require extraordinary means. In this, the creative arts can be a healing balm, a profound exploration and opening, a pure transmission from the greater-than-self. The chapters in this book teach us how to use music, dance, poetry, storytelling, art, journaling, and self-awareness practices so that, according to Davies, "the neglected imagination is watered and flourishes." She further observes, "The arts can also contribute in acquiring...interpersonal skills, emotional literacy, team skills, problem-solving, lateral thinking, flexibility and adaptability." These skills are foundational not only for the work of midwifery, but for life. Thus this astute and practical compilation of ideas may well serve other providers and educators in the healing arts, providing a blueprint for innovation and change. As Davies makes clear in every aspect of this work, "Art has the power to confront and challenge dogma and ideology." In this, there is hope for the renaissance of true midwifery, for care of women and their families that is holistic and therefore genuine: care that is really caring.

Although we may not consciously remember life in the womb—for most of us, a time and place of comfort and security—we spend our lives trying to recreate that magical, nurtured feeling in our primary relationships. When cultural values are at odds with this, we may give in, forget, and end up feeling empty and despondent.

But with midwifery holistic and restored to its full capacity, there is hope that women may bring the beauty of gestation and the lessons of birth to life, strengthening the role of the feminine in culture so that our focus on materialism and conflict may be brought into balance by qualities of nurturing and peace-making.

Many thanks to each of these wonderful contributors for the groundbreaking work they have done towards this end, and may they inspire you as deeply as they have inspired me!

Elizabeth Davis, B.A., C.P.M.
Author, *Heart & Hands: A Midwife's Guide to Pregnancy & Birth (4th edition)*
Co-director, National Midwifery Institute, Inc.

ACKNOWLEDGEMENTS

I would like to acknowledge the following people for their help, support and love. My husband Tom and children Alex, Helen and Joe for allowing me the time and space to work on what was for me a huge undertaking. My friend and colleague Sara for her counsel and advice, and for putting the whole process into perspective at times. To Mary Seager at Elsevier for giving me the opportunity to achieve my long-held dream of producing a book around the arts and midwifery. To Rebecca Nelemans, for her endless patience and support throughout the development of the book even when I was travelling in South America and Australasia. To the wonderful group of creative and dynamic women who have made the book possible with their talents, skills and wisdom. Lastly, to all the artists, writers, poets, musicians, dancers and craftswomen mentioned within the book, who confirm for us that birth is much more than a mere physical event.

CHAPTER ONE

Introduction

>——————————(•)——————————<

LORNA DAVIES

The Art and Soul of Midwifery is essentially a book about creativity and how the arts may be used as a catalyst to inspire creativity within the sphere of midwifery. It will explore how music, dance, storytelling, poetry and other forms of artistic expression may be used to enhance practice, inform within education and add new perspectives within research.

Concept of creativity

The concept of creativity is currently a hot topic in many areas of life. It is referred to with enthusiasm by big business magnates, educational consultants and politicians alike, and is heralded as a key factor that will encourage growth and development in the decades to come. It is impossible to read a company report, political manifesto or university prospectus without encountering theories on encouraging inventiveness, developing resourcefulness and the value of ingenuity. But what does creativity really mean?

Whilst carrying out a research study in 2003, Australian occupational therapist Therese Schmid discovered that creativity as a phenomenon has a multifaceted structure that makes it very difficult to define, and as I began to write the introduction to this book, I reached an impasse when attempting to define 'creativity'. So I armed myself with coloured pencils and drawing paper and, in the style of creativity guru Tony Buzan (1996), I sat down to carry out a mind-mapping exercise, in an attempt to create some order from my scattered thoughts. I dutifully wrote the title in a little sketched cloud placed strategically in the middle of the page. Each word was carefully colour coded to help to develop the web of ideas that I imagined would flow. However, the thought that kept wandering through my mind was 'why did I want to create this book?'. So I fought off the desire to follow the colour-coded set of words, which was after all far too logical and left-brained, and just went with the flow, allowing my right brain to create whatever it wanted to. The result was a spirographic explosion of colour where layer upon layer of swirls and curves tumbled and spiralled over the centre of the sheet of paper, where I had written the title of the book.

Franken (2001) defines creativity as:

'the tendency to generate or recognize ideas, alternatives, or possibilities that may be useful in solving problems, communicating with others, and entertaining ourselves and others.'

What I had been doing whilst drawing was creating an alternative way of expressing how the words and concepts contained within the title of the book are interconnected. By imaging the looping and crossing of ideas, I was representing the interrelatedness of the core concepts of art, creativity and midwifery. By utilising an alternative approach, I had identified the main objective of the book and my problem had been solved. It enabled me to communicate my ideas in a succinct if abstract way that also gave me entertainment value as it was fun.

On reflection, it struck me that the activity embraced a definition of creativity that suddenly worked for me: that is, the translation of our own special talents and vision into an external reality that is new and useful (Dacey et al 1998). It is about taking something that everyone can see but doing something different with it, thereby offering the opportunity for an alternative or new interpretation.

The stifling of creativity

As human beings, we are members of a creative species. We are all born with a creative capacity that may be nurtured and encouraged to develop or be allowed to wither through lack of love, care and attention. Picasso once observed, 'Every child is an artist. The problem is how to remain an artist once he grows up'. Offer 3-year-olds a selection of poster paints and a piece of paper and they will proudly present you with their masterpiece without a bit of self-consciousness. If you offer an adult the same tools in higher education, the majority will feel at best challenged and at worst, patronised. Ask 5-year-olds to dance to any given piece of music and they will generally willingly oblige. Ask the same of a 12-year-old and you are likely to be met with a prepubescent scowl.

Just what has happened in the intervening years to provoke this change of heart? We have already acknowledged that creativity is now recognised as a valuable asset in many quarters, yet paradoxically many people appear to believe that creativity is something that belongs to the 'gifted' and equate the arts with high culture and therefore not readily accessible. Many critics would suggest that our mainstream educational system continues to elevate the status of the scientific and undermines the value of the aesthetic during our developmental years (Whittaker 2004). Literacy, science and numeracy are the core features within the national curriculum and although some teachers may use creative methods to teach within these core areas, these hard academic components may compromise the inclusion of the more aesthetic elements of life and learning. In these important early developmental blueprint days, when children are most receptive to new ideas and free thinking, we suppress them by enforcing a focus on the perceived academic subjects with their taxing targets and achievement levels. Although primary school children may be 'allowed' to spend time using art, this time becomes increasingly rationed throughout the school years. Whittaker (2004) writes that between the ages of 5 and 14, the arts are mandatory but they are not monitored in the same way as maths and science. When the basic competence of schools is judged on academic teaching and results, the arts become a target for cutting resources when the purse string is tight. By the time they are 'streamed' for GCSE courses, the vast majority of children have chosen to 'drop' art, unless of course they have 'talent' and have opted for a 'specialist' art-based programme in order to pursue a career in an arts-based area.

Multiple intelligences and whole-brain thinking

We are increasingly recognising the fact that there are many different forms of 'intelligence'. Howard Gardner (1985) talks about multiple intelligences that include logico-mathematical, literary (the two forms of intelligence that are probably most valued by Western industrialised societies) spatial, bodily-kinaesthetic and musical. To suggest that one form of intelligence takes precedence over another is to undermine the other, perhaps less concrete ways of thinking and knowing and may inadvertently lead to gross discrimination, in education and in life generally.

Speculations are being made by psychological and neurological research about the specialisation of the two cerebral hemispheres of the brain, and the suggestion that the arts and the sciences 'belong' to different hemispheres. It is known that the two hemispheres do not have identical functions. Most memory for language is stored in the left hemisphere whereas certain processes associated with visual imagery are held in the right hemisphere. The right hemisphere governs to artistic creation while the left is responsible for logical and rational activities such as mathematics. The right brain, it would appear, also has prominence over the emotions. This is not to suggest that the activities within the hemispheres are totally separate or that a tendency to left or right brain thinking separates us as individuals (Simon 2001). It has been demonstrated that the hemispheres do have similarities and that in cases of early brain damage in one half, the other can equally be affected.

The creative processes for the arts and the sciences are not mutually exclusive, otherwise Leonardo da Vinci, Escher and many others would not have been able to leave both their artistic and scientific legacies for future generations. These exceptional beings were indubitably what we would now term whole-brain thinkers. In education, if we can stimulate the individual to utilise both of these spheres of influence, then we may help to develop a 'whole-brain thinker'. However, this would mean reviewing all our education systems from preschool through to higher education to ensure that a balance is achieved between the arts and the sciences, the left and the right hemispheres.

The arts as a catalyst for change

The arts can be used for empowering self and others as catalysts for change. Albert Einstein once said:

'Imagination is more important than knowledge: knowledge is limited.
Imagination encircles the world.'

When using music, poetry, theatre, handicrafts and any of the other expressive arts, the neglected imagination is watered and flourishes. The arts can also contribute in acquiring skills such as communication and interpersonal skills, emotional literacy, team skills, problem solving, lateral thinking, flexibility and adaptability. These are qualities that employers in every sphere of employment would look for and value in an employee (Anderson & Davies 2004).

Arts in health and healthcare education

In many areas of healthcare, the healing power of the aesthetic has begun to achieve mainstream recognition. Artists and poets in residence are now found in many hospital departments and artworks adorn the walls of clinics, surgeries and other venues where healthcare is offered. The once marginalised arts therapies are now heralded as a valuable form of complementary if not primary therapy. The National Network for Arts in

Health coordinates projects and initiatives within healthcare, including arts in hospital, arts and health in the community, and art therapies. In the UK, this trend is recognised at governmental level as having huge public health benefits, a point raised by the then Minister for Public Health Hazel Blears, in a speech entitled 'Capital Investment in the Arts, Regeneration and Health' (DoH 2003).

However, although it is laudable that the value of the arts as therapy is gaining credence, there is equally a need to equip healthcare practitioners with the values and skills that may be enhanced with a greater arts-based input in healthcare education. There is some evidence that some educationalists are taking the arts versus science debate in healthcare seriously. There are first-class examples of the arts and humanities being incorporated into medical education in an attempt to add a humanistic dimension (Calman & Downie 1996).

Some nursing programmes are introducing modules relating to the arts and health. MA courses in Arts in Health are now appearing in a number of prospectuses. These initiatives are not, however, in my opinion, widespread enough and there is still a heavy weighting in favour of science in healthcare, to the detriment of the arts and what they have to offer.

Arts in maternity care

If we look at the area of maternity care, it would seem that the potential of the aesthetic to facilitate the transcendental journey from womanhood to motherhood is only just beginning to gain recognition. During pregnancy, women, and equally their partners, are going through enormous changes in their lives. These changes will indeed affect every aspect of their being and not simply their physical state, as we are sometimes led to believe. How do we get them to explore the emotional, psychological, social and spiritual dimensions of becoming a mother or a father? We talk about 'holistic care' a great deal in midwifery practice and education. Yet if we are not truly 'with woman' on this journey that she is undertaking, then talk of holism becomes merely rhetoric. In order to help the woman to achieve her very individual needs in this period, we need to meet her with an open heart and equally open mind. This requires the adoption and integration of a different range of skills from the clinical skills which are currently given priority in midwifery.

As Clarke (1996) states:

'We seem to have lost touch with what authentic woman centred midwifery is and how it differs from the obstetric model. There are more than just the simplistic normal/abnormal health/ill health definitions of difference. There is the unspoken promise of midwives themselves, to nurture and respect other women in ways which are relevant to the cultural and spiritual meaning of motherhood in the social context of their lives. Within the obstetric model, this type of midwifery is difficult to foster.'

So how do midwives begin to reconstruct their role? How do they bridge the divide between technician and nurturer? Sound knowledge and competence in practice are clearly essential. Midwives need to understand what specific blood results will mean for the woman or how to carry out a specific manoeuvre in the face of an emergency situation. Yet it is perhaps not surprisingly the compassionate and caring qualities that women positively value in their midwife – qualities such as the ability to listen, to respond in a non-judgemental manner, to demonstrate empathy and to offer genuine support. There is much discussion amongst midwives about challenging the medicalisation of childbirth but if we are going to successfully challenge the dominance of the scientific, we need to give value, space and time to exploring alternatives ways of expression, thinking and being. Creative expression is one way in which we may begin to draw upon such alternatives (Anderson & Davies 2004).

The purpose and structure of the book

The Art and Soul of Midwifery intends to provide relevant theory and practical tools to enable midwives to begin to bridge this divide and explore alternative ways of thinking and being. The majority of the writers are midwives and midwife teachers who have spent several years exploring these issues in theory and practice, frequently from a unique perspective. The chapters address the major forms of expressive arts and explore their application to midwifery and birth.

There are three chapters that deal with the subject of art within the book. The first chapter, 'The last taboo: representations of childbearing in art form', examines the representation of pregnancy, birth and the period of new motherhood in artwork from different ages and cultures and explore some of the issues arising from a feminist perspective. The second chapter, authored by Mary Grehan, explores the impact of such projects on environment, employees and clients. Mary Grehan is an arts project coordinator and researcher who has led a number of arts projects in maternity settings. The third chapter, 'Birth art as a timeless avenue to a soulful birth', is an account by Pam England, author and driving force behind the 'Birthing from Within' movement, who has used art in prenatal sessions for many years with sometimes staggering effects.

In her chapter 'Weaving the fabric of life', Sara Wickham examines the value of handcrafts in midwifery. Traditionally crafts were used to provide a layette for the baby but the value of allowing the mother to focus on her newborn may have had much greater significance by promoting bonding with her baby and possibly even helping to facilitate an easier birth by allowing her 'broody' hormones to flow. Additionally, the tradition of the midwife and crafting would appear to have slipped away without anyone noticing. What significance did the knitting needle or crochet have in relation to the philosophy of midwifery? Is craftwork something that we could consider reclaiming for the period of birth, and how would we go about doing so?

There is now a recognition in healthcare practice that stories can be used for many different purposes. They may be used to instil a sense of integration, understanding and pride in family and culture. The telling of stories can foster healing, offer new perspectives on one's own place in the world and demonstrate a willingness to appreciate and celebrate the cultures of others. The chapter on storytelling by Nessa McHugh explores the use of story telling in midwifery practice as a means of making the experiences within midwifery meaningful.

Poetry is a valuable form of communication because of the continued cultural value placed upon it by society and its continual impact upon society. It also offers the capability of expressing complex human emotions and encloses the quality of inviting moral and social enquiry. In her chapter 'Poetry and childbirth: "A light by which we may see". From technician to midwife', Tricia Anderson analyses some of the poetry that has been produced around the subject area of childbirth and create a context for this form of self-expression within midwifery education and practice.

Theatre is a very powerful form of expressive art and Kirsten Baker, as both actress and midwife, is ideally placed to explore the use of theatre in midwifery. In 'Looking at ourselves: using theatre to examine structures around birth', she shares some of the ways in which theatre can be used to analyse and reflect on the role of the midwife, and in particular the work of Progress Theatre, a midwifery theatre group who use theatre to work with midwives and their stories of clinical life.

In her chapter on literature and birth, Terri Coates addresses the ways in which the role of the midwife and representations of childbirth period have been portrayed in literary works throughout the centuries. From the disparaging view of the midwife by Chekhov and Dickens to the contemporary reflections of childbearing by Rachel Cusk, the examples cited offer insight into social attitudes and mores pertaining to childbirth around their time of publication.

Janice Marsh-Prelesnik is an American midwife and musician who co-authors the chapter on music and birth. Music is a powerful medium which can induce multiple responses: physiological, emotional, cognitive and behavioural. Scientific reports show that music can reduce anxiety and perceived pain levels, as well as reducing drug dosages required. Music can also elevate mood, regulate vital signs, boost the immune system and improve focus. It can also have a positive effect on the baby's development before and after birth. This chapter examines the benefits and applies the findings to practical ways of utilising music within the midwifery curriculum and practice areas.

On a similar note, can the use of dance enhance the experience of pregnancy, child-birth and the postnatal period for a woman, her baby, her family and the midwife? Could the synchrony achieved during the 'dance of birth', when a woman moves in time with her birthing supporters and companions, make a difference to outcome? Carol Bartle, midwife and dancer, explores these questions in her chapter and reveals that dance may have a very valid place in the childbearing period.

Midwife and educator Janice Bass set out to explore the issue of creativity in midwifery education by focusing on the educators identified as 'creative' by students. The findings from her study identified that creative teaching involves whole-brain think-ing and is embedded within a continuum of creative dimensions and that teachers who utilise creative approaches appear to have values and beliefs that fit with a humanistic education model and holistic midwifery model. She acknowledges that the findings are not intended as a definitive list but they do provide the basis for further study.

In the chapter 'Feeling the fear and doing it regardless', Lorna Davies and Sara Wickham join forces to draw on theory generated by earlier chapters in order to develop ideas to take forward to inform practice in midwifery education. The chapter contains suggestions and ideas, as well as practical advice on making such ideas work. The chapter also suggests ideas to use in parent education and other similar group activities.

The creative arts have been successfully used to identify and make meaning of the spiritual element within a holistic model of healthcare. The period of new parenthood, including pregnancy and birth, offers enormous potential for providing parents-to-be with a vehicle to address this somewhat nebulous area that does not necessarily fit com-fortably within a pseudo-scientific medical model. In the last chapter, Jenny Hall will explore ways in which this can be achieved within midwifery practice for the benefits of mothers, babies, midwives and even society at large.

Conclusion

According to Edward de Bono (1992), adults are too afraid of failure to allow their creative side to flourish and later in life, people start believing that the most important thing is to be right all the time. Creativity is risky because there are often no right or wrong answers. This means, perhaps, that an arts-based approach may not sit comfortably within the current dominant trend of risk management where it is believed that we can predict risk and thereby prevent negative outcomes. However, we know in our hearts and our intellects that this belief is flawed, just as we realise that medicine is a very imprecise science and one that doesn't necessarily have all the answers, particularly when it comes to the inimitable world of the new mother and her baby.

In the last few decades, some important groundwork has been carried out in the prenatal and perinatal fields, with the likes of Verny & Kelly (1988) and Odent (1999) establishing new and frequently astonishing perspectives. The recognition of the fetus as a sentient and intelligent being is leading us to comprehend that what happens to us during our very earliest stages of development can have profound effects on our subsequent development as a person. Federico & Whitwell (2001) believe that the windows which have now been opened are growing larger, to include the exploration of our spiritual selves, and that as our knowledge of this largely uncharted territory expands, we may discover that science, art and even religion will converge into a greater understanding of consciousness and a harmony that we have yet to experience.

In *The Art and Soul of Midwifery*, perhaps we can assist in creating such a paradigm shift, by acknowledging that there is another way and that by utilising the creative arts in practice, education and research, we may help to enhance the physical, emotional, psychological, social and spiritual well-being of the childbearing community and may even help to put the 'soul' back into birth.

References

Anderson T, Davies L 2004 Celebrating the 'art' of midwifery. Practising Midwife 7(6):22–25

Buzan T 1996 The mind map book: how to use radiant thinking to maximize your brain's untapped potential. Plume, New York

Calman K, Downie R 1996 Why arts courses for medical curricula? Lancet 347: 1499–1450

Clarke R 1996 Minding our own business. British Journal of Midwifery 4(4): 209–211

Dacey J S, Lennon K, Fiore L 1998 Understanding creativity: the interplay of biological, psychological, and social factors. Jossey Bass, San Francisco

de Bono E 1992 Serious creativity: using the power of lateral thinking to create new ideas. Harper Business, New York

Department of Health 2003 Speech by Hazel Blears MP, 25 February 2003: Capital Investment in the Arts, Regeneration and Health. Available online at: www.dh.gov.uk/NewsHome/Speeches/SpeechesList/SpeechesArticle/fs/en?CONTENT_ID=4031624&chk=MkC5rT

Federico G F, Whitwell G E 2001 Music therapy and pregnancy. Journal of Prenatal and Perinatal Psychology and Health 15(4): 299–310

Franken R E 2001 Human motivation, 5th edn. Wadsworth Publishing, Florence, KY

Gardner H 1985 Frames of mind: the theory of multiple intelligences. Basic Books, New York

Odent M 1999 The scientification of love. Free Association Press, London

Schmid T 2004 Meanings of creativity within occupations therapy practice. Australian Occupational Therapy Journal 51: 80–88

Simon H A 2001 Creativity in the arts and sciences. Kenyon Review 23(2). Ebsco-host database. Available online at: www.ebsoc-host.com

Verny J, Kelly J 1988 Secret life of the unborn child. Time Warner, New York

Whittaker D 2004 Visual literacy – art in education. ABX Library. Available online at: http://epe.lac-bac.gc.ca/100/202/300/artsbusiness/html/2001/05-05/library04012001.html

CHAPTER TWO

The Last Taboo:
Representations of Childbearing in Art Form

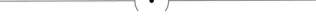

LORNA DAVIES

'The representation of the maternal experience and the acknowledgement of our ambivalence towards it remains taboo, screened from us by the culture's stereotyped and popularised images, both of idealised and denigrated women.'

(Reed 1997)

In 1931 when Jacob Epstein created his resplendent representation of fecundity in the form of his notorious sculpture entitled 'Genesis', it was treated by many within the art world, as well as those with less immediate insight, as an affront to civilisation. The critics in the 1930s could be forgiven for being closed in their worldview, particularly in relation to the subject matter of pregnancy. Victorian values still loomed and childbearing was felt to be a matter that women had to tolerate stoically but certainly not celebrate. Epstein's majestic sculpture, fashioned on traditional African tribal art, was undoubtedly a confrontational piece that aimed to challenge the values and beliefs of the interwar period. Epstein believed that womanhood was earthy and robust and this view seriously challenged the traditional notion of beauty as being synonymous with sexual modesty.

In 1940, Epstein stated that:

'At one blow whole generations of sculptors and sculpture are shattered and sent flying into the limbo of triviality, and my "Genesis", with her fruitful womb, confronts our enfeebled generation. Within her, Man takes on new hope for the future.'

However, the optimism expressed by the sculptor was not as far reaching as he may have imagined. The continuing censorship of images of women around the childbearing period ensured that other comparable images remained rare and, in many cases, vilified for decades to come.

As recently as 1991, the Annie Liebowitz photograph of a heavily pregnant Demi Moore on the cover of the popular women's periodical *Vanity Fair* provoked public outrage and led to some American shops refusing to sell the publication unless it was placed in a paper bag. Incredibly, the idea of subjecting a maternal figure to a gaze that had tones of eroticism challenged the liberal mores of many of those living in the last decade of the 20th century.

If pregnancy in a visual form has the potential to create a furore, what of the even more transgressive concept of representing the woman in labour or giving birth?

Jonathan Waller is an artist who was prompted to pursue the theme of birth in his work as a result of the long and difficult birthing experience of his wife. The ordeal left him feeling raw and exposed but also in awe of women undergoing the process of birth.

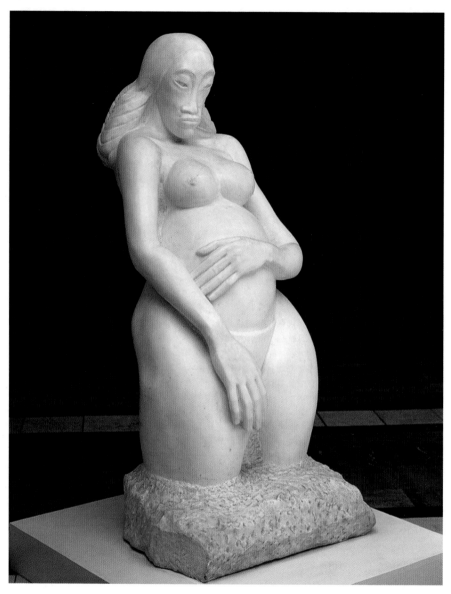

Figure 2.1 Genesis, Jacob Epstein. © Whitworth Gallery/Tate Enterprises.

The cathartic experience of creating works that celebrated the strength and wonderment of labour and birth led to a series of larger-than-life paintings depicting the event in detail. In 1996, on the eve of an exhibition where one of his birth studies was to be hung, Jonathan discovered that the gallery (where he regularly exhibited) had removed the painting from view. Ironically, the incident brought major publicity and some acclaim for his birth works.

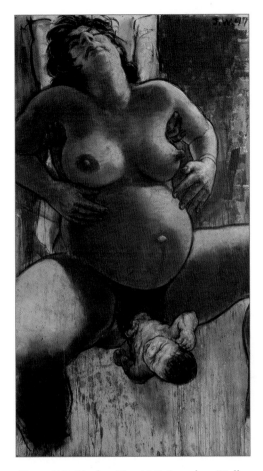

Figure 2.2 Mother No. 44 © Jonathan Waller

However, during a major exhibition in Cheltenham 2 years later, amongst the more positive comments in the guest book were included others which were less complimentary, such
as, 'These pictures are not suitable for children walking by. If we must have them, put them
in the other room. Why are there so many? One (or two at most) would suffice'.

Waller's artwork continues to have the potential to shock because the image of a
woman giving birth is so incredibly rare. However, one might imagine that his paintings
would be treated with greater understanding by midwives at the 'coalface'. These are
the people who observe the phenomenon of birth on a daily basis and must be all too
familiar with the sensations and heightened states of emotion that Waller attempted so
hard to represent in his paintings. Several years ago, Waller was generous enough to
offer the maternity unit in a provincial UK hospital a painting of a labouring woman
languishing in water with her pregnant abdomen surfacing from the pool. When one
looks closely enough, one is able to see that the head of the baby is gently crowning
below the surface of the water. Some viewers might say that the expression on the
woman's face is analogous to that of someone achieving orgasm. The woman appears

to be free from both pain and fear and looks as though she is on a 'natural high'. The painting was due to be unveiled at a special ceremony but on the day that it was delivered to the maternity unit, a massive furore broke out. It was claimed that the nature of the painting had not been made clear and that its 'explicit' character made it unsuitable for display in a hospital maternity unit. There were even accusations of the painting being pornographic. It was eventually sited in a quiet and dark corridor, away from the gaze of a potential audience who may have been affronted by the image of a brave, bold birthing woman, in a painting that was compared to 'The Birth of Venus' by an important figure officiating at the unveiling. Eventually, when the unit was refurbished, it was 'discovered' that there was nowhere even remotely suitable for the painting to hang and it was duly removed and eventually found refuge at the local university.

What is it about these works of art that provokes such emotional responses and feelings of discomfiture for many viewers? Perhaps it is the evident strength of the women who are portrayed that creates the challenge. I would suggest that all three of the images in question represent empowerment, the strength and power of the pregnant and birthing woman. They directly confront the viewer, defying them to avert their gaze, challenging them to deny them their autonomy and control. In a world where control of birth is denied to many women, the images may make people feel out of control. Perhaps they were denied control within their own birthing experience and find such images to be too potent a reminder.

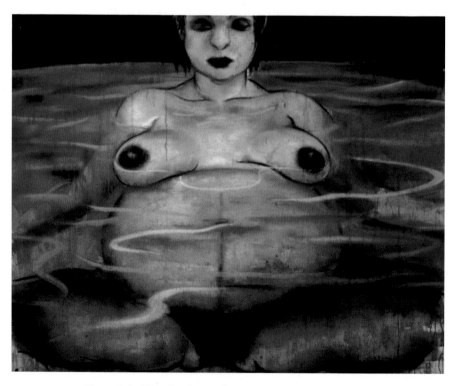

Figure 2.3 Waterbirth (Mother No. 5) © Jonathan Waller

The images could be interpreted as implicitly, or explicitly in some cases, sexual in nature, which may have made their adversaries feel uncomfortable. When does a candid and confrontational image become pornographic? Perhaps the quasi-orgasmic expression on the face of the woman in the Jonathan Waller painting was more than some could bear. For too many years we have worked at eradicating the sexuality of childbirth, forgetting that pregnancy is the product of a sexual act, babies are the product of a sexual act, and that birth is in fact a sexual act, utilising the same reproductive organs and hormonal benefits. It is possible that such revulsion at the recognition of birth as a sexual act is the net result.

Is gender at the root of the problem? Chicago & Lucie-Smith (1999) suggest that the experience of birth is so overlooked in art because it lies within a woman's sphere and therefore is not considered important enough to be worth representing. They also ask whether men undermine the significance of birth artistically, because it is fundamentally the greatest creative act ever to be undertaken and one which, by virtue of their sex, they are necessarily denied. Essentially, is this all about uterus envy?

Some may feel for religious or spiritual reasons that the public exposure of such frank material is unacceptable. Some religions hold the view that women in the throes of giving birth are ritually unclean. Others may be of the opinion that artists should not be intruding on territory of such sanctity and that a piece of artistic representation could never hope to truly represent the profundity of the event.

Alternatively, from a physiological perspective, should we be subjecting an act which relies on a primal response to the public gaze in any way, shape or form? Michel Odent (1999) believes that any interference may disrupt the flow of birth and therefore preconceived ideas formed from any media may have the effect of preempting a woman's expectations and responses. Should we stop intellectualising and simply allow women to be 'in the moment' whilst giving birth? If this is the case then perhaps no images of childbirth should be made public.

Regardless of the reasons why the images may not be acceptable to some, who is to say that the Epstein sculpture, the Leibowitz photograph and the Waller painting did not lead the critics to consider their own values and beliefs around birth? Art unequivocally has the power to confront and challenge dogma and ideology in a way that is unique and I like to suppose that the images may have served as a catalyst for change, by provoking a reaction in the minds of some of their opponents, leading them to question their attitudes relating to birth.

In order to contextualise the place of birth within art, it may be useful to look way back at prehistory, in order to view how our forebears dealt with this subject within their respective cultures and societies.

Ancient history

The earliest evidence that we have available indicates that the role of the mother in neolithic and palaeolithic times was greater than at any time during history. Their nature was more fully expressed, their contributions to their society were more valued, their creativity was celebrated and their impact on civilisation was highly influential (Thurer 1994). The earliest deities were goddesses and motherhood was viewed as a divine state of being. The Great Mother did not attempt to disguise her pregnancy and the very earliest known religious icons were naked female figurines, often in an advanced state of pregnancy (Ehrenberg 1989). The Venus of Willendorf, a statuette about 11 cm in height, is one such example of the reverence of the maternal state. When she was first discovered in Austria in the early 20th century, it was believed that she dated to approximately 15 000–10 000 BC. However, in the 1990s, a study on the stratigraphic sequence of the archaeological layers comprising the sculpture led the researchers to surmise that the Venus of Willendorf was produced around 24 000–22 000 BC (Dobres 1996).

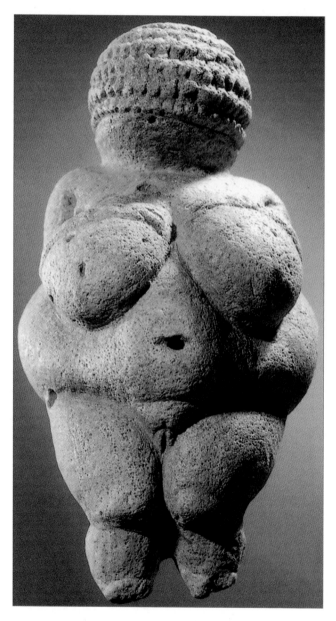

Figure 2.4 Venus of Willendorf

Inanna was the most important goddess of the Sumerian pantheon in ancient Mesopotamia. As the Queen of Heaven and Earth, who ruled as Mother of All, she was also viewed as the goddess of fertility, birth and nature. Her most famous myth centres on her journey to the underworld. As part of the descent into the underworld she has to pass through seven gates, leaving jewellery and garments (representing worldly goods and values) at each gate until she is naked. She eventually encounters her sister Ereshkigal, the Queen of the Underworld, the dark goddess who kills Innana and hangs her on a hook for 3 days. She is saved by the god Enki, who sends two creatures who symbolise wisdom to liberate her. Pam England (2002) has adapted the myth of Innana and her descent for use with 21st-century couples in preparation for parenting. The legend of Innana is used as a metaphor for the stages that a woman must go through on her journey to becoming a mother. She analogises the character of Erishkegal as that of the alter ego of the woman, and the death and hanging scene as the rebirth of the new mother. The Queen of Heaven and Earth and goddess of fertility still reigns in Birthing from Within sessions, quite a feat for someone who predates the birth of Christ by 4000 years.

Egyptian historical evidence also bears testimony to the sacred value of childbirth in that ancient civilisation. The Egyptians also held many deities in reverence during the period of pregnancy and childbirth and again, they were by and large female goddess figures. The Westcar Papyrus (circa 1650 BC) includes the tale of Reddjedet, a woman giving birth to triplets (using a birthing stool) who was assisted by five goddesses: Aset (Isis), Nebt-Het (Nephtys), Heqet, Meskhenet and Khnum. We are informed that they sealed the room and 'Aset placed herself before her, Nebt-Het behind her, Heqat hastened the birth'. The five then cut the umbilical cord, washed the baby and told the fortune of the child (Jonsson 2005).

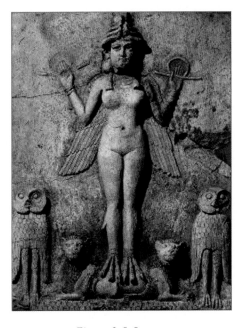

Figure 2.5 Innana

Hieroglyphic evidence shows us that women delivered their babies kneeling or sitting on their heels or on a delivery seat. Archaeologists have also unearthed platforms which appear to be related to childbirth and can be seen in hieroglyphic images. The platform was a rectangular mud brick construction, partially enclosed but with an opening on its long side, and a couple of steps leading up to it (Tyldesley 1995). An account of giving birth by standing on the bricks is well described in the novel *The Red Tent* by Anita Diamant (2002).

In pre-Columbian art, we may witness the deification of the birthing state, with statues of goddesses as birthing woman, squatting in an upright position. Tlazolteotl (c.1300–1521) was known as the goddess of earth, sex and childbirth. She was also known as 'the eater of filth', a title arising from the legend that at the end of a man's life, she would come to him to allow him to confess his sins which allowed her then to cleanse his soul, thereby eating its filth. The association of birth and death as dual roles in the work of a goddess is not something confined to Aztec folklore. Isis the Egyptian moon goddess was the creator, mother, nurse of all, but equally she was the destroyer. There seems to have been an acceptance in ancient culture that birth and death were interrelated.

Artemis is another example of how motherhood was given goddess status in ancient Greece. Bes is just one example of African mother deities and the Celtic divine being Morgawse was given the title 'goddess of mothers'. In fact, it would appear that in the vast majority of pre-Christian cultures and societies, the concept of the birth goddess was essentially a universal phenomenon.

Ehrenberg (1989) believes that the first signs of the decline of motherhood as divine eminence began to appear in ancient Rome in around 600 BC. Terra Mater, the Roman counterpart of Artemis in Greek culture, held goddess status in ancient Rome but according to Ehrenberg, the 'mother as goddess' was replaced with the firm establishment of a patriarchal paradigm in Roman society around this period. In this paradigm, in contrast to the experience of our palaeolithic and neolithic foremothers, maternal power was viewed as something which rendered women culpable, and thus less worthy and capable of effecting social influence. To a greater or lesser extent, this appeared to remain as the prevailing ideology throughout history in the so-called civilised world thereafter.

Christianity and its consequences

The advent of Christianity can be seen to have perpetuated the idea that birth was something that should not be publicly acknowledged. It was begrudgingly referred to as a necessary evil, the 'Curse of Eve'. Christ is acknowledged in theological terms as the product of an immaculate conception and this has led to a persistent iconic representation of his mother as the 'Virgin' Mary. The virgin birth legend is by no means unique to Christianity as, like many other traditions within the Christian Church, it was borrowed from other cultures and religions. According to legend, Cybele, Aphrodite, Demeter, Isis, Astarte, Hathor, Inanna and Ishtar were all recorded as being both mother and virgin who gave birth to a half-human, half-divine child who died and was reborn (Jennings 2004). However, the mother of Christ was not formally accredited with goddess status by the Christian Church, although some would argue that the cult that has followed her throughout the centuries would give her that most holy state of sanctity, particularly within the Roman Catholic Church.

Her depictions in art are many and varied. There are many representations where Mary is shown to be in a pregnant state, notably in paintings and sculptures around

'The Visitation' where Mary meets with her cousin Elizabeth who is also pregnant. There are also a number of paintings where the Christ Child is being breastfed by his mother. However, although images of Jesus and his mother abound, an image of the actual 'blood and guts' birth of Christ is, to my knowledge, non-existent.

The Madonna and Child image has influenced Western art enormously and the representation is almost without exception idealised. In the same way that contemporary magazine images present women with an almost impossible model of perfection, the image of the Virgin Mary has been used as a way of perpetuating the servitude of women and making them feel guilty if they are not able to reach the proposed level of perfection. Because of this, the everyday reality of women can only be seen in some of the art that focuses on a narrow interpretation of the role of women. The depiction of the woman as self effacing wife and mother, poor second in relation to her man, does indicate how women were traditionally expected to behave. It has also been argued by many feminist critics (Daly 1979, de Beauvoir 1949) that the 'Virgin and Child' idealisation may have contributed to and perpetuated the concept of the Madonna/Whore complex or paradox, a psychological dysfunctional state where a man can view a woman either in terms of absolute purity or absolute degradation but is unable to reconcile that a woman can be both lover and mother.

This dualism has pervaded the representation of women in paintings and other art forms for centuries and it has been argued that such misogynistic iconographic imagery has served to maintain the phallocentric status quo. Feminists have battled against this myth for decades and reflect the sentiment that is enshrined in the words of Cyndi Lauper:

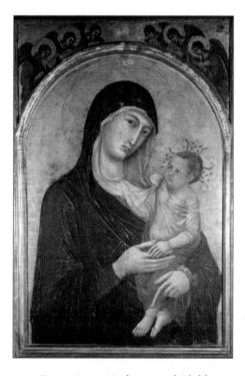

Figure 2.6 a Madonna and Child

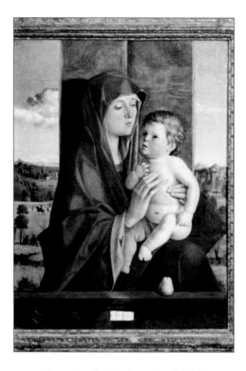

Figure 2.6 b Madonna and Child

'Every woman's a Madonna; every woman's a whore
You can try to reduce me but I'm so much more
I don't want to be your mother; won't be shoved in a drawer
cause every woman's a Madonna, every woman's a whore, that's right'
(Lauper & Wittman 2001)

Chicago & Lucie-Smith (1999) suggest that as one of the most fundamental of all human processes, birth itself has no need of any particular framework to give it an aura of the sacred. Yet it could be said that at an artistic level, the potential of the subject has been hijacked by a religion that has denied us access to a discourse for centuries.

Social context of birth in art

There are quite a number of paintings that illustrate the setting and context of birth throughout history, and these give us considerable insight into the celebration of the event within different times and cultures. Some of these are biblical in origin, such as the subject of the birth of Mary, mother of Jesus. In the many paintings that depict this event, the artists tell us as much about birth in their own period and culture as they do about the period in which Mary was allegedly born. 'The Birth of Mary' by Ghirlandaio, c.1485–90, is one such example. The artist invites the audience into the birthing room where the women servants are engaged in attending to the needs of the mother and her newborn child whilst the 'ladies of the household' gather to greet the baby. The artist presents birth firmly within a social context and as would befit the traditions of both eras, there are only women present.

Jan Steen's painting 'The Christening Feast' is a delightfully lively account of a birth in which the whole of the community appears to be involved. It may on initial inspection seem odd that the family are celebrating the baptism of the child whilst the mother lies in bed looking to all intents and purposes as though she is recovering from the demands of giving birth. However, it is documented that sometimes the christening presents were made on the day of the birth or a few days afterwards. These festivities sometimes lasted 6 weeks, one christening feast following another. In the meantime, the husband neglected his business or his work and debts often resulted (Singleton 1909). There are many metaphors, analogies and subplots in evidence when the painting is studied carefully. The broken eggs, for example, would represent infidelity. The sausages being held aloft are an overt phallic symbol. The alleged father of the baby is shadowed by a character who is making what would have been instantly recognisable as the sign of the cuckold. This work illustrates the social nature of birth in 15th-century Holland and reminds us of a time when the event was more than the medicalised procedure that it has become for most of us in Western industrialised society.

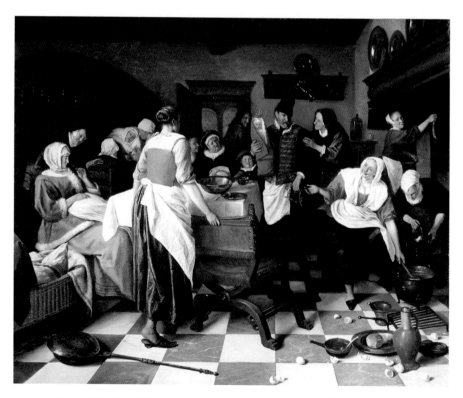

Figure 2.7 The Christening Feast, Jan Steen © The Wallace Collection

Early 20th-century male perspectives

The 20th century produced far more images relating to the childbearing period than the preceding centuries but these still tend to focus more on the gestational and postnatal periods and the actual business of birth is by and large seriously underrepresented. Even where artworks relating to pregnancy and birth do exist, they are frequently overlooked in favour of works that could be said to lie within the male domain. Artists such as Egon Schiele, an Austrian painter and disciple of Gustav Klimt, acquired a somewhat notorious reputation for his erotic portraits. However, his heartrending representation of pregnancy in 'Pregnant Woman and Death' (1911) is given much less consideration, in spite of the fact that the painting prophesied the death of his wife in late pregnancy as a result of contracting Spanish influenza.

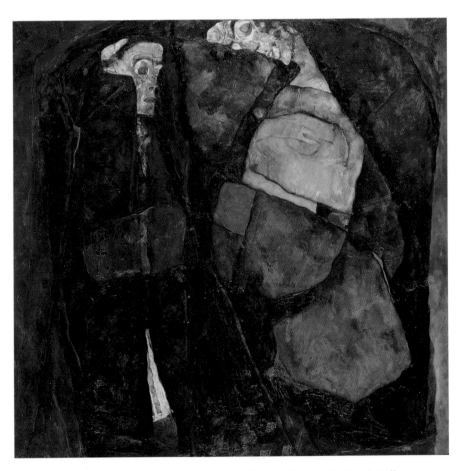

Figure 2.8 Pregnant Woman and Death, Egon Schiele © National Gallery in Prague 2005

Likewise, Otto Dix is often identified as the artist who painted the horrors of the Great War whilst his studies of pregnant women and even the image of his newborn son Ursus ('Newborn Baby on Hands', 1927) held aloft in the hands of a midwife, would seem to be given far less recognition. The realism of this painting in the style of the Neue Sachlichkeit movement can be interpreted as quite jarring. His son Ursus, portrayed directly following his birth, is held aloft by gnarled and aged hands. The baby sports a bluish-red swollen nose, perhaps as a result of a perinatal injury, and no-one could accuse Dix of sentimentalising the birth of his son.

Social realism

In the early years of the 20th century, the German art world produced two female artists of notable acclaim, Kathe Kollwitz and Paula Modersohn Becker. Both of these women sought to represent the life of women in Germany in the early years of the 20th century. They were part of the expressionist movement, whose participants rebelled against the time-honoured conventions of representative art and experimented with new ways to capture the essence of humanity.

Kollwitz was a social realist and her imagery is marked by poverty-stricken women barely able to nurture or provide nutrition for their children. Her art resonates with compassion and serves as an indictment of the social conditions in Germany at that time. She produced several works illustrating the hardship of pregnancy and childrearing for the working-class women of the time. The woodcut 'The Widow' (1922–23) presents a woman who is clearly burdened with the weight of poverty. She is slumped against a wall and, one can presume from the title of the piece, mourning the loss of her husband. Her belly is swollen with child, her shoulders are hunched as she stares aimlessly ahead with little if any hope for the future of her child. Contrasting with this image, Kollwitz, a prolific artist, also produced images of impoverished people in stark settings but with an air of hope.

Modersohn Becker painted women in the childbearing period but they were presented in a more robust and less deprived manner. Her painting 'Mutter und Kind' serves as a contrast to the idealised Madonna and Child images, discussed earlier. The nude mother and child lie together in a complete state of unity and to me, the image radiates 'mother love'. Nudity in this picture conflicts with feminist ideas of the female nude as an object of public consumption, because Modersohn Becker uses the state in such a way as to obliterate notions of sexuality (Betterton 1996).

In the painting 'Self Portrait', Modersohn Becker represents herself as pregnant when she was not. It was at the precise point when she had decided to abandon her husband, Otto Modersohn, in northern Germany to remain working as an independent artist in Paris. Some critics interpret the painting as 'looking forward to motherhood'. Becker was 30 when she painted her self portrait and 31 when she died as a result of complications after childbirth, which was relatively old to bear a first child in the first decade of the 20th century. The following words from her journal demonstrate her longing for a child and make the self portrait of her phantom pregnancy all the more poignant.

'There are times when this feeling of devotion and dependence lies dormant...
Then all at once this feeling awakes and surges and roars, as if the container would nearly burst. There's no room for anything else. My Mother. Dawn is within me and I feel the approaching day. I am becoming something.'

(1902, in Modersohn Becker 1980)

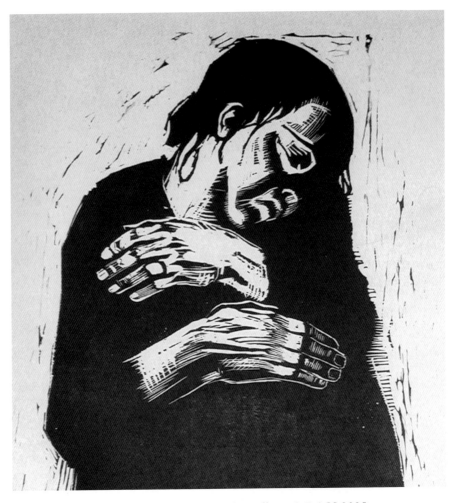

Figure 2.9 The Widow, Kathe Kollwitz © DACS 2005

Frida Kahlo, a Mexican artist, began to paint in 1925 whilst recovering from an accident that left her permanently disabled. It also left her unable to bear children, a fact which haunted her during her turbulent marriage to fellow artist Diego Rivera and which was a theme that dominated many of her paintings.

Although paintings such as 'Henry Ford Hospital' depict the sense of loss, betrayal and loneliness that she must have felt at the time of her three or more miscarriages, other self portraits explore issues about her own early childhood and identify her personal construct of mothering. The images in paintings like 'My Birth' (1932) and 'My Nurse and I' focus heavily on a fragmented and incomplete relationship with her mother.

In 'My Birth', the knees of the woman on the bed are bent and spread in the position of giving birth. Frida's head is newly born but fully grown and adult in feature. It

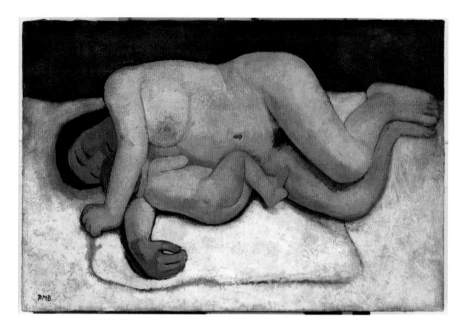

Figure 2.10 Mutter und Kind, Paula Modersohn-Becker
© *Paula Modersohn-Becker Museum*

is difficult to establish whether she is dead or alive. Above the bed hangs a portrait of the Virgin of Sorrows bleeding and weeping, stabbed by two daggers. The image seems to underline an understanding that Kahlo had perhaps had between herself and her mother, that her birth had been a kind of death for her mother (Herrera 1998). Metaphorically speaking, Kahlo could only have been born after her mother died and consequently the experience of bonding between them never took place. Without a consistent primary caregiver, attuned to provide the mirroring she needed to thrive and develop adequately, she had in a sense given psychological birth to herself (Grimberg 1989).

Her painting 'My Nurse and I' (1937) shows Kahlo still working on the issue of a faulty attachment and its consequences. Kahlo considered this work a companion to 'My Birth' (Herrera 1998). The painting depicts her as half infant, half woman. She appears in the arms of her Indian wetnurse and presumably because she could not remember the features of her nurse, she covered the face with an Aztec mask. The mouth of the infant/adult drips milk, though she is not actively engaged in suckling. She looks directly at the viewer, making no eye contact with her nurse.

American Alice Neel (1900–84) was a figurative painter who worked during the decades of realism, postwar abstract expressionism, 1960s pop and 1970s minimalism. She persevered in her work in spite of a turbulent personal life, that impacted on her working life, until the 1960s. Although she produced some landscape work during her career, her primary focus was on portraiture. Her subjects were usually family and friends and she represented them as human beings, in real-life situations with true emotions. In fact, she deplored the term 'portrait' and described herself as a collector of souls (Neel 1985).

Neel's work is remarkable for including at least eight pregnant nudes and she thought the whole picture of woman without pregnancy was trivial.

'It's treating woman as sex object. But you know, sex results in something.'

(www.uam.ucsb.edu/Pages/pregnant_woman.html)

Feminists and images of birth

Griselda Pollock (1999), a feminist art historian, believes that in order to achieve success, feminists have to concern themselves with exposing the biases of art history as a whole and not simply focus on the work of women artists. An initial response may validate that belief, given the relative rarity of artworks by women and relating to women. However, on closer inspection, the oft-cited question 'Why are there no great women artists?' (Nochlin 1988) can be seriously challenged. There have in fact been many great women artists but they also are frequently overlooked, particularly when the subject matter with which they are dealing lies outside the mainstream catalogue of acceptable material, such as that relating to pregnancy, birth and the realities of early motherhood. Feminist art critics and historians have been instrumental in recovering information about contributions of women artists and patrons that have failed to receive acclaim or even acknowledgement by previous male art critics and historians (Borzello 2000).

The latter half of the 20th century saw the advent of the second wave of feminism, which was heralded by a marked increase in artworks that represented the lives and experiences of women. The Marxist art critic John Berger (1972) proposed that Western art mirrored the unequal relationships that existed in society generally, and that 'Men look at women. Women watch themselves being looked at' (Berger 1972, p.45). The feminist art backlash unleashed a series of works that represented subjects relating to women. They explored vaginal imagery and menstrual blood, amongst other 'taboo' subjects. Mary Kelly, for example, produced an extensive work entitled the 'Post Partum Document', a six-part work that charted the relationship between the artist and her son over a period of 6 years. By drawing on contemporary feminist thought, and in particular on psychoanalysis, in the work (which included controversial items such as soiled nappies) Kelly was able to explore the contradictions for a woman artist between her creative and procreative roles (Kelly 1998).

Some of the second-wave feminist artists defiantly flaunted the theme of birth in an attempt to demystify and normalise this universal human experience. When Monica Sjoo exhibited the notorious 'God Giving Birth' in 1968, many women recognised the painting as an attempt to create a powerful symbolic image of one of the realities of femininity and women's lives (Hopper 2001). 'God Giving Birth' was inspired by the home birth of her son in 1961. The painting depicts a female deity boldly straddling the earth whilst in the process of giving birth, with the universe as a backdrop. Interestingly, the image can be seen to hark back to the neolithic and Pre-Columbian representations of female divinities. It may be that the image embodies the need for an alternative spiritual perspective, which many modern women feel. Ironically, when the painting was exhibited at Swiss Cottage library in London, as part of an exhibition of women artists, it was widely rebuked by both public and critics and Sjoo came very close to being prosecuted under the blasphemy law (Hopper 2001).

Judy Chicago (1985) decided to approach the subject area by inviting women to participate in the production of an amazing collection of needlework art, which collectively became known as the Birth Project.

'Since there were so few images, I decided that I would have to go directly to the women, ask them to tell me about their birth experiences.'

(Chicago 1985, p.6)

The pieces were created from quilting, appliqué, patchwork and other traditional needlework forms. Chicago, a controversial feminist artist of notoriety, had rocked the art world with her 'Dinner Party' exhibition, in which she displayed sculptures of the genitalia of influential women in history. Likewise, Birth Project brought Chicago both acclaim and disapproval in equal measures. In addition to ensuring that the neglected subject of childbirth was represented in the 80 pieces that made up the collection, Birth Project made a further valuable point about gender and art. Chicago recognised that needlework was considered to be 'women's work' and was not valued as a medium for art making. The magnificent Birth Project, with its raw and powerful imagery, defied that assumption and may have contributed to a renaissance in traditional women's crafts, but with the recognition that these are now valued as art and not just handicrafts.

Helen Chadwick was an avant-garde British artist who died prematurely at the age of 43 in 1996. Much of her work is said to be simultaneously beautiful and disquieting (McKellar 2005). In 1995, she produced 'One Flesh', an iconographic representation of the Madonna and Child created from a collage of colour photocopies, in some parts consisting of very small fragments. The production of such an image might at first glance appear to be an unusual choice of subject for a contemporary artist to engage with. However, the content of the image when closely observed is unlike that of any other Madonna and Child representation (Hearles 1997). The very medium in which

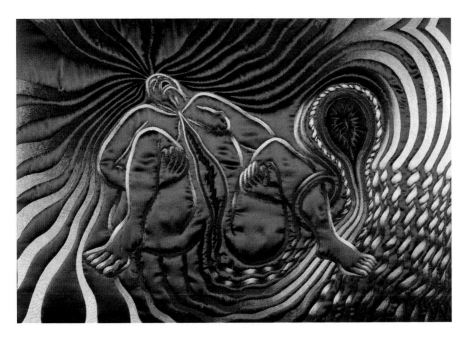

Figure 2.11 Birth Tear, Judy Chicago © Through The Flower

it is created contemporises it and leads the viewer to recognise that this is no classic portrayal of Mary and the Christ Child. The floating object, hovering halo-like above the Madonna's head, is on closer scrutiny seen to be a placenta. According to Hearles (1997), Chadwick described the placenta as forming a kind of biological trinity together with the two characters in the picture. When one looks even more closely, the eye is drawn to a smaller golden area where pierced genitalia, complete with jewellery, is in evidence. Chadwick described this as 'taking up the usual lofty position of a cherub or perhaps an allegorical sun and moon' (Hearles 1997). The Madonna is pointing to the genitalia of the baby, which is female, and she is cutting the umbilical cord with her other hand. Chadwick is said to have embarked on the work with the intention of creating a classical Mother and Child piece of 'corporeal reality'. However, she realised that such a reality would require the baby to be male. This shocking revelation of implicit sexism led her to deliver 'One Flesh' depicting the child not as Christ but as an earthly and female human being (McKellar 2005).

The future of birth art

An even more contemporary and potentially more disturbing image of pregnancy is that portrayed in 'Introspection' by Canadian artist Heidi Taillefer. For me, this painting represents the hijacking of the social event of childbearing by medicine and technology.

The mother figure has been transmogrified by the artist into a cyborg, which is defined by Donna Haraway (1991) as a hybrid of machine and organism. Haraway goes on to say that:

'Modern medicine is also full of cyborgs, of couplings between organism and machine, each conceived as coded devices, in an intimacy and with a power that was not generated in the history of sexuality.'

(Haraway 1991, p.149)

'Introspection' reminds us that we need to consider one last crucial issue in this debate. That is, what effect has the medicalisation of childbirth had on artistic representations of pregnancy, birth and early motherhood? This is a considerable area of deliberation and one which we can only expect to scratch the surface of within this chapter. It has been argued on many counts that medicine objectifies women and that the medicalisation of pregnancy and birth reduces the function of childbirth from a transformative and life-enhancing event to a risk-filled potential medical emergency. Regarding women as objects deems their everyday experiences theoretically insignificant. If the whole episode is placed within a pseudo-scientific framework, it begins to lose its humanity. By pathologising childbearing, it is implied that women will make incompetent decisions regarding the health of both themselves and their unborn children. Hence, to ensure safety of mother and unborn child, obstetricians rely exclusively on a discourse that disregards women's experiences. Until doctors, and society at large, begin to recognise that women's lived experiences of childbearing are worthy and reliable sources of knowledge, women will be denied an experience of childbearing that is meaningful and life enhancing. We can only assume that the commandeering of childbearing by the medical authorities has impacted on the work that potentially could have made women feel more positive and have led to a greater sense of autonomy.

I for one have no desire to see the 'cyborg' mother become the 21st-century iconic representation of childbirth and yet, at this time, birth in Western industrialised society

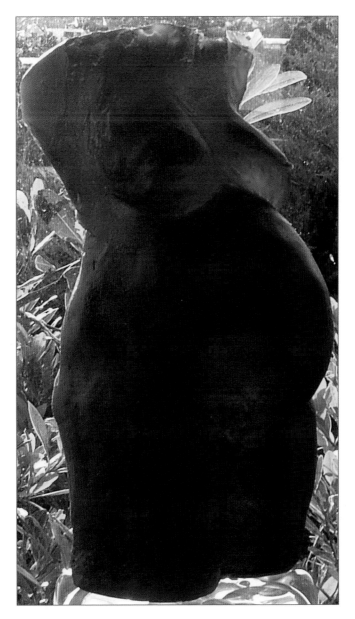

Figure 2.12 Llew Summers sculpture

is in something of a crisis and maternity care is in chronic need of a reconstruction. Caesarean section rates are rocketing; midwives are leaving the profession in droves and it feels as though women have lost the belief in their bodies to grow and bear babies without the intervention of increasing technology. There is no doubt that if birth is to be reclaimed by women and midwives as a primarily social event, then we need more positive affirmations of the essential mystery, primacy and wonderment of women's bodies, and of women's ability to 'know best' about the things their bodies require and the choices which they need to make.

We need to be able to access and utilise images that contrast with the stark and clinical glimpse of the future of birth that we are offered in the work of Heidi Taillefer. My spirits were recently lifted after being introduced to the popular and prolific New Zealand sculptor Llew Summers. Summers has fashioned a series of works around the subject of maternity. The piece illustrated in Figure 2.12 is cast in red lead crystal and when backed with a light source, it creates a depth of intensity that embraces the 'heart and soul' of pregnancy, the essence of life. For me, the Llew Summers sculpture represents the sense of connection and energy that flows between a mother and her unborn child. It manages to convey an experience of the universality of birth without sentimentality or cliché.

I believe that the work of artists like Llew Summers and others could be used to promote the importance of normal birth in society. We know from the work of art therapists that art can have profound effects on the physical, emotional, psychological, spiritual and social well-being of individuals, and that the universality of art and its ability to relate one human being to another through visual form are vitally important. According to Ryder (1987), art provides us with one of the most potent proofs of the basic unity of all people. The rapid advances of technological intervention that we are currently being subjected to may have serious implications for the future health and well-being of society (Odent 2004). If we are to curtail this trend and raise awareness of what it is to be fully human, then we need to change both public and professional perception and attitudes. Perhaps by increasing the use of art in healthcare settings; encouraging the use of beautiful artistic illustrations in birth-related textbooks in addition to anatomical drawings; inviting artists in residence to work with women and their families during pregnancy; and by continuing to increase use of art and humanities within both midwifery and medical education, we can begin to create a greater sense of equilibrium between the 'arts' and the 'sciences' which may hold at bay the 'cyborg culture' that denies women access to their own unique experience of childbearing.

References

Berger J 1972 Ways of seeing. Pelican, Gretna, LA

Betterton R 1996 An intimate distance: women artists and the body. Routledge, London

Borzello F 2000 A world of our own: women as artists. Thames and Hudson, London

Chicago J 1985 Birth Project. Doubleday, New York

Chicago J, Lucie-Smith E 1999 Women and art – uncontested territory. Weidenfeld and Nicolson, London

Daly M 1979 Gyn/ecology: the meta-ethics of radical feminism. The Women's Press, London

de Beauvoir S 1949 The second sex (Vintage Classics 1997). Vintage Press, New York

Diamant A 2002 The red tent. Pan, London

Dobres MA 1996 Venus figurines. In: Fagan BM (ed) The Oxford companion to archaeology. Oxford University Press, Oxford

Ehrenberg M 1989 Women in prehistory. British Museum Press, London

England P 2002 Innana's descent: inititation and return. Birthing from Within Books, Albuquerque, NM

Epstein J 1940 Let there be sculpture. Michael Joseph, London

Grimberg S 1989 Frida Kahlo. JG Press, Emmaus, PA

Haraway D 1991 Simians, cyborgs, and women: the reinvention of nature. Free Association Books, London

Hearles E 1997 Helen Chadwick – One Flesh. Exposure Magazine. Available online at: http://members.lycos.co.uk/exposuremagazine/helen.html

Herrera H 1998 Frida: a biography of Frida Kahlo. Bloomsbury, London

Hopper G 2001 Women in art: the last taboo. Journal of Art and Design Education 20(3): 311–319

Jennings S 2004 Goddesses. Hay House Publishing, London

Kelly M 1998 Post Partum Document. University of California Press, Berkeley, CA

Lauper C, Wittman W 2001 Madonna whore. Rellla Music/Sony Publishing (BMI) and Weedy Wet Songs (ASCAP)

Martin JR 1985 Reclaiming a conversation: the ideal of the educated woman. Yale University Press, New Haven, CT

McKellar L 2005 The word made flesh: re-embodying the Madonna and Child in Helen Chadwick's One Flesh: the sacred and the feminine. AHRC CentreCATH, Leeds

Modersohn Becker P 1980 The letters and journal of Paula Modersohn Becker (trans. J Diane Radycki). Scarecrow Press, Lanham, MD

Neel A 1985 Paintings since 1970. Pennsylvania Academy of the Fine Arts. Available online at: www.uam.ucsb.edu/Pages/pregnant_woman.html

Nochlin L 1988 Why have there been no great women artists? In: Women, art and power and other essays. Harper and Row, New York

Odent M 1999 The scientification of love. Free Association Press, London

Odent M 2004 The caesarean. Free Association Books, London

Pollock G 1999 Differencing the canon: feminism and the histories of art. Routledge, London

Reed L 1997 The Last Closet in Make 76. Journal of Women's Art April/May: 9

Ryder W 1987 The role of art in self-realization. Art Education 40(21): 22–24

Singleton E 1909 Dutch New York. Dodd, Mead, New York

Thurer S 1994 The myths of motherhood. Penguin, Harmondsworth

Tyldesley J 1995 Daughters of Isis: women of Ancient Egypt. Penguin Books, London

Waller J 1998 Birth visitors comments book. Axiom Gallery, Cheltenham

CHAPTER THREE

Birth Art as a Timeless Avenue to a Soulful Birth

)————————————(•)————————————(

PAM ENGLAND

Almost everyone loves to hear birth stories. Even more moving and engaging is seeing the story teller's image, one they drew or painted to portray some part of their story.

For the past 15 years I have been showing countless expectant and postpartum parents and birth-related professionals how to use drawing, painting or sculpting as a powerful tool for self-discovery and holistic preparation for childbirth. Parents also gain profound insights using the birth art process to help resolve birth trauma.

Quite by accident, I began studying the images and art of expectant and postpartum parents in 1988 while earning my Masters in counseling psychology. As a nurse-midwife and artist, I thought it might be interesting to compare the images of ancient and modern pregnant women. So I designed a small study for my thesis in which I collected images made by 18 pregnant women in their first and third trimesters.

The result was so compelling that I introduced the process of making birth art during my prenatal visits and childbirth classes, and have been continually fascinated ever since. This chapter lays the foundation for creating a space for parents to make and explore their own images.

While the primal power of the mother and child relationship has been expressed by Western artists in the past two centuries, less common are images associated with the experience of giving birth. Although common to ancient and indigenous peoples, birth-related art (both folk and professional) has been lost to modern Westerners.

Birth is a universal experience that literally touches everyone, so why in the past few centuries has there been almost no art devoted to the mystery of pregnancy and birth? Patriarchy's oppression of women debarred them from education, reading, writing, making art or the practice of medicine, and eventually midwifery. As a result, the artistic and historical account of women's lives and experiences was limited to that which sprang from the consciousness of men.

By excluding the work of women artists from history, men maintained control not only of women themselves but also of their worldview. Women were socialised to define themselves and their relationships to the world only through men's perception of reality. Women learned to validate their perceptions according to the dominant male view, including the medical model's perception of birth (Chicago 1979, p.159).

The absence of folk art, sacred birth art or the practice of making birth art as a part of antenatal preparation creates a void which is filled by the culture's dominant images of birth: medical images. Thus, from childhood, a woman unconsciously adopts medical images of birth, without ever exploring her own images of *being* pregnant or *giving* birth. Yet it is her own images, whether ignored or acknowledged, that

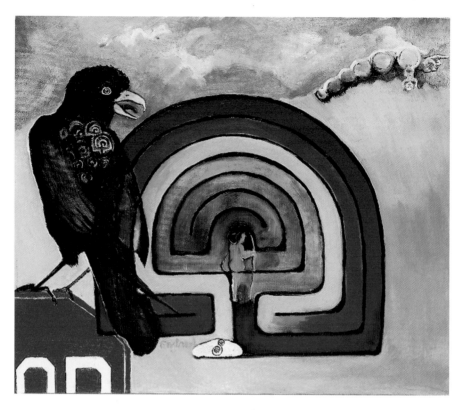

Figure 3.1 Raven

determine how she prepares for and thus experiences her transitions during the childbearing year.

This is made clear in Sara's story. After a normal pregnancy, Sara's first labour was induced with pitocin (syntocinon) but the induction failed. After 2 days, her cervix had only dilated to 3 cm and her baby became distressed. She gave birth by caesarean section.

Several years later, pregnant with her second child, Sara was receiving routine antenatal care from a midwife. She worried about having another labour that did not progress and she was terrified of the pain. Her plan was to avoid pain by learning self-hypnosis and to avoid medical intervention by having a home birth.

Even after being proactive and taking precautions, Sara was still anxious and fearful. Her preparation had consisted of obtaining information from the experts as if it could be used as ammunition against her fears.

I asked her, 'How do you envision your cervix opening in labour this time?'

Her head cocked to one side, she stared at me with a dazed look. 'I don't know, I don't see my cervix.' What she meant was, 'I don't see my cervix opening'.

Sara *was* still carrying a frozen image of her cervix 'not opening' with all that pain and work last time. She was about to go into this labour with an image of her cervix not opening foremost in her mind. If there is a connection between mind and body, this would not be in her best interests.

Sara's holistic antenatal preparation required her to paint a series of images of her cervix opening, softening and releasing her baby, and of how she saw herself *coping* with the intensity of labour.

Scientific, medical images of birth inform the cerebral but they do not connect us to our own mother-knowing; they do not connect us with our ancestors or living community; they do not awaken our maternal instincts.

Medical professionals must rely on accurate scientific images of the human body. Nonetheless, medical birth images objectify the body; they fragment our continuous, subjective experience of pregnancy, birth and the postpartum period into parts, trimesters, stages, organs, cells, hormones and a host of microscopic measurable values.

Photographs, illustrations and the language in medical textbooks, and even some consumer books on birth, reduce the birthing woman to a 'patient', often positioning her on her back and draped in sterile sheets. These images are not benign for women or their 'caregivers'; images like these shape everyone's expectations, beliefs and behaviour.

Without an introspective process like birth art, parents tend to ignore or even discount their own imagery, especially if it differs from the expert's representation. In preparing for birth and motherhood, it is of critical importance that pregnant women explore their own images. Both the *process* of making birth art as well as their *reflection* on the process (not the product) give mothers and fathers insights they could never have in an ordinary classroom experience (listening to a teacher, taking notes or watching videos).

Art and ambience in the clinical setting

'Art in the community has a subtle, unconscious, refining influence... True art strikes deeper than the surface. There is that which we call the subconscious. We do certain things and are influenced by certain things without knowing why. We hear a band play a military selection, and, though we may not be at all martially inclined, we suddenly become conscious of the fact that we have walked in step to the music.'

(Robert Henri 1923)

And so it is with 'maternity patients' who, upon entering the clinical environment loaded with symbols that non-verbally entrain them, unconsciously begin to 'walk in step' with the unspoken values of their 'caregivers'.

Most people are aware that their mood and health can be immediately altered by the environment, decor, lighting or music. Midwives and other healthcare professionals trained and working in the healthcare system gradually become impervious to the clinic environment, until eventually the symbols and messages embedded in everything from health posters to the general interior decorating go unnoticed by the conscious mind.

An expectant mother, as a visitor to a clinic environment new to her, will notice everything. What will she see? What meaning will she unconsciously give it? How will the environment affect her sense of well-being or happiness or motivate her to self-care as a mother?

Unfortunately, antenatal clinics and birth room decor are typically 'denatured', a mirror image of the impersonal, objective and harried world of medical care. Clinic spaces are designed for the staff to function efficiently. Waiting and examining rooms, birthing and recovery rooms are not designed or decorated with the patients' emotional or psychological well-being in mind. When prenatal clinics and birth rooms are completely devoid of nature and nature symbols, sacred symbols and folk art, what non-verbal message does the ambience send?

'A single mental picture can have a far more potent effect on
the body than a dictionary of words.'

(Jaffe & Bresler 1980)

Imagine a labouring mother walking slowly down the long, brightly lit public corridor in a labour and delivery ward. It is lined with at least 20 huge photographs bordered in identical ornate, antique-gold painted frames. Photo after photo, flawless models (who have never gained an extra pound or lost an hour of sleep!) pose as mothers in ridiculous white satin and lacey dresses; each model holds a baby dressed in white satin, a perfectly content baby smiling or sleeping peacefully on the model's lap. Each time the labouring mother looks up as a contraction fades away, her eyes rest for a moment on one of these soulless, deceptive photos selling the myth of motherhood. What is this all about? How is this art inspiring or informing the mother?

Redecorating without Martha Stewart

Art isn't just a framed picture on the wall, it's expressed in a thousand ways from the colours we wear or use to paint our walls, to the way that tea is served. A small gesture can make a huge difference; consider a small water fountain or bouquet of fresh flowers.

Instead of commercial art, consider displaying birth art made by parents with a brief written description of what the drawing inspired in the parent. Not only does this validate the parent who made the art and inspire the parents who see and read about the art, but it breaks down the hierarchy of learning and invites parents to learn from one another.

Creating a space for parents to make birth art

First, you will need to provide a few supplies and prepare the space. You can offer one medium at a time. Experiment to find out what you and your clients like best.

Drawing

Given the opportunity, tools and an assignment, most parents eagerly begin to draw. A few parents hesitate, worrying that they don't know 'how to draw'. Achieving realism is not the object of making any art, especially not birth art. Birth art is for the parent (not the midwife or anyone else) to see what she or he has not seen before, to take a moment to reflect on what's going on.

'Drawing is energy made visible,' explains Pat Allen (1995) in her book *Art is a Way of Knowing*. 'Drawing is a way to contact the energy of the subject matter ... or an inner state of being' (p.21).

What you will need

1. *Soft chalk pastels or oil pastels*. Soft chalk pastels make drawing an image effortless (avoid the cheap, waxy-hard ones found in office supply); the process is relaxing and colours blend easily. Chalk pastels leave dust behind so you will need to protect carpet with a plastic or muslin dropcloth. Instruct parents to spill the loose dust on their drawings into a waste basket before holding it up.

    With oil pastels, colours blend well, but it is a greasy medium that requires effort to apply. Especially if the image will be dense with colour, sturdy paper (not newsprint) will be required. Oil pastels won't leave dust but you don't want toddlers writing on the walls or furniture with them.

    Advice about crayons, pens and pencils – if you must protect the walls and furniture from toddler-art, crayons, pens and pencils may be a solution; however, be aware they are the worst media for parents. The hard waxy quality of crayons requires a lot of work to create a strong image, they do not lend themselves to detail, and because they do not blend well, 'mistakes' feel permanent. Pens are permanent and 'unforgiving'; both pens and pencils are typically used to write, so the left brain will be instantly activated. Pencil drawings invite the temptation to erase, fix, 'get it right', completely undermining the purpose of making birth art. All these obstacles ultimately discourage the novice artist.

2. *Plain white paper*; butcher paper will do. Offer typing paper and larger sheets, 17" × 24".

3. *A drawing surface*. A small table or a firm board to rest on the lap, i.e. a clipboard or cardboard.

Painting

Painting calls for sensuous strokes with a big brush or fingers. Parents use more colour and make bolder images. Painting seems to allow the image to emerge, layer over layer, and without question, parents become more relaxed and introspective with painting than with other media.

What you will need

1. *Paint brushes*. Soft natural hair (squirrel hair), size 8–10.

2. *Container of clean water*.

3. *Tempera paints*. Five colours will suffice: black, white and the primary colours (red, blue and yellow). Use small wide-mouthed jars to hold the paint, so that you can cover them air-tight at the end of the day and preserve them. Add a little water to thin if they begin to dry out.

4. *White paper* on the table or taped to the wall or a cardboard that leans against the wall; paper should be 17" × 24" or larger and 60# weight or more.

5. Plastic or muslin *dropcloth* beneath the painting.

Sculpting

The oldest birth art was made in clay or carved in the limestone walls of caves 200 000 years ago. Our prehistoric ancestors' awe at the mystery of pregnancy and birth is reflected in the exquisite form and power found in their sculptures of the Great Mother.

Clay gives three-dimensional form to our images. It gets us in touch with the earth and the earthy part of ourselves, the messy part of life and birth. It's the medium of choice if parents want to get in touch with their gut instinct or feelings. Clay is malleable, taking and losing form, following and giving shape to one's thoughts. Using clay, parents can carve or construct an image. Clay is a great medium for carving a LabOrinth (see below) and for sculpting a handheld sculpture of a power symbol or an animal that reminds them of easy birthing and good mothering. The small sculpture can be fired and later held in labour as a focal point.

You can create a workspace covered with a plastic tablecloth on the table and one on the floor to prevent drips or chalk dust from damaging rugs or fabric.

Some sculptures last only as long as it takes to witness them; then they can be crushed and thrown back in the clay bag. Other sculptures want to be kept dry.

What you will need

1. *Various sculpting materials* to choose from: bee's wax, Sculpey or earth clay. Wax and Sculpey are more expensive and they are not messy (which is not necessarily a plus for birth art). Sculpey comes in colours and it can be baked in a home oven to make it permanent. Grey or red clay can be bought inexpensively from art or ceramic supply stores.

2. *Dropcloth.* Canvas is optimal as it absorbs fluid from the clay as it's worked. Roll up the canvas to store it. You don't need to wash it, just shake the clay dust out occasionally.

3. *Small sponge.* Putting a wet sponge in a bag of stiff clay remoistens it. Also, a small sponge can be used to smooth clay sculptures.

4. *Tools* (optional). Clay sculptures can be built solely by hand. However, you can provide a few simple clay sculpting tools from the art store or kitchen, e.g. garlic press, ice pick, knives and forks. In making labyrinths (described below), you will need a rolling pin, an object to draw the pattern into the clay, and one to gouge or smooth out the corridors.

How much time does this take?

You do not have to sit with the parents while they make birth art; it's an introspective process and they go deeper and feel more relaxed about it when they are not being watched. The time parents would otherwise idle away in the waiting room is constructively used to make art or perhaps write a journal.

Just create the space and provide the materials and assignments – parents will do the rest. Most parents work best from suggested assignments (see below). If you are inviting parents to make birth art while they sit in the waiting room for an appointment, write a birth art 'assignment of the week' on a whiteboard or leave a list of ideas posted on the wall. Even a brief prenatal visit is enriched when you talk about what they learned from the *process* of making the image.

Childbirth classes provide another opportunity to make birth art. Give parents an art assignment in class. While they work for 15–20 minutes, you can have a cup of tea and relax. Before talking about their art in the group, suggest they journal what they learned from the process or the image; give them another 5–10 minutes to do this. Because we are more accustomed to writing, journaling helps us gather our thoughts before sharing in a group. Not everyone will want or need to share but by journaling for a few minutes, parents capture and reflect on what was important for them.

Talk to the mothers (or fathers) about their *process* while making the art, not about the *product*. As a midwife, you will enjoy seeing the colourful images. Avoid the temptation to focus on the art, to ask questions about the art (product). That is equivalent to looking at the electronic monitor in labour to get information without looking at or talking to the mother. Here are a few questions that help parents learn from their art or art-making process.

- Was there a moment while making this picture/sculpture when you were surprised?
- Was there a moment when you didn't know what to do next? What did you do then? (Some people, when they don't know what to do next, will simply quit. They are afraid of making a mistake or getting disapproval so they quit 'while they are ahead'. It's not so important what you actually did when you didn't know what to do; it's more important that you *notice* your habitual tendency when you face the unknown. You can learn to 'know thyself', to disrupt the habitual mind and cultivate a resourceful, solution-focused mindset. Part of holistic prenatal education is to develop personal skills, not just get information from measurements and books.)
- Sometimes we get attached to the painting at a certain point, thinking it looks pretty good and if we keep going, we'll mess it up. So we quit to look good. (Kind of like taking the epidural in labour before we embarrass ourselves by making too much noise.)
- What do you know now that you didn't know before making this image, or before taking time to reflect on it? Was there something you've been thinking about or trying to avoid that showed up in the drawing?
- What needs to be done next? This process is not a psychological assessment of the artist; it is a living process, allowing her to see what she has not seen before and to take action. Thinking about something is not action. She must *do* something.

A few birth art assignments

Being pregnant
What is *being* pregnant like for you? Go beyond what others tell you it is or should be. It could be a physical experience, social event, emotional or spiritual feeling or an abstract image.

Womb with a view
Imagine you could take a peek through a window in your womb. What is your baby doing in his/her womb all day? What does your baby look like? What does he/she see, feel or hear?

Strongest image of giving birth
When you think of being in labour or giving birth, what image comes to mind first and most strongly? It can be positive, negative, scary, spiritual; take a good look and include as many details as you see or feel.

Birth in our culture

Pretend you are an alien on a mission. You must send back one picture that captures the way humanoids in this culture give birth. Include as much detail as you can to communicate our rituals, beliefs and feelings about childbirth.

Clay sculpture assignments

1. If using earth clay, first 'work the clay', i.e. squish and fold it to work out the air bubbles so your sculpture won't blow up during firing in the kiln.
2. Sometimes a form will emerge out of the lump of clay, and you can work the clay to bring it out. Sometimes an image will just come to mind as you are working the clay.
3. You can also bring and sculpt from the clay an image of:
    *   an animal that reminds you of easy birthing or good mothering
    *   a symbol that connects you to your spirituality, to your ancestors or personal power.
4. Sculpt a hand-held LabOrinth.

Seeing our way: labyrinth becomes LabOrinth

Here's a simple birth art project that teaches parents about the psychological and spiritual stages of labour they are likely to encounter. They can hang their LabOrinth on the wall during labour as a focal point that induces a state of relaxation.

Labour graph as a symbol

An object or abstraction that represents something else is a symbol; symbols send non-verbal messages to the right hemisphere of the brain, where they are felt instantly throughout the body and emotions.

The tools a birth attendant relies on to monitor labour are not necessarily going to be as helpful to the labouring mother. A classic example is the (controversial) labour graph (also called partogram or Friedman's graph), on which the watchful birth attendant plots a labouring mother's cervical dilation and the descent of her baby against a 'normal labour progress' timeline. This aids in early detection and treatment of an abnormal labour pattern.

The labour data graph depicts how medical people see labour – *from the outside*. While this tool helps birth attendants, it is an oversimplified and confusing *symbol* for parents who often internalise the straight line of progress as an expectation that labour will progress in a straight line!

Expectant parents need a different symbol or tool to navigate birth from their perspective – *from within*. Most mothers and fathers agree that their experience of labour is better depicted as a labyrinth.

The labyrinth is a universal, sacred symbol of life. It's universal (as opposed to personal) because it's been found across the globe on cave walls, pottery, weavings and even in centuries-old European churches.

A labyrinth represents the roller-coaster drama in our lives, our back-and-forth decision-making process, and the body itself. The labyrinth resembles organic patterns

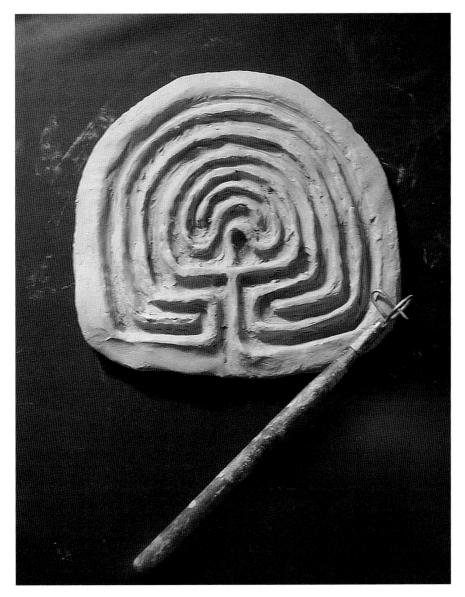

Figure 3.2 Lab O rinth

we see in a human brain, intestines and circulatory system; a structure in the inner ear is called the labyrinth. The first journeys we make from our father's body to our mother's womb, and from the centre of our mother's body into the world, are labyrinthine.

Unlike a maze, which has many dead ends and wrong choices designed to trick the mind, a labyrinth is a design with a single, winding, unobstructed path from the outside of itself to the centre. The labyrinth user makes no choices in direction; therefore, the labyrinth path naturally fosters mental relaxation and introspection, and is frequently

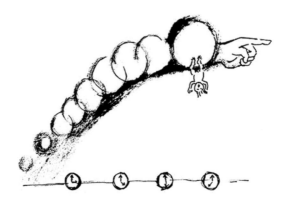

Figure 3.3 Partograph. Cervical dilation is represented by successively larger circles, beginning at 1-2 cm dilation and openning gradually, until – at the end of the line – the cervix is completely dilated. The baby falls out and the mother is discharged (represented by pointing finger), and that's, that.

viewed by its users as a metaphor for our spiritual 'life' journey. In other words, like life, labyrinths contain many twists and turns but no dead ends (Artress 1995).

From the moment a woman discovers she is with child, she inevitably crosses an invisible threshold and enters a psychic labyrinth as a maiden. Through her ordinary life, taking one step, one day and one contraction at a time, she will reach the centre, where she gives birth not only to her child but to herself as a mother. She cannot linger in the centre, nor can she exit quickly by crossing the lines of the labyrinth. She must return along the same path, slowly and patiently, allowing her the time she needs to process her birth experience and integrate her new status as a mother.

As an antenatal teaching tool, the ancient labyrinth becomes a LabOrinth. Could there be a more fitting compass for mothers in the childbearing year?

Ancient peoples and healers knew empirically what modern research has confirmed. Whether we are walking a labyrinth on the ground, finger-tracing a handheld labyrinth or tracing a wall-hanging labyrinth with the eye, within minutes we experience a profound sense of calmness, well-being and effortless, creative problem solving. While walking or tracing a labyrinth, blood pressure and pulse lower and EEGs show changes in brain waves.

We rely on the neurons in our brain to fire rapidly when we assimilate new information or need to concentrate, make quick decisions or be coordinated (in motor skills). When beta waves in the brain fire rapidly, between 13 and 40 Hz, we are in a *beta* state. When attending a labour, midwives should be in a beta state, i.e. wide awake, alert and attentive.

On the other hand, labouring mothers do not labour well when their brain is in a hypervigilant beta state. A woman in active labour is likely to experience a slowing of brain waves, ranging between 7 and 12 Hz. This is called the *alpha* state; it is a place of deep relaxation but not quite meditation. It is important to cultivate this state during labour preparation exercises as mothers will experience it when they are in the normal endorphin-trance of labour.

In the alpha state, a mother is aware of what's going on around her but she notices objectively, without judgements and mental chatter. Imagined fears fade into the background while a sense of peace and well-being occupies the foreground of consciousness. This allows her to access creativity, intuition and insights that were just out of her reach in beta state.

Going deeper into relaxation, she enters the *theta* state where brain activity slows almost to the point of sleep, but not quite. Theta waves range between 4 and 7 Hz. In this state, a mother would experience flashes of dreamlike imagery and a sensation of 'floating'. Because it is an expansive state, she may feel her mind expand beyond the boundaries of her body. It is nature's design for mothers to experience active labour (without medication) in alpha and theta as a way of coping with the intense physical work and the need for intuitive knowing.

In the alpha or theta states, the activity in the left and right hemispheres becomes balanced. This is called brain synchrony and is associated with enhanced learning, flashes of insight and intuitive awareness (Ayres 1979, Fehmi & Fritz 1980).

How to make a seven-circuit labyrinth

What you will need

1. *Soft pastels or coloured pencils.* These media can be smudged or erased should you make a mistake (whereas magic markers are permanent). Using two colours helps beginners stay on course by using one colour to draw the template and another to draw the arcs. Once the labyrinth is complete, you can go over it with one colour or blend in many colours.

2. *Paper.* Any size will do for practice or finger-tracing. However, if parents want to hang their LabOrinth on the wall as a focal point for labour, they should make it on a large sheet of paper.

Directions

- First, draw the template (Fig. 3.4). Labyrinths 'grow' upwards, so place the template in the lower third of your paper. If you place the template in the centre of the paper, you will run out of room at the top before you finish drawing all the arcs.
- Next, draw the arcs.
- Think of the tip of each line and each dot as a 'point'. You will be connecting a point from the left side in sequence to the next available point on the right (see Fig. 3.4).
- Begin with the centre point (i.e., the upper point on the vertical line in the cross) and draw an arc to the first point on the right (the vertical tip on the 'corner'). Ironically, the first line you drew formed the centre, the 'end' of the labyrinth's path.
- Continue making arcs from left to right until the labyrinth is complete. You will have to extend the lines and dots horizontally to make the labyrinth's

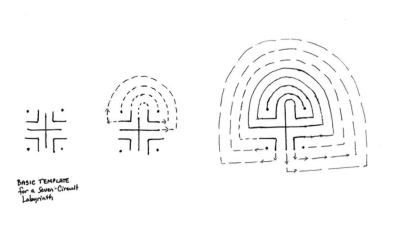

BASIC TEMPLATE
for a Seven-Circuit
Labyrinth

Figure 3.4 Basic Template for a Seven-Circuit Labyrinth

corridors fairly uniform. (You can also make a labyrinth making arcs from right to left.)

- Give your labyrinth a trial run. Finger-trace the path from the entrance to the centre to be sure the path is continuous. Sometimes it takes more than one try but the process of making the labyrinth is not unlike the patience required to find your way through labour.

How to make a LabOrinth

- Draw the seven-circuit labyrinth.
- Draw a Threshold Stone, an essential step in making a LabOrinth. The threshold stone for the LabOrinth was inspired by the impression made by the daunting threshold that marks the narrow entrance to the ancient burial chamber at New Grange in Ireland. A massive threshold stone, elaborately decorated with geometric designs, forced the seeker coming from the mundane world to stop and reflect, if only for the moment it took to figure out how to climb over it. When leaving the tomb, facing the monolithic threshold prevents a mindless reentry into the world.

  As a sacred symbol, thresholds remind us (or force us) to pause, to bring our attention to this blessed moment in which we are leaving one way of being or of knowing and entering into the unknown. Every threshold represents death and rebirth.

  We cross countless thresholds every day. There are invisible thresholds between the inbreath and the outbreath; the infinitesimal wave between not-knowing and knowing, not-seeing and seeing; waking and sleep. With attention, we can notice the moment of crossing the subtle, felt threshold from a sense of well-being to being out of sync – which enables us to respond to a situation or problem as a ripple, rather than wait until the flood.

There are ordinary visible thresholds, too, such as the doorsill at the front door which takes us from the private sanctuary of our home into the world, thresholds over subway doors, elevator doors, and the doorway from the corridor into the birthing room.

In Zen training, students are instructed to cross door thresholds with the left foot. It's not that the left foot is more special than the right; it's that being aware of which foot is crossing the threshold serves as a wake-up call. Any threshold practice is an invitation to be present, to acknowledge within one's own mind the end of one activity and the beginning of another.

There are countless thresholds in the childbearing year, emotional, physical and social. Passive waiting becomes active expulsion. Incubation becomes emergence, from darkness into light. A mother needs to be aware of these thresholds as part of birthing-in-awareness.

The Threshold Stone is an ancient and profound symbol reminding us to bring our full attention to the work at hand. Ancient people gave ordinary objects symbolic status by decorating them. Draw your Threshold Stone; make it big enough to cover the portal to your LabOrinth. Decorate the Threshold Stone with symbols that send a message to you.

- Now draw two little footprints in front of the Threshold Stone to represent you standing on the ground of everything you know and believe before you embark on labour or another upcoming life transition.
- Nothing should be drawn in the corridors or the centre of a labyrinth. However, some parents add drawings or write messages in the empty space outside the LabOrinth.

Metaphorical food for thought

Whether or not she feels 'ready', with her first contraction or when her water breaks, every mother crosses the threshold and enters her LabOrinth. Once in the LabOrinth, all a mother needs is steady determination to take one step at a time until she gives birth (symbolically represented by the centre of the labyrinth).

A mother cannot get lost in a labyrinth but in a maze she could lose her way and become disoriented. A maze has more than one entrance or exit and hidden cul-de-sacs, which means you have to make decisions, remember where you were, what did and didn't work, and think your way through to avoid getting lost. In a way, the maze is a fitting symbol for negotiating the many choices everyone must make in the managed medical-surgical model of birth.

There is no need to study the path before entering a labyrinth. In a similar way, women do not need to overplan labour; rather they need to feel and intuit their way through it. You could be blindfolded and still reach the centre of a labyrinth by feeling your way through the path. There is no time course or deadline.

One of the strict rules is to never look for a shortcut or exit the labyrinth by crossing over the lines. You must leave the same way you came, step by step through the seven circuits.

The Postpartum Return is beautifully aligned with the labyrinth. Soon after the birth, the mother is likely to be reflecting about the labour and birth, talking about it, writing about it; others will be asking her about it, bringing her food and presents. In the early postpartum weeks, the corridors are closely wrapped around the birth. But in due time, the corridors are further from the birth, longer like the long sleepless nights,

Did you know that Hindu midwives in India hang a yantra in the birth room? A yantra is a wall-hanging labyrinth. According to tradition, the parents should hang their labyrinth or yantra on a wall facing north or east, placing the centre of the labyrinth or yantra at the level of the mother's eyes. This may change as her position changes from standing to sitting or lying down.

The mother looks steadily into the centre of the yantra, trying not to blink a lot. She is instructed to focus on the centre while observing the whole yantra at once without looking at particular details.

As part of prenatal preparation, a mother can practise this exercise for at least 15–30 minutes every day. This practice will slow her brain waves down to alpha or theta and the experience will give her a sense of well-being.

the months of feeling isolated, misplaced, missing your old life... It takes 3 years to adjust as a couple.

The midwife's work as a labyrinth

While the expectant mother is traversing her LabOrinth, the midwife is navigating her own labyrinth-of-life. At any given moment, a midwife is moving through more than one labyrinth-of-life: one labyrinth represents her love relationship, another her career path, another represents the path unfolding moment to moment as she works alongside the labouring mother. In the Tao of Birthing, imagine that the mother, father, baby and midwife are arising together and moving together, at their own speed, in their own corridor but in the same LabOrinth.

Opening

From many books and childbirth class charts, mothers learn to envision cervical dilation as rigid concentric circles. Every midwife knows that a ripe, dilating cervix rarely feels rigid like the raised rigid circle on the plastic chart! But mothers don't know that, so they envision dilation as a rigid sensation.

What would mothers experience if we described the cervix as juicy, soft, stretchy and yielding as the baby pressed against it with every nudge from the contracting uterus?

Make a visual and visceral dilation image You can make this image for parents as a teaching demonstration and/or have them make one for themselves for experiential learning. Here's what to do: First, take down the rigid dilation charts. Throw them away. Put away your ruler. Mothers don't need to be scientific and specific about dilation (midwives do).

Next, get a big, big sheet of paper. Hang or prop it up on the wall. Get it wet with a sponge or spray bottle.

Give your big 5 cm (2") paintbrush a good long drink of water, then dip it in tempera, acrylic or water colour.

Paint a loose, not too perfect, circle representing the cervix when labour begins. Leave an opening in the centre of at least 3–4 cm.

Then, give your brush another big drink of water and, using a little different colour, make another juicy 'cervix' that has dilated more. Allow the edges to be a little irregular or wavy to illustrate its capacity to stretch.

Then grab a bigger paintbrush (8 cm or 3"), let it take a big drink of water first and dip it into a new colour and make a juicy, yielding, opening wide-and-loose cervix. Let the paint drip and run down the paper, like amniotic water running down the mother's legs.

Parents will be amused at your antics but they will also be adopting new felt-imagery. Let this demonstration portray the living quality of labour.

You could also let the mothers make their own juicy-opening cervical dilation charts and bring them to labour where they can hang on the wall and invoke that feeling within.

Opening in labour When we talk about opening in labour, we usually think of cervical dilation but we know that 'opening' in labour is much more than that. This birth art process begins by asking the parents that if the *activity* of labour could be described in one word, what would that word be? ... Opening.

Parents are asked to get comfortable and close their eyes as they are guided with a visualisation that takes them from head to toe, envisioning a psychological, emotional and physical opening in labour of the mind, throat, heart, pelvic bones, cervix and vagina. Upon opening their eyes, parents are invited to paint their new, expanded image of 'Opening in Labour'.

These images are among the most colourful and celebratory among the birth art assignments. Parents often hang these images in the birth room as a reminder to open their entire being to the powerful work of labour.

Conclusion

As midwife, you bear witness not only to the baby's emergence but to the emergence of the mother, father and family. What is expressed during the birth art process and journaling also need to be witnessed, without being interpreted, judged or evaluated. The witness affirms the birth of the insight, the emergence of clarity and intention.

Few images stand the test of time and hold a universal truth, such as the Venus of Willendorf. As the image is being expressed, it is a living statement. Once the image is finished, it often becomes historical statement because the person who made the image and had insights is already a 'changed' person. So, it is important that neither the parent nor the midwife becomes attached to the image or its story.

The overall response from mothers and fathers who make birth art is positive. They appreciate the opportunity to be creative, to be heard, to get in touch with what is really going on inside them.

Over and over, women report that they never thought about how they envisioned their own pregnancy and that in reflecting on their images, they encountered a whole range of new experiences. One mother said, 'Being in the work world, I felt like denatured alcohol. Making birth art brought nature back into my pregnancy. All women should do this'.

Often parents feel increased awareness of their unborn child or they get in touch with issues that need to be addressed to be fully prepared to give birth or become parents. One first-time mother said, 'I became aware of my fear of looking primitive or needy. I knew it vaguely before the drawing, but I knew it definitely after making the painting'. After this fear was made conscious, she explored her biases and created new beliefs that would not inhibit her natural behaviour in labour.

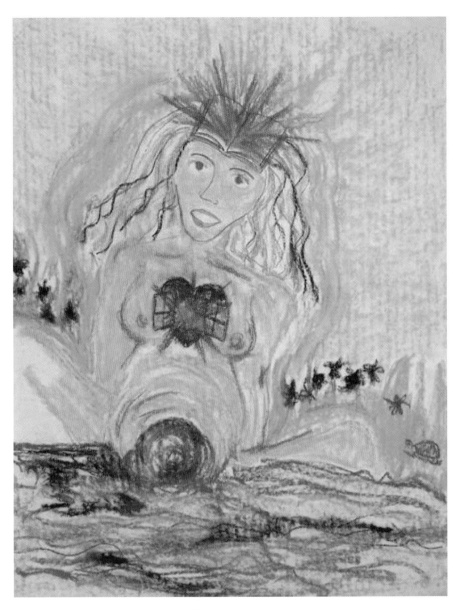

Figure 3.5 Jennifer

'My image came to me while Pam led the class through a visualisation exercise on opening in birth. The [image of the] open book in my mind represents the acceptance of both learned knowledge and internal, natural wisdom. Moving downward, my eyes and mouth are open, mirroring my opening cervix as it prepares for the birth of my baby. My heart's a wide open window that reveals a shining light and lets in light as well. I am in nature, surrounded by a calm blue sky, lushness speckled with blooms and swirling, flowing water. Each area holds the others' colours, the energy that moves through the whole image is the same energy that will birth the child and the mother.'

— 46 —   (Jennifer, first-time mother; Fig. 3.5)

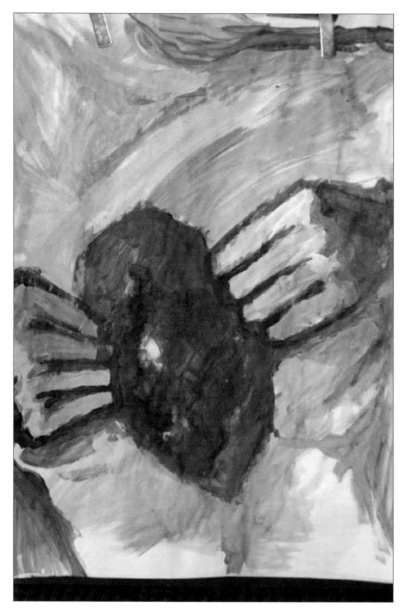

• *Figure 3.6 Jimmie*

'I am told that birth will change my life, and I know part of me will try to fight that. This drawing is about the strength I will need in order to open myself and accept the change, to allow myself to become a father.'

(Jimmie; Fig. 3.6)

The process of making birth art can be viewed as an analogy for the process of giving birth. When parents hesitate because they don't know 'how to draw or make art', it is analogous to not knowing how to have a contraction or take care of a baby; it is analogous to wanting to do it right, to let experts make art or deliver them. By stretching past their comfort zone and meeting some kind of success, they are building confidence to meet the unknown in labour and parenting.

References

Allen PB 1995 Art is a way of knowing. Shambhala, Boston, MA

Artress L 1995 Walking a sacred path: rediscovering the labyrinth as a spiritual tool. Riverhead Books, New York

Ayres AJ 1979 Sensory integration and the child. Western Psychological Services, Los Angeles, CA

Chicago J 1979 The Birth Project. Doubleday, New York

Fehmi L, Fritz G 1980 Open focus: the attentional foundation of health and well-being. Somatics 2: 34–40

Henri R 1923 The art of Spirit. Westview Press, Boulder, CO

Jaffe DT, Bresler DE 1980 The use of guided imagery as an adjunct to medical diagnosis and treatment. Journal of Humanistic Psychology 20(4): 45–59

CHAPTER FOUR

The Delivery of Art in a Maternity Hospital

MARY GREHAN

The field of arts and health has, to a large extent, emerged from a perceived relationship between art and healing. This has been realised not only by the arts therapies and participatory arts activities in healthcare contexts but also by the creation of healing environments (Kirklin & Richardson 2003) in which the placement of visual art plays a role. However, this rationale for art in hospitals may not have the same currency in a maternity hospital in which, despite the medicalisation of pregnancy and childbirth, most of the clients are not medically ill. If the therapeutic benefits of art in maternity hospitals are made redundant by the context, art in maternity hospitals needs to be considered under alternative agendas. In art terms, the process of placing art in a hospital is driven by recent trends to bring art out of galleries and museums and to integrate it into the fabric of society. This is being done through community arts, site-specific public art, artists' residencies and through curating exhibitions in non-traditional contexts.

As a curator, I have explored all these ways of delivering an arts experience in hospitals and in so doing, have walked a tightrope between the culture of the maternity hospital and that of the art world. In this chapter, I will categorise this curatorial work into two approaches for the purposes of reflecting on the challenges, rewards and unexpected outcomes that are specific to placing art in maternity hospitals with reference to specific examples. I will draw upon my own experience of curating art in hospital contexts over the past 11 years, interviews with professionals in the fields of midwifery and arts and health, relevant literature and my research around the experience of viewing art in hospitals.

One approach to placing art in hospitals is in line with gallery curatorship. Art that fits the physical environment and perceived needs of the audience is installed, often taking the form of temporary exhibitions and permanent collections. The artwork is not produced specifically for the hospital context and equally could be found in a gallery context. The relationship is directly between the artwork and its viewer and there is divergent thinking around the most appropriate art for this kind of intervention, which this chapter will consider.

An alternative and more contemporary approach is contextual art practice in which the artist engages with the physical, psychological and social dimensions of the hospital, which in turn becomes the very stuff of the artwork. The artist is afforded the opportunity to forge a relationship, and in some cases collaborate, with the hospital community.

'What exists ... is an unknown relationship between artist and audience, a relationship that may itself become the artwork.'

(Lacy 1995, p.20)

Contextual art practice is explored here through examples of site-specific commissions and residencies. While not advocating one approach over another, this chapter will consider how each determines the nature of the relationship between the viewer and the artwork.

In 1994, I curated an extensive, multidisciplinary arts programme for the National Maternity Hospital (NMH), Holles Street, Dublin, the impetus for which came from the hospital's celebrations of its centenary and its desire to raise its public profile in the context of a perceived competitive climate between the three main maternity hospitals in Dublin. The programme comprised a major exhibition on the themes of maternity, fertility and regeneration, participatory arts workshops for staff members and the children of patients, an outreach community arts programme which engaged a women's group in the area, a writer's residency with poet Eavan Boland, a play commission with playwright Marina Carr and a programme of seven site-specific artworks produced in response to the hospital context and installed throughout the building. The latter had the greatest impact on the various strata of the hospital community.

'Probably the most dramatic thing was the [site] visit of 60 artists to the hospital. Once you let all of those people walk all over the hospital, things would never be the same.'

(Matron Maeve Dwyer, interview, 1995)

The artworks generated a stream of responses from patients, visitors and staff, and from the wider community, most of which could not have been anticipated at the commissioning stage. People engaged with them often as something other than art, in a way that illustrated very forcibly how we bring our personal experiences to bear on the process of viewing art. Through these responses, which were often unexpected and always revealing, the artworks raised issues about the nature of the institution which up to that point had not been articulated. This is demonstrated by '100 Names and Dates', the first of the site-specific commissions, in which artist Áine Nic Giolla Coda sign-wrote 100 names and years of birth of babies born in the NMH or delivered by NMH nurses, over the previous century, throughout the building. Each name denoted all the babies born in the hospital that year (Figs 4.1, 4.2).

Approximately 2500 names and dates were offered to the project by the users of the hospital and members of the public. Many of these came with special requests and anecdotes relating to the birth, some of which were of social and historical significance. The artist selected the 100 names, one for each year since 1894, at random. However, the question of selection of names became a highly contentious one among members of staff, as many asserted a right to have their name on the wall. The names were seen as some kind of reward or accolade. Up until that point, the only names on the walls were those of the Masters, emblazoned in gold in the front hall. Unlike the Masters' names, the only achievement that was celebrated through '100 Names and Dates' was, quite simply, the achievement of being born.

'The Mastership system of management which was expressed in the charter [of the Rotunda Hospital, Dublin of 1752] was subsequently adopted by the Coombe and National Maternity Hospital [Dublin] and appears to have stood the test of time. This system ensures that one person is responsible for any policy decisions and for the day to day running of the hospital over a seven year period.'

(Mary Robinson, cited in Browne 1995, p.x)

In some cases, the project called people to draw upon their personal histories. One woman, whose name had been included in the artwork, travelled from Co. Donegal in the north west of Ireland to see it and attend the coffee morning we organised to

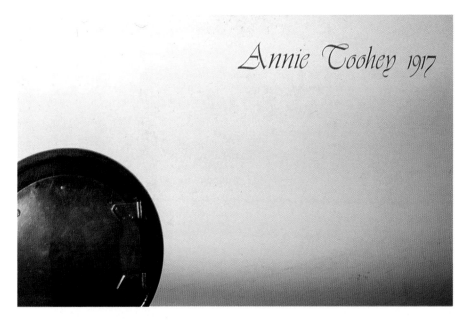

Figure 4.1 Anne Toohey © Aine Nic Giolla Coda

celebrate the completion of the project. She was the only survivor of triplets and she brought with her memorabilia relating to her birth and the birth of her siblings, such as receipts from the B&B her father stayed in on the night of the birth. This project was a testament to the birth of the siblings she never knew.

In looking at maternity hospitals as places for positioning art, this project reminds us that they do more than house and enable the process of childbirth. They also form an important part of people's history and identity. The place of birth has a significance for us for life. It is written on our birth certificate and becomes part of our formal identity. It can determine a number of socioeconomic and cultural factors in our lives. We are born *into* places. They are part of our inheritance.

'I think that the Names and Dates project challenged people to consider who the hospital is here for, who matters and who has power in this institution. Every time you pass one of these names, it's a very strong, powerful message coming across ... that this person matters.'

(Matron Maeve Dwyer, interview, 1995)

Like many site-specific artworks which explore and excavate a site, the democracy of '100 Names and Dates' was a catalyst for something greater than the artwork itself. In this case, the project created a debate about issues of ownership, control and power within the hospital. Art became 'the leveller', facilitating points of contact and dialogue between the various strata of the hospital hierarchy and contributing to a sense of community in which no viewer is an expert and every viewer is an expert.

Another NMH site-specific artwork was 'Viewer' by Kate Malone which took the form of a series of photographs presented on light boxes and placed throughout the hospital – the special care unit, the gynaecological clinic, the gynaecological ward,

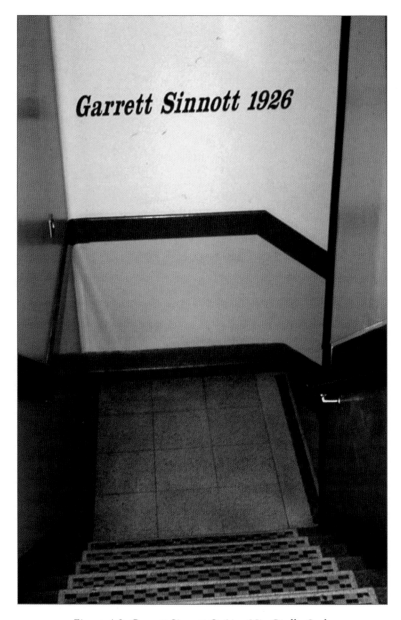

Figure 4.2 Garrett Sinnott © Aine Nic Giolla Coda

the mother and baby room, the delivery ward, the private postnatal ward and the fetal assessment unit. These were produced over a period of 6 months which Kate spent in the hospital, meeting staff, parents and babies, and photographing the hospital environment and its babies. Kate was particularly taken with the special care unit and the question of dependence and independence of the premature baby.

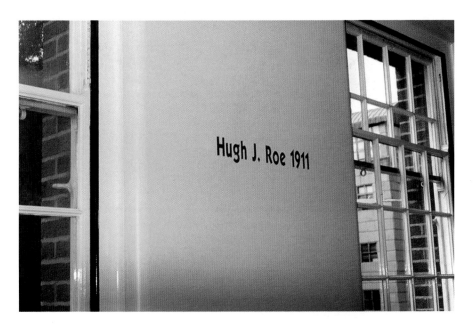

Figure 4.3 Hugh J. Roe © Aine Nic Giolla Coda

Despite a considered and sensitive placing of images, they generated strong responses from the users of the hospital. The nursing manager of the fetal assessment unit asked Kate to remove the image of a woman's naked pregnant abdomen which had been placed in the unit, which she said was not liked by the women waiting for their ultrasound check-up. She requested instead, on behalf of the women, that Kate replace the image with a photograph of an ultrasound scan Kate had taken, which suggests that the expectant women were more comfortable with images of the interior of their womb than the exterior of their abdomen.

Likewise, Kate's image of an empty cot in the private wing, although ambiguous, was interpreted as ominous by staff. Psychological tests have shown that perception is influenced by the viewer's expectations (Coren et al 1979, p.362). Expectations are in turn determined by the context in which images are viewed. The request to remove the image reflected patients' fears that their pregnancy might not reach full term or that they may not give birth to a healthy baby. One visitor had taken the image to be a 'baby snatching warning device'. (Baby snatching had been in the news at that time.) Once again Kate replaced this image. Through this negotiation with the audience about the artwork, she recognised the maternity hospital as an emotionally loaded environment which impacts on how art is viewed.

The boundaries between the various types of contextual art practice are becoming increasingly blurred as artists explore the relationship between their work with its audience. Áine Nic Giolla Coda's and Kate Malone's projects began as public art commissions and evolved into residencies, in which the artists had a visible presence in the hospital and built a working relationship with the hospital community. This model of residency can accommodate the sort of dialogue and negotiation we experienced in Kate's project, 'Viewer'.

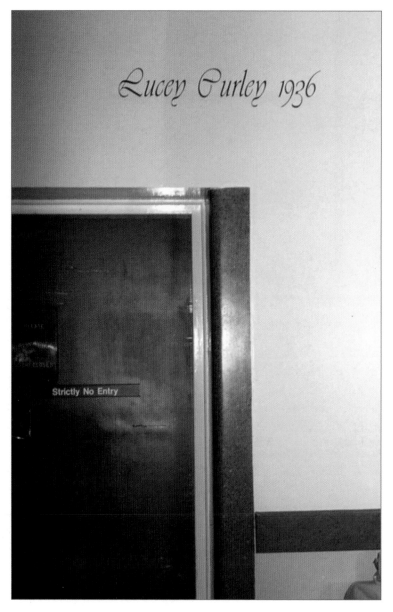

Figure 4.4 Lucy Turley © Aine Nic Giolla Coda

In 1999, Gabriella Sancisi was artist-in-residence for 2 weeks in Dorset County Hospital as part of a public art commissioning scheme. During this time she produced a series of six large, dramatic portraits of naked babies newly born in the maternity unit which went on permanent display on a main corridor of the general hospital. The maternity unit subsequently requested that a series of 20 smaller photographs by Gabriella of babies taken during her residency be placed in the labour ward.

Although the display of images of babies in maternity hospitals can be controversial, the response to these images in Dorset County Hospital has been overwhelmingly positive. Alex Coulter, the hospital's Arts Coordinator, attributes this to the culture of the hospital in which an arts programme has played a significant role over the last 15 years and therefore sustains a greater level of openness by staff, patients and visitors towards its art. She also sees the hospital layout, whereby the gynaecological ward is separate from the maternity unit, as a factor in reducing potentially negative responses from woman who may be distressed by images of babies (interview, 2005).

The rapid turnover of patients and short duration of the residency prevented Gabriella from developing a relationship with the mothers whose babies she would photograph over a period of time. The residency was therefore dependent on her ability to achieve the trust of the maternity staff in order to be allowed to approach mothers shortly before they gave birth, which was symptomatic of the 'here and now' culture of the maternity unit. The interest with which the final artworks were received by the staff is due to this relationship of trust and the staff's own involvement in the production of the artwork. This involvement is critical in avoiding the kind of resentment staff can experience when art is anonymously imposed on their working environment. Where an involvement in the production of the artwork cannot be facilitated through a relationship with the artist, good mediation materials such as artists' statements can compensate for this, offering the viewer an insight into the context in which the artwork was made.

The notion of an artist's residency in a maternity hospital was pioneered in 1992–93 when Ghislaine Howard was artist-in-residence for 4 months at St Mary's Hospital maternity unit, Manchester. Throughout the residency, Ghislaine worked like a war artist, quickly recording scenes from every aspect of hospital life, before returning to the studio to develop these into more finished works (Fig. 4.5). She forged relationships with a number of patients and charted part of the journey of one particular expectant woman through her pregnancy right up to and including her caesarean section. These experiences led to a series of emotionally powerful and intimate paintings.

Ghislaine felt 'a weight of responsibility together with a strong sense of privilege' in recording 'a place where the fragility as well as the urgency of life can be keenly felt, where for some the struggle for life may be hard' (Howard 1994). However, unlike Gabriella Sancisi's residency, she was not developing art for exhibition within the maternity hospital and was therefore liberated from some of the constraints associated with placing art in hospitals. Rather, the body of paintings she produced were shown in an exhibition entitled 'A Shared Experience' in Manchester Art Gallery in 1993. This ground-breaking exhibition signified a move to reconnect art to human experience in a celebration of childbirth.

> 'It is a salutary thought that an experience that all humans have shared is so
> rarely seen in art galleries.'
>
> (Howard 1993)

Critic Robert Clarke attributes the absence of images about birth and new life from Western art to '...the comparative exclusion of women's subjective experience from the art arena ...' (Clarke 1993). Thus, although Ghislaine Howard's residency did not produce artworks for exhibition in St Mary's Hospital maternity unit, it was significant in presenting the work of the maternity hospital on a public platform and validating childbirth within the art world.

Contextual art practice in the form of residencies and site-specific artworks is not unique to a hospital context. Artists are now working in schools, factories and even

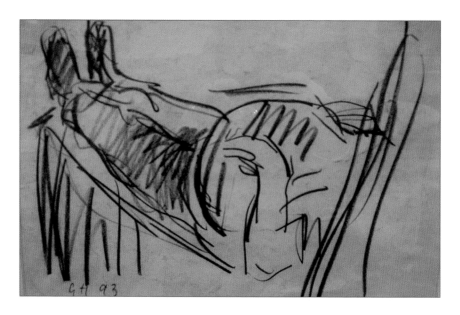

Figure 4.5 Woman waiting, Ante-natal Unit © Ghislaine Howard

police stations. This can be attributed to a '...shift of attention from what an [art] object is to where it is (and how the two are inseparable)' (Huberman 2005, p.56). Almost like a documentary film maker, through the residency the artist casts an independent eye over the institution, innocent to a large extent of the internal politics, the tensions, the hierarchies and the power play. Also, like a documentary film maker, it is the process of observing the institution and all its members as one unity that can create a sense of collective identity, where one may not previously have existed.

'As a temporary "resident", the artist still remains a "stranger". But the presence of a stranger may be just what it takes for the rest of us to feel at home.'

(Buchler 1999, p.45)

Unlike contextual art practice, the curatorship of art in hospitals in line with gallery curatorship is not based on the presence of the artist in the hospital. Art is introduced to a hospital through loans, donations, acquisitions and temporary exhibitions. This is not a new activity. For example, Paintings in Hospitals has been lending original art-works from its extensive art collection to NHS hospitals, hospices and other healthcare facilities in England, Wales and Ireland since 1959. Within the field of arts and health, this approach to art in hospitals is seen to fulfil a number of diverse and sometimes conflicting functions, including diversion for patients (Ulrich 2002), enabling patients to deal with their experience by reflecting it through art (Moss 1987), and humanising the institution and enabling it to build relationships of trust with the wider community (M White, interview, 2002).

Roger Ulrich's study on the impact of different types of artworks on the recovery and health outcomes of postoperative coronary care patients demonstrated that patients who were shown an image of a nature scene of still water surrounded by trees were less anxious within 2 days after surgery and handled pain medicine better. This led Ulrich to prescribe images he considers suitable for hospitals such as smiles, grassy fields, blooms, foliage and verdant vegetation, which he claims are positive distractions across different cultures and personality types and which have in scientific terms 'hard wired biological preparedness' (2000, p.51). Ulrich says that an ambiguous stimulus produces a projection of the emotion the viewer is experiencing. 'If we are happy, we see happy. If we are sad, we see sad. If fearful, we see frightening' (p.53). Ulrich concludes that only the 'unambiguously positive image seems therapeutic' and differentiates between art which is suitable for the gallery and that which is suitable for the hospital.

'...even if art is good or great in a critical sense – a Pollock, a Picasso, a Renoir, a Van Gogh – it will be bad art if it adversely affects health outcomes.'

(Ulrich 2000, p.51)

However, positive visual distractions for patients could be created with equal or greater efficacy by exterior views, good landscaping and interior design.

Contrary to Ulrich's position, art historian Linda Moss states that:

'The intention of using the arts in hospital is almost never to distract people from the medical or personal problems that they face in hospital. Rather it is the opposite: to allow people to face their problems, sort their experience through the arts as a personal, private alternative to the more defined communication of conversation.'

(Moss 1987, p.29)

Curator Mary Jane Jacob believes that art which addresses critical life issues of direct concern to the viewer will engage its audience (Jacob 1995, p.54), unlike art which has no direct relevance to its viewers. However, images which may be acclaimed in a gallery context could be provocative to women who were expecting, or had lost, a child. During my time at the National Maternity Hospital, Dublin, I was asked by the Nursing Manager of the miscarriage and infant death unit to remove a photograph of a baby being bathed which the arts programme had placed on a ground floor corridor leading to the mortuary. It appeared that to women who had lost a child, the display of this image of a baby was more provocative than other images promoting breastfeeding on display in the hospital, or even a real baby, possibly because it was seen as an insensitive action of one person or a group acting on behalf of the hospital. Perhaps the removal of the photograph was also perceived as something that could be determined by the hospital users, unlike many other aspects of the hospital environment.

It is argued that in the case of images evoking emotions of distress among women who have lost a child, the hospital can provide a supportive environment for the woman. In the Women's Centre of the Oxford Radcliffe Hospital Trust, a baby doll lay in an old-fashioned cot in the foyer of the hospital. Despite receiving a request to remove the doll and cot on the grounds that it could be distressing to women who have lost a child, Senior Midwifery Manager Janet Knowles decided that both should remain (interview, 2002). She believes that if such images are upsetting to women who have lost a child, it is best that this happens within the maternity hospital where they can access support from staff to help them to deal with their grief. Janet believes that while a hospital does not want to be either provocative or antagonistic to its clients, emotions around child loss and images which draw these up should not be hidden away. Rather, they should be given the space to be dealt within a supportive hospital environment.

Art has the potential to trigger many latent emotions, including grief, but unless appropriate supports are in place for the grieving patient, it is irresponsible to knowingly curate art which will evoke such responses. However, the creation of a specific art-viewing experience through curatorship is not an exact science. According to Stephen Martin (1990, p.175), 'Meaning [in an artwork] is like a braid in which culture, personal history, and archetypes are interwoven'. Meaning is therefore personal to the viewer and may be determined by his or her experience and projection and the context in which the artwork is viewed.

In reality, the relevant decision maker, whether it is a curator or arts committee looking for artistic quality or a medical professional looking for clinical benefits, will determine the choice of art for a hospital. While careful consultation with the users of the hospital must pave the way for any arts-in-hospital programme, given the high turnover of women passing through a maternity hospital, such consultation often does not reach further than the staff. The staff become the spokespeople for the patients. An arts programme is therefore reliant on the staff to take on a feeling of ownership towards the art. Once this ownership is taken, the hospital community can support art choices that are far from being simply decorative.

Involving staff in the selection of artwork in the early stages of a project is one way to develop their sense of ownership of the artwork. For example, in 2003, the Waterford Healing Arts Trust, in partnership with the maternity unit of Waterford Regional Hospital, invited artists to submit artworks on the theme of new life into an open submission competition for a group exhibition entitled 'Arrival'. The exhibition was linked to the health promotion work of the unit by promoting positive and culturally diverse images of parenthood. The exhibits were selected from 170 art submissions received by a panel comprising representatives from the fields of midwifery and art. The discussion of the submissions oscillated between an assessment of the quality of the art and an assessment of the medical condition of the mother and babies featured in the artworks. As a facilitator of the selection process, I encouraged the panel not to dismiss artworks on the basis of the medical condition of the subjects but to consider the aesthetic qualities of the artwork. The aim of the exhibition was not to portray perfection but to reflect reality, or many different realities. When the content of the artwork is of special interest to the viewers, in this case, the midwives on the selection panel, it can override the aesthetic qualities of the artwork and dominate the viewing experience.

The final exhibition did present different views of childbirth and parenthood. Artist Sharon Kelly's image of a child's bonnet in one of the 'Arrival' exhibits was a personal symbol of memory and loss. The artist had experienced child loss through both miscarriage and infant death, in the early 1990s, and much of her subsequent work had explored that theme. The image was sufficiently ambiguous not to upset viewers. However, it was significant that child loss had a role in the story of parenthood that was painted by this exhibition which otherwise risked alienating parents who had experienced child loss.

In addition to securing staff support, such as that of midwives, a curator working in a maternity hospital must develop a keen sense of timing and place. In 2002, as Arts Coordinator of the Waterford Healing Arts Trust in Waterford Regional Hospital, Ireland, I received a request from the nursing staff to remove a photograph of a young mother and her toddler by Mary Beth Meehan from the antenatal outpatients waiting area. I was reminded that not all women will reach full term and hence the image of mother and child could reinforce the expectant mother's fears rather than celebrate her impending arrival. A woman's anxiety about the impending birth of her child can reduce her willingness and even ability to engage with art. In some cases, art may be an unwarranted intrusion. The curator walks a tightrope between presenting art that is relevant to the context and 'avoid[ing] imagery, which could upset people' (Moss, 1988, p.1). In placing a painting of a healthy baby entitled 'Well Breasted Baby' by Berna Lawton in the maternity unit of the same hospital, the staff opted to locate the image in the labour ward near the entrance to the delivery suite at which point birthing was imminent. The curator must attempt to understand the viewer's experience at the time and place of viewing based on the given context and apply this understanding to the placement of the artwork.

The distinctiveness of a maternity hospital as a context for art was illustrated most forcibly in a group exhibition I curated entitled 'Mind Where You Look', which featured 15 diverse artworks by 13 artists and was the basis of a comparative study between an acute hospital and a gallery as sites for viewing art. The exhibition was placed in Fairfield General Hospital, Bury, Lancashire, in April 2005 and in Gallery Oldham, Lancashire, in May 2005.

'Mind Where You Look' featured 'Pregnant Self Portrait, July 1984' by Ghislaine Howard which was painted just before the birth of the artist's first child. She had been working on a series of pregnant self portraits and planned this as a preliminary study for a larger work, but her son's unexpected birth 4 weeks early stopped her in her tracks.

'The painting has a tremendous significance for me as it set the agenda for the work I have done ever since which centres on recording and celebrating "the dark joy" of our shared human experience.'

(Ghislaine Howard, artist's statement, 2005)

This seminal work was selected for the antenatal outpatients department of Fairfield General Hospital by the Nursing Manager who 'recognised the body language' of the pregnant subject. However, many of the staff and clients of the department described the impact of the painting as depressing. In Gallery Oldham, viewers stated feelings of sympathy and nostalgia in response to the same painting. The contrast in responses to this painting in both sites, and in particular the strong responses to it in Fairfield General Hospital, could be interpreted as an illustration of Roger Ulrich's view that an ambiguous stimulus produces a projection of the emotion the viewer is experiencing (Ulrich 2000, p.53). If we accept that 'Patients in hospital are frightened of pain, of the unknown, of being out of control ...' (Noble 1999, p.25), the projection of fear and anxiety is particularly relevant to how artworks are viewed in hospital. The presence of the artwork in the hospital, particularly a controversial artwork, can create something much greater than viewing experience. It can bring preexisting, and often unstated, attitudes and assumptions into sharp focus. It can bring to the surface the ideology of the institution and the fears and anxieties of patients that underpin the day-to-day interactions between patients, visitors and staff.

It can be argued that placing art in a hospital as if it were a gallery does not take account of the involuntary nature of the art-viewing experience, and that a greater degree of dialogue is needed between the artist and the hospital community if art in hospitals is to be a meaningful experience for staff, patients and visitors. It seems therefore that contextual art practice which facilitates a relationship between the artist and its audience has an advantage over more traditional styles of curatorship in this case. However, in the long term, art cannot depend on these personal relationships alone to engage its audience. It must be able to work on its own, as each encounter with a viewer represents a new relationship. Therefore the route of art into the maternity hospital is secondary to some simple principles of good practice in curatorship.

The hospital-based curator considers the viewer and his or her experience at the time of viewing as well as the subject of the artwork. This can be done through consultation with the hospital staff, which can also result in a sense of ownership by the staff towards the artwork. The mediation of the relationship between the maternity hospital and the artwork can be facilitated by a direct relationship with the artist through a residency programme or, in the absence of this, by public talks, workshops or written statements.

Placing art in a maternity hospital is not dependent on the presence of a dedicated curator. The process can be curated by staff members and/or a voluntary arts committee. However, an understanding of the full potential of the art experience to engage its viewer and stimulate a response is needed in order to maximise the benefits of art in hospitals. Only decorative art is required to create a pleasant environment, a visual distraction for patients or a system of way-finding in hospitals. While these may be valid applications of art in hospitals, without also curating art which takes into account the hospital context, as in the case of '100 Names and Dates' and 'Viewer', the potential of art to fully engage its audience may be lost.

In addition, an overly prescriptive curatorial practice, which in the case of the maternity hospital might, for example, recommend that images of babies be avoided, limits the creative potential of an art intervention. Creativity and innovation are central to art and curatorship. Creativity, innovation and responsibility are the cornerstones of arts and health practice. According to artist Nigel Rolfe, who sat on the selection panel for the site-specific commissioning programme in the National Maternity Hospital:

> '...the placement of one world [art] in another [the hospital] was at once sensitive and often difficult. Often times as artists we are too image interested. Perhaps to be expected, we pursue how work looks more than the job it does. The context here [the National Maternity Hospital, Dublin] would not allow this, no grey areas, work made must take into account its subject and audience in one.'
>
> (Rolfe, cited in Grehan 1999, p.246)

In summary, the curatorship of art in a maternity hospital, as a means of reintegrating art into the fabric of society, is a careful balancing act between presenting art which engages and stimulates the viewer and avoiding provocation at a time when viewers may be emotionally vulnerable. This balancing act is informed by an understanding of the social and psychological life of the maternity hospital.

References

Browne A (ed) 1995 The masters, midwives and ladies in waiting. The Rotunda Hospital 1745–1995. A and A Farmar, Dublin

Buchler P 1999 Other people's culture. In: Curious: artist's research within expert culture. Visual Art Projects, Scotland

Clarke R 1993 A shared experience. Guardian 29 March. Available online: www.ghislainehoward.com

Coren S, Porac C, Ward L M 1979 Sensation and perception, 2nd edn. Academic Press Inc, Orlando, FL

Grehan M 1999 The National Maternity Hospital site-specific art programme In: Arte e hospedale. Fondazione Michelucci, Italy

Howard G 1993 A shared experience. Available online: www.ghislainehoward.com

Howard G 1994 An artist's diary. Art Review March. Available online: www.ghislainehoward.com

Huberman A 2005 The sound of space. Art Review LVI, UK

Jacob M J 1995 An unfashionable audience. In: Lacy S (ed) Mapping the terrain. Bay Press, Seattle, USA

Kirklin D, Richardson R 2003 The healing environment: without and within. Royal College of Physicians, London

Lacy S 1995 Cultural pilgrimages and metaphoric journeys. In: Lacy S (ed) Mapping the terrain. Bay Press, Seattle, USA

Martin S 1990 Meaning in art. In: Barnaby K, D'Acierna Pallegrino (eds) Towards a hermeneutics of culture. Routledge, London

Moss L 1987 Art for health's sake. Carnegie UK Trust, Fife

Moss L 1988 Art and healthcare: a handbook of hospital arts. DHSS, London

Noble A 1999 Needs of clients and patients in hospital buildings. In: Haldane D, Loppert S (eds) The arts in healthcare: learning from experience. King's Fund, London

Ulrich R 2000 The effects of viewing art on medical outcomes. In: Turner F, Senior P (eds) A powerful force for good: culture, health and the arts – an anthology. Manchester Metropolitan University, Manchester

Further reading

Cork R 1989 For the needs of their own spirit: art in hospitals. In: Miles M (ed) Art for public places: critical essays. Winchester School of Art Press, Winchester

Haldane D, Loppert S (eds) The arts in healthcare: learning from experience. King's Fund, London

Kaye C (ed) 1997 The arts in healthcare: a palette of possibilities. Jessica Kingsley Publishers, London

Lelchuk Staricoff R 2004 Arts in health: a review of the medical literature. Arts Council of England, London

NHS 2002 Improving the patient experience: the art of good health – using visual arts in healthcare. Stationery Office, London

Electronic sources

Arts at Dorset County Hospital. www.arts-dch.org.uk

Paintings in Hospitals. www.paintingsinhospitals.org.uk/

Waterford Healing Arts Trust. www.waterfordhealingarts.com

CHAPTER FIVE

Weaving the Fabric of Life:
Women, Birth and Craft

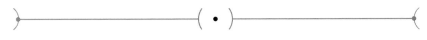

SARA WICKHAM

When I was 7, my grandmother taught me to knit and sew and whenever my grandparents arrived at our house (usually on Sunday afternoons), I would usually be waiting for her guidance and approval on my latest project. I would sit at her feet and spread out my things, happily sewing small animals from brightly coloured felt, knitting scarves for bears and then combining my knitting and sewing ability to make stripy bumble bees, to which I would attach safety pins and sell to my family and friends for a few pence, thereby starting my first small business. My whole family encouraged me in this endeavour, although it wasn't until I was much older that I realised this probably arose less out of a desire to nurture my creativity or entrepreneurial talents than because it kept me from talking over the football, which I thought was very boring and pointless. Craft, on the other hand, I perceived as both interesting and useful.

Three aspects of these early experiences are still with me today. I remain a floor-dweller by preference, having not yet found a piece of furniture which can enable me to properly spread out the ingredients for my projects. I can still be persuaded to quietly 'watch' the football or other TV programmes I am not interested in, as long as I am able to amuse myself amidst fabric, thread, wool, beads, buttons and other exciting things from which I can create small masterpieces. But perhaps most importantly of all, I still gain immense happiness from my craft activities, as well as relaxation, satisfaction, a sense of peace, joy – especially when creating something to give as a gift – and time and space in which to think, reflect, dream or switch my brain off completely.

These things led me to bring crafts into my work as a midwife, midwife teacher and workshop facilitator, and to reflect on the relationships between women, craft, birth and midwifery. In this chapter, then, I plan to weave together several different strands of theory, practice and experience with craft: how craft is grounded in women's stories and heritage, how craft relates to health, birth and midwifery, and how craft can be used in a practical sense by women and midwives. This chapter includes a number of quotes from midwives; these are all women who have kindly talked to me about their own experiences with craft, and feelings about this area.

Laying out the pieces and feeling the fabric

I offer no apology for the fact that this chapter is predominantly based upon my personal experience in this area, as opposed to being a largely theoretical piece; the very nature of craft activity means that it is a practical and personal journey and I have attempted to reflect that here. However, it is customary to begin any kind of discourse with a definition of what one means when using a term like 'craft'. Perhaps because

I see craft as located in personal and individual experience, I find myself balking at the idea of confining a concept like craft within a linguistic box. This also stems from being somewhat weary (and wary) of the debates around the differences between arts and crafts, which include the questions around whether midwifery is an art, craft, science or a combination of all three. I feel it matters less what we call it than what we actually do. A third reason for my hesitation to settle on exact definitions stems from a conversation I had with Lorna Davies when this book was still at the discussion stage. Lorna made a comment about me being the one to write this chapter because I was 'more crafty' than her, on the basis that I make things from fabric and wool. However, in mid-sentence, she realised that, actually, she did have a creative process which she loves and which she gets energy from – cooking and baking. I suspect that many other people may have a craft which they might not yet think of as a craft, and for this reason I would rather be inclusive about this concept than exclusive.

Having said all of that, I see no problem with laying out some of the very broad elements that link different crafts, as long as these are regarded as flexible. Crafts do tend to be essentially creative, where this describes the making of something new. Crafts also tend to involve the use of the hands, feet or other parts of the body (rather than simply the brain) and, generally, craft involves a level of skill – which does not mean that there aren't crafts which can't easily be done by someone with no prior skill or experience but that, in general, time and experience tend to lead to improvement. So, while my own interest in craft as expressed throughout this chapter tends to lead me to focus more on the kinds of craft that involve fabric, thread and needles, I certainly don't believe that crafts have to involve these things. Box 5.1 lists 50 examples of crafts (as they are described by some of the people who do them); there are probably hundreds more – by the loose characterisation that I've offered here, pregnancy, birthing, mothering and midwifing could all be considered crafts!

There is something quite interesting about the things listed in Box 5.1; most of the words used to describe crafts are verbs, and describe a process rather than an end product. Linguistically, this might sound obvious, yet it immediately highlights one of the key aspects of craft which will recur as a theme in this chapter; it is as much about the journey as the destination.

Selecting a few interesting historical beads...

There is little doubt that crafts have greatly enhanced human lives for millennia. As I was researching this chapter, I heard anthropologist Robbie Davis-Floyd talk about

---

Box 5.1

Expanding the possibilities: the range of craft

Knitting, crochet, sewing, weaving, spinning, farming, fishing, beading, woodwork, metalwork, patchwork, baking, appliqué, cooking, cake decorating, painting, quilting, cross stitch, tanning, needlepoint, ceramics, basket making, candle making, butter churning, brewing, tatting, macramé, embroidery, sugarcraft, felting, book binding, model making, writing, song writing, herbalism, gardening, stencilling, wine making, glass blowing, pottery, sculpting, whittling, carving, smocking, rug making, lace making, dress making, flower arranging, belly casting, drum making

how women were responsible for one of the major movements in human development – the creation of the 'carrying sack' which enabled women to bring home the food they gathered. It made me think about how very crucial the development of craft knowledge was to the survival of the human species. Before you could go out to the shops and buy clothes, someone had to spin the wool or other material, weave it into cloth and then sew it into a shape which you could wear. Irregularly shaped animal skins might be great for keeping you warm, but there is little doubt that much was gained from the cutting, shaping and fixing of these and other fabrics into shapes which gave warmth and protection while allowing freedom of movement. Similarly, the crafting of clay into pots, pans, bowls and other cooking and eating equipment meant that families had the freedom to store and carry food and water. If it were not for the development of craft in ancient times, we might still all be gathering around the local stream several times a day.

If we unpick some of the seams in old stories and books, we can see that crafts have been a key theme of stories for thousands of years. Similarly, crafts have been used to depict stories for thousands of years, for example in tapestries. Many ancient cultures depict the Goddess as weaver or spinner; she often appears as a spider, for example as Spider Woman (Navaho), Nut (Egyptian), Atargatis (Sumerian) and Freya (Norse). In a modern description of ancient goddess-related images that, for her, describe the 'Sorting Moon' of Samhain, or Hallowe'en, Annette Hinshaw includes:

> 'The Norns, three old women who weave the thread of our lives and dwell beside Mimir's Well under the roots of Yggdrasil, the world tree. The three Fates – Clotho, who spins, Lachesis, who measures, and Atropos, who cuts the thread – weaving the web of human life in strands of dark and shadow.'
>
> (Hinshaw 1999, p.222)

Originating in predualistic times, these stories and images reflect women and their crafts in ways which are simultaneously creative and destructive; life-giving and life-taking, embracing both darkness and light. This idea was not challenging in ancient times, when people had very different worldviews from our modern dualistic perspective.

Crafts remained a key aspect of people's lives, stories and art as dualistic, male-based religion took over from a matrifocal worldview. Women were still depicted as the weavers and spinners of life; Mohammed's daughter Fatima is known as the 'weaver of knots' and Jesus' mother Mary has been depicted in paintings as a spinner, with the thread running through her child, visible in her pregnant womb. When men first began to write their stories and poems down, they included women's crafts and some aspects of their ancient meanings. Homer described Helen weaving at the beginning of the *Iliad* and Circe and Calypso are weaving when Odysseus arrives in the *Odyssey*, while in the Latin *Metamorphoses*, Ovid (1955) tells of Arachne and Athena's weaving competition. These stories have been revisited a number of times; Arachne later appeared in Dante's *Divine Comedy* and her representation has more recently been debated by a number of feminist writers who see a trend which concerns them – that of the increasingly negative depiction of women and their crafts (e.g. Maharaj 1991). It seems that the changing worldview may have caused craft, as a woman's activity, to become vilified along with other aspects of feminine power.

Fairy stories also contain many references to crafts and, like ancient stories, they seem to depict both women and their crafts as negative and positive; creative and destructive; empowering and disempowering; empowered and disempowered, which perhaps links back to predualistic goddess mythology. In some fairy stories, women are the heroines. In others, mothers, stepmothers and older women are depicted as evil, as in the example of the old woman in *Babes in the Wood*, who baked toxic cakes to poison children. Other stories which could be said to depict crafts in a negative way include *Cinderella*, who was forced to sew and mend endlessly, as befitted her lowly station; *Rumplestiltskin*, in which the miller's daughter was set the impossible (at least for her) task of spinning straw into gold; and *Sleeping Beauty*, who was sent off for an extended siesta by a spinning wheel.

Yet in others it is possible to see the threads of craft activity in a different light. In *Spindle, Shuttle and Needle*, a dying mother gives these three items to her daughter and they help her both to work and to 'catch' her prince (which, even if not the goal of a modern woman, would have been deemed a positive and successful result when it was written!). Similarly, in *Six Swans*, a girl has to combine her spinning talents with a great deal of determination in refraining from speaking while she weaves the six vests which will restore her six brothers to life (the men had been turned into swans following their father's curse). This story can be viewed as a negative representation of women, in that it may be suggesting that women should 'spin and not be heard', yet also as a positive one, where the sister's skill and determination lead to her becoming the heroine who saves six men.

Over time, the changes in religious and moral doctrines through which societies have moved have led many stories to metamorphose and it is now difficult to see the bones of the stories without extensive research. Even when noting that 'many women's teaching tales about sex, love, money, marriage, birthing, death and transformation were lost', Clarissa Pinkola Estés (1992, p.16) suggests that people can often make sense of these stories in ways which fit their own lives and journeys. My re-reading of these stories has led me to feel that, while it is not inaccurate to suggest that crafts, along with women, have become denigrated in some circles, the threads that describe the strengths of women and their crafts do still exist. Further, I would argue that the co-existence of the two attests to the continued existence of a more complex worldview than offered by a few generations who have focused on dualism, while concurrently allowing each of us to view these things in whichever light we personally choose to focus on.

For me, these stories evidence that the ancient, more egalitarian mythology which allows us to understand the co-existence of good and evil, darkness and light, is still present today. Their contrasts and paradoxes allow me space to wonder. Sometimes I wonder if Cinderella, in the midst of her sewing, enjoyed the opportunity for dreaming that often characterises craft-time, and it matters less to me that Thumbelina's weaving ultimately led to her meeting and marrying the Flower King than that she so lovingly wove a coverlet of hay to gently cover the body of an apparently dead bird. We take from stories what we need and perhaps the reason why many of our stories detail craft is that for so long craft has been so integral to our lives. Craft has never been absent from our stories and there is something beautifully circular in the way in which so many fairy tales themselves involve spinning or weaving, while we talk about spinning or weaving a tale.

Yet craft is not limited to stories in our modern era; the rate at which hobby shops are springing up in town centres suggests something of a resurgence in our interest in craft. Craft is a practical tool – one which Gandhi put to excellent use when encouraging the people of India to spin and weave in order to gain independence from England – yet it has other dimensions which may, if we are not careful, be overlooked; dimensions which make it truly enlightening, effective and emancipatory for women and midwives.

Weaving the threads: linking craft, birth and midwifery

Midwives have different reasons for loving craft. I asked three midwives who either spend their spare time doing craft work or who seemed to especially enjoy a midwifery craft workshop to tell me what it was that they enjoyed so much.

'I spin in my spare time. Spinning is so ... it's multidimensional. It's creative, but also an orderly process. It involves thinking but you can also do it mindlessly. I love the textures, to feel the rhythm, to feel the process of the natural fibres passing through my hands. It's a whole texture thing, that whole feeling thing. It's become my biggest passion.' *Theresa*

'Sewing herb pillows [at a herb workshop] reminded me of how much I enjoyed making doll's bed clothes as a little girl.' *Liz*

'I think anything in the creative process brings us closer to our deeper space, which is exactly where we want to be as a midwife or a labouring woman, in that intuitive self.' *Xena*

Although these midwives are describing something quite deep in their attraction to craft, there is a very obvious thread linking midwifery and handcraft: the level of manual dexterity needed in both. Midwives' hands are perhaps their greatest tools so, as midwives are dextrous and craft requires dexterity, it is unsurprising that many midwives already enjoy knitting, sewing or other crafts.

'I have known (and do know) lots of midwives who have previously worked/ studied arts or crafts before becoming midwives, or whose hobbies involve crafts. I definitely believe that there is some sort of "womanly" connection between the two – perhaps "wisdom" is a collection of skills, both practical and on other levels?' *Genevieve*

The skills of feeling through our fingers and being in control of our hands are essential to both midwifery and craftwork.

'When I learned to repair perineal wounds, I loved how my previous skill with a needle and thread enabled me to actively enjoy completing this important skill. Having the physical skill allowed me to focus my attention on communicating with the new mother, explaining the process to her, observing her responses and offering care, advice, reassurance and a little humour!' *Liz*

But these midwives are also talking about something deeper than manual dexterity; they are talking about the process of creation itself and about a deeper level of wisdom. They mention creation, create their own circles of reminiscence and link these journeys with deeper kinds of knowing than are found in your average midwifery textbook or evidence-based practice guidelines. Although both of these topics are explored elsewhere in this book, there is something almost poetic or musical about their words and the feelings that they are expressing.

They are not the only midwives to make links between craft and birth.

'Jean Sutton describes the influence of the nesting instinct on the way a woman's body prepares for birth; women who take time out of their lives towards the end of their pregnancy to knit baby clothes and ponder on their experience may be better prepared physically, and perhaps mentally for labour. She explains that knitting helps to produce the "marshmallow cervix", which is no longer a common finding of vaginal examination...

Naoli Vinaver, a Mexican midwife, feels that modern women need to be more "juicy" in late pregnancy and labour, and knitting may be a way to achieve this. This is not to suggest that all women need to stay at home during pregnancy and knit baby clothes, but rather that the space which women may find in spending time on handcrafts may be beneficial.'

(Wickham 1999, p.6)

Crafts are also about giving birth to ideas in a practical sense and there is another very clear parallel here. The journey of birth is also a journey of creation and midwives share this journey with women. Alongside their hand skills, many midwives possess the same kind of imagination needed when doing craft; the kind of imagination which enables seeing what might 'become'. Here, I see a strong parallel between the crafters' ability to imagine what can be made from the raw ingredients in front of them and midwives' ability to imagine the size and position of the baby or the way she is wriggling through her mother's pelvis on her journey of birth.

There are links between craft and birth from the perspective of the woman as well as the midwife. I have worked with a number of women who have used the space created by handcrafts during pregnancy to help them to meditate, get in touch with their babies and come to terms with the journey they are undertaking. For all of these reasons, I was saddened when I heard recently that, when one of my teaching colleagues discussed the use of craft around birth with a group of midwives, two of the midwives told her how they had been sent a memo asking them to stop taking their knitting into practice on night shifts during the move from a cottage hospital to a larger unit because it was deemed 'unprofessional'. Thus, while the links between craft, birth and midwifery are manifold, the context of modern midwifery practice may be such that it is difficult for midwives to bring these threads together in their work.

Just as midwives searching for literature on music in health have had to turn to music therapy, I looked to the occupational therapy literature to find out what was going on in the world of theory. It appears that it is not only midwives who are deemed unprofessional in their attraction to craft; Tessa Perrin (2000) suggests that occupational therapists may be turning away from the 'arts and craft' aspects of their work, asking:

'Have [we] become so preoccupied with assessment and with the provision of prosthetic environments that we are losing the art (and the heart) of what it means to use occupations in healing? ... In our thrust towards ever-increasing scientific credibility over the past 40 years we have lost something very fundamental to the roots of occupational therapy.'

(Perrin 2000, p.129)

Perrin goes on to discuss some of the benefits she sees in using craft as therapy. She describes creativity as 'part of the therapeutic dynamic' (p.130) and tells of being able to help an elderly man out of deep depression by enabling him to focus on making a wooden tractor for his grandson. She argues that craft is able to both anchor us in the here and now and enable us to use the external (hands and senses) to influence the internal (thoughts and emotions).

The therapeutic potential of craft is echoed by Allart Wilcock (1999) who, in reflecting on the concepts of doing, being and becoming, tells the story of her Aunt Maggie. Learning to knit had taken Maggie out of the space where she saw herself as a disabled woman with few skills and transformed her, primarily by engaging her in an occupation with meaning and purpose.

> 'She became an occupational being, rather than an occupationally-deprived being. She became a person in her own right. The imbalance between her doing and being had inhibited her becoming a contributing social being.'

(Allart Wilcock 1999, p.6)

Box 5.2

Recipe for knitting a hat for a baby

Take a ball of soft baby wool and a pair of knitting needles (old size 10 or metric size 3.25 mm) and settle down with a cup of tea or glass of wine in an environment which you find relaxing, whether this is a blanket on the lawn with a CD of soothing music, an old armchair in front of the fire or parked in front of your favourite film or soap opera. Turn off the phone and disconnect the doorbell. Cast on 73 stitches and stocking stitch (knit a row, then purl a row) six rows. Don't be afraid to let this bit of the knitting curl around, as these rows are supposed to form a natural curl which will be a little border to the bottom of the hat.

Hold the knitting away from you so that you can admire your work, take a sip of your tea or wine and, when you feel like it, change to size 8 (metric size 4.0 mm) needles by knitting the next row on to one of the new needles. Purl the next row (remembering you need to swap the needle you have just knitted the stitches off with the other new needle before you do so!) and then continue in stocking stitch, taking regular sips and dreaming about the newborn baby until the work measures about 10 cm. If you are a midwife, marvel at how your body easily knows how to measure this distance with your fingers. If you are not a midwife, 10 cm is roughly the diagonal width of a woman's palm, from the bottom of the little finger to the bottom of the thumb. If you are a mother-to-be, you may like to marvel at how your womb will open to about this width in order for your baby to be born. Like the petals of flowers, women's wombs open gently, yet with a powerful, ancient force.

Begin the decreasing rows (to make the crown of the hat) when you are ready. Knit one stitch, then knit two stitches together, then knit six stitches. Continue the 'knit two stitches together, then knit six stitches' pattern along the rest of the row. Purl a row, knit a row, purl a row again and then stop to daydream a bit.

When you feel like it (and only when you feel like it), begin another decreasing row by knitting one stitch and then follow a pattern of 'knit two together and then knit five' for the rest of the row. Knit a row, purl a row and knit another row, remembering to relax and daydream as you go. Who taught you to knit? Did you knit when you were small? Has it been a while since you knitted something? If so, how does it feel to be doing it now?

Have a little think about whether it is time to make another cup of tea or find something to nibble on while you work. Give your fingers a little stretch and admire your creation-in-progress.

For the next decreasing row, knit one and then 'knit two together and then knit four' for the rest of the row. Purl one row. Follow the decreasing pattern by doing a

---

Box 5.2 (Continued)

decreasing row where you knit one, then 'knit two together and then knit three' for a row, purl a row, and then knit one and 'knit two together and knit two' for a row, before purling back. By now, you probably don't need reminding to daydream about the baby who will wear the hat, and you may find yourself unexpectedly coming up with insights and answers to some of the questions which had been racing around your mind and bothering you before you sat down to knit. Don't worry that you only have a few stitches left and seem close to the end – you can always remain in this space by making another hat, perhaps to give away.

'Knit one stitch and then knit two stitches together' across the whole of the next row, and then purl a row. For the last row, knit one stitch and then 'knit two stitches together' across the whole row. You can then cut the wool about a foot (or 30 cm) from the end, threading the end onto a sewing needle and then thread this through all the stitches, gathering them up, pulling them off the knitting needle and fastening the gathered bit with a couple of stitches. Don't cut the thread, though, as you can use this to sew the two sides of the hat together, remembering that it may be neater if you turn the hat inside out first. Secure the wool at the base of the hat by stitching three times in the same place, and then cut the wool. Turn the hat the right way around, perhaps helping the base to curl a little more, and admire your work. Close your eyes, take a deep breath and reflect on how you feel, and whether you feel differently to the way you felt before you sat down to knit. Can you feel a sense of connection to all the other women who have ever knitted a hat for their baby?

It is possible to vary this hat in many ways, by changing the wool every few rows to make stripes (if you are new to knitting, it is easier to remember how many rows in each stripe if you always change at the beginning of a 'knit' row) or by knitting the first six rows in a different colour from the remainder of the hat. If you don't know how to do 'purl' stitches, then just do 'knit' stitches throughout.

There are endless possibilities for using craft as therapy for pregnant women, either individually or in groups. There is nothing like learning to knit to improve your patience, or encouraging the creation of something like a quilt square or dreamcatcher to cause people to pause and think about what is important to them. With the caveat that this is not going to suit every woman, would the incorporation of craft into preparation for parenting sessions help women to focus on the baby and what might happen after the birth? Would midwives supporting bereaved women find value in running groups where women could get together to make quilts to remember their babies by?

Dropped stitches: a brief pause for reflection

I have to confess to feeling quite incapable of expressing some of the things I want to say about craft through the written word. It would be much easier if, instead of only being able to read about it, you could choose to press a button somewhere on the cover of this book and be instantly transported to a quiet space where you could try out a craft workshop (as described in the next section) and perhaps feel it yourself. I have a partial solution to this problem in the form of the recipe above, which offers directions for a personal craft experience. This recipe continues my use of metaphor to explore this area; although we usually talk about using patterns to guide our sewing or knitting, I've chosen the word 'recipe' for the guide above. The main reason for this is my feeling that there is more to knitting (and every other craft) than the mathematical instructions, which I have attempted to convey in my recipe.

It makes me feel slightly better about my own literary inadequacies that a number of other people, including Schmid (2004), have also described the phenomenon where complex and multifaceted creative processes generally manifest in practice in a far richer way than can be revealed through literature. One possible explanation for this difficulty can be glimpsed in the words of psychologist and story teller Clarissa Pinkola Estés.

> 'The "craft of making" is an important part of [my] work. I work to empower my clients by teaching them the age-old crafts of the hands ... The craft of questions, the craft of stories, the craft of the hands – all these are the making of something, and that something is soul.'
>
> (Pinkola Estés 1992, p.15)

Catching dreams: using craft with midwives

Because of my personal fascination with craft, and for many of the reasons I have already described, I have been attempting in small ways to bring craft, birth and midwifery together in my work. While I had possessed craft skills for most of my life, and had written about craft and birth in the midwifery press (Wickham 1999), it was not until a number of things serendipitously came together around the same time that I saw the potential for leading midwifery craft workshops myself. During my first visit to The Farm in Tennessee, I learned of the 'healing garden' of quilts that patients at one hospital had made – the quilts were displayed on a wall and were a testament to all that can be therapeutic about craft. Another turning point came after I had attended a 'dreamcatcher' workshop; I saw the profound and positive effect this had in enabling participants to find space to reflect on where they were in their lives, and draw meaning in relation to their work as midwives and teachers.

Since then, I have facilitated a number of craft workshops, where midwives have made (among other things) quilt squares, herb pillows, cloth dolphins, lotus flowers and dreamcatchers. I have woven many midwives and women into huge human dreamcatchers, so that they could learn the principle of weaving the web and go on to create their own. I ask them to stand in a circle and hold hands, becoming the circle on which the dreamcatcher is woven, and I weave a web from a large ball of thick wool. As I weave, I tell them the story of Grandmother Spider and explain the significance of the circle of life, the web of life and the beads and trinkets which are woven in to represent prayers. Telling the ancient stories and making dreamcatchers – which are often given to new babies – remind women and midwives of the connections and origins of life, enabling them to muse on whichever of the metaphors have meaning for them at that point.

When leading craft sessions, it is quite common to hear a number of midwives say at the outset that they are not creative. Yet I have never experienced a situation where someone chose not to participate. This is in contrast to singing sessions, where a few midwives feel self-conscious at first, the majority get over this feeling quite quickly but one or two might never reach the point where they want to join in. It is almost as if, once someone has 'cleared' it with the group (or perhaps with themselves) that they will not produce a masterpiece, they then give themselves permission to play anyway, often surprising themselves with what they are able to create.

After giving the group whatever instructions and help they need to be able to understand how to complete their project, I then invite them to select what they need to make their own version of whatever we are creating. I learned not to simply take along the fabric and threads that I liked when I realised that the vivid orange-striped fabric, which would have lain at the bottom of my craft hamper for years, was another midwife's idea of aesthetic perfection. There is generally a noisy and unladylike stampede while midwives pile into the offerings of the day, each looking for the perfect ingredient for her project.

The stampede lulls slightly as those decisive midwives who spotted what they wanted from the other side of the room capture their prey and take it back to their corner. As they begin their work, you can watch other people hesitating around the pile, carefully feeling different pieces of fabric, comparing colours and textures and eventually selecting things that are meaningful to them. Soon, there is almost complete silence, broken only by requests to pass scissors, enquiries as to whether the rest of a piece of fabric is available for sharing and mumbled apologies as someone decides they need to return to gather more materials but, in the process, has to negotiate her way over a pile of midwives who are now all lying sprawled across the floor, intensely focused on their blossoming creations.

Sometimes, the silence continues and those who finish early leave the room to preserve the sense of peace for others. At other times, the silence evolves into the sound of midwives sharing stories of their lives, reflection on their work and discussion of many of the issues I have talked about here. The depth and intensity of the space which people enter during this kind of workshop mean that it simply cannot be followed by a lecture or any kind of noisy activity; people want to drift around, have a drink or perhaps go off by themselves for a walk afterwards.

After allowing time for these things to happen, I try to make space for the group to share their work and feelings about it. There is something childlike about holding up your finished creation to have it admired by others; the 'show and tell' that brings a sense of pride, also not unlike the feelings of pride experienced by parents showing their new baby to family and friends. Here, I am reminded of the poem that says '...We did it ourselves', highlighting both the need for midwives to enable parents to realise that they are the creators of their child's birth and the sense of pride that can have a hugely positive impact on self-esteem. Likewise, the loss that sometimes accompanies birth can occur, albeit on a far lesser scale, with craftwork.

> 'I cried when a glass of water was accidentally spilt and ruined a design I had spent all day working on, from frustration, from sadness and from the knowledge that there was nothing I could do to bring my work back.' *Imogen*

Midwives can gain some very obvious personal benefits from this kind of workshop, including capturing the sense of well-being that often arises when with groups of women, yet which is often absent when working in our often difficult everyday environments. I assisted British midwives to make cloth dolphins on a Florida midwife's porch and several years later, their dolphin still reminds them of the tranquillity and community they experienced there. I know of at least one midwife who carries something she made at one of these workshops into the labour ward where she works; she says it reminds her that, whatever goes on around her, all is well.

In the summer, being outdoors in a quiet space where nature can be heard brings a special kind of energy to the experience, which can feel fresh and liberating, while indoor workshops in the winter bring feelings of cosiness and comfort. By separating out time (from 'normal' activities) to work on craft, people can gain a sense of the passage of time and of the location of the present moment within the seasons of the year and the calendar that is meaningful to them. Luboshitsky & Bennett Gaber (2001) explore the therapeutic value of craft in preparing for holidays and celebrations, suggesting that this can be one way of bringing a sense of spirituality into practice – something which, despite our understanding that this is a positive and vital aspect of midwifery, we generally find hard to do.

I have been stunned by how much midwives enjoy craft workshops, of all different kinds, and the depth of reflection that often ensues. There are plenty of other examples of learning about emotions through crafts, from my own experience and that of others; I don't think it would be overdramatic to suggest that many of life's lessons can be experienced on a micro-level from making things. One midwife found, while making a dreamcatcher, that she became incredibly frustrated when the thread kept slipping around the hoop she had chosen.

'It was partly because we'd been in this lovely dome, in a circle of postmenopausal women, that was really good and I didn't want to come out! Sara was showing us how to make dreamcatchers and, being a practical person, I should have found it easy – but it wouldn't go the way I wanted … I nearly screwed the thing up, I was outraged! At a birth I'm totally patient, I sit and wait, whereas with that [dreamcatcher], I just … well, I had to start again!'

At a later workshop, the same midwife again experienced frustration when she felt rushed by other participants into finishing her quilt square so that all the squares could be placed on the floor, patchwork-style, before the end of the session.

'When we did the quilt thing I felt really cross that I hadn't done it fast enough … I wanted to do it on **my** time. I was cross … I was last, I got sick and thought of this society all moving too fast, leaving me behind … it was like a feeling of being rushed into decision-making, which is not what I do as an independent midwife. I thought, did that have something to say to me?'

During a couple of herb workshops, which were in themselves very practical, I showed midwives how to make and fill magical herb pillows while they listened to the speaker. In offering craft work during another session, as opposed to leading a craft workshop that was solely a craft workshop, I was initially slightly unsure about whether this would mean that people would be less able to take in what was being said because they were concentrating on their craft activity. In reality, the opposite occurred and most of the midwives at these workshops found it easier to listen to what is being said.

'It was great because it wasn't the kind of workshop where you needed to write things down, and it meant I had something to do with my hands.' *Lisa*
'It actually had the effect of concentrating me on the words I was listening to – the intensity was surprising.' *Genevieve*

A midwife teacher who has attended some of these workshops wrote the following reflection.

'The craft sessions I have attended have often been part of a day of learning about some other non-craft subject and I always feel a kind of peace associated with them. A group of women focused on a simple task (usually) of creating something – sometimes individual items, sometimes a group project – there is a sense of peaceful togetherness and focus – it's not the same feeling as actively trying to relax, but more of a time to fit pieces of a puzzle together, to make sense of the day so far. It sometimes makes me think of "women's work" and regret the togetherness we have lost since we don't gather as a group of women to talk and make things any more.' *Abigail*

Sewing up

Craft, to me, appears to be an area full of potential for both women and midwives. Craft is grounded in our history and our stories, embodied in our hands and hearts and carries the potential to give us time and space to dream, reflect and process our journeys. I once wrote that my childhood view of a midwife was someone who sat on the end of a woman's bed, or in the corner of her bedroom, and knitted (Wickham 1999). Nowadays, I carry a small, unfinished tapestry in my birth bag, which I work on while women are on their journeys of labour, and I realise that I have become one of those midwives. As I think about the connections that midwives have always found on their own journeys, the webs and spirals that we often use as metaphors and the desperate need that we face to bring birth back into the hands of women, I wonder if part of the answer to reclaiming birth might lie in the reclaiming of craft...

Acknowledgements

I would like to thank a few people who have nurtured and inspired my own journey with craft: Peggy Lee and Rita Wickham, my grandmother and mother, who taught me to knit and sew; my father, Robin Wickham, who (usually) tolerated having tiny bits of discarded felt and wool littering the back seat of the car as I journeyed around as a child making my small creations; my partner Ishvar who continues to tolerate the mess and patiently hoovers it all up; Jenny, who taught me to make dreamcatchers; Janice Bass, who created the space for us to make dreamcatchers, and Lorna Davies, who has supported me so well in exploring this area with women, students and midwives.

References

Allart Wilcock A 1999 Reflections on doing, being and becoming. Australian Occupational Therapy Journal 46: 1–11

Hinshaw A 1999 Earth time, moon time: rediscovering the sacred lunar year. Llewellyn, St Paul, MN

Luboshitsky D, Bennett Gaber L 2001 Holidays and celebrations as spiritual occupation. Australian Occupational Therapy Journal 48(2): 66

Maharaj S 1991 Arachne's genre: towards inter-cultural studies in textiles. Journal of Design History 4(2): 75–96

Ovid (1955) Metamorphoses (trans. R Humphries). Indiana University Press, Bloomington, IN

Perrin T 2000 Don't despise the fluffy bunny: a reflection from practice. British Journal of Occupational Therapy 64(3): 129–134

Pinkola Estés C 1992 Women who run with the wolves: contacting the power of the wild woman. Rider, London

Schmid T 2004 Meanings of creativity within occupational therapy practice. Australian Occupational Therapy Journal 51: 80–88

Wickham S 1999 Reclaiming the art in birth. Midwifery Matters 83: 6–7

CHAPTER SIX

Poetry and Childbirth:
'A Light by Which We May See'. *
From Technician to Midwife

TRICIA ANDERSON

'...and the end of our exploring
will be to arrive where we started
and know the place for the first time.'

(TS Eliot, Little Gidding, Four Quartets)

Introduction

There is little food for the soul in modern midwifery. Most midwives have been educated within the medical model of childbirth which values science and the intellect above all. This model preaches objectivity and dispassion; working in this environment over time can separate midwives from themselves, both as women and mothers. Yet midwifery espouses a holistic philosophy, in which we nurture women's hearts, minds and souls by meeting them with our own. Emotionally literate and compassionate in a range of the deepest human emotions we may never have experienced; the loss of a baby, fear of pain and death, the break-up of marriage, betrayal of faith, the loss of fertility, the celebration of life, the exhilaration of birth, the joy, the doubt and despair ... Childbirth is perhaps the most intense time in a woman's life, in which the dull rush of modern life is suspended and large dark questions and truths hang exposed; all human life is there.

Yet the medical world in which we are educated and largely work is but a poor, two-dimensional slice of this multidimensional world, and we are left wanting. We are taught how to unblock an occluded intravenous line but not how to calm a disquieted soul. The overarching theme of this medical worldview is 'separation': separation of mind from body, of health professional from human being. Here, the pregnant body is a machine in line waiting to be fixed; it has no emotions, no capacity for self-healing, no self-determination, no faith, no hope, no pain. The midwife is merely a uniformed and faceless technician on the production line: cataloguing, processing, fixing, sending on.

---

*'The poem ... is a little myth of man's capacity of making life meaningful. And in the end, the poem is not a thing we see – it is, rather, a light by which we may see – and what we see is life.' Robert Penn Warren, *Saturday Review*, 22 March 1958

Yet a good midwife – for women – emerges time and time again from the qualitative research literature as compassionate, empathetic and respectful. As well as being technically competent, she is fully 'present' and genuinely interested in each woman as an individual, autonomous and self-determining human-being. She 'understands'.

So how can we understand things that we may never experience ourselves, to enhance our care of others and enrich our own lives? How are we to develop our understanding and compassion, our empathy and sensitivity, to become whole people ourselves? There is no module in any midwifery education programme for us to develop and enhance these attributes that women value in us so highly. Many believe that these things can't be taught, but I disagree. Ways do exist to reawaken the heart to the power and beauty of birth and connect back that which the medical model has torn asunder, but because of our society's supervaluation of science they are often dismissed out of hand. However, as William Hazlitt wrote in 1818:

'Poetry is the universal language which the heart holds with nature and itself. He who has a contempt for poetry, cannot have much respect for himself, or for anything else.'

One way to connect is to use literature and poetry. 'For those among us who have never had a miscarriage or an abortion … poems bring us into direct contact with those who have. For a few moments, their anguish, their uncertainty, their pain is ours' (Otten 1993, p.xxvi).

Birth poetry - a historical sketch

'A poem is a window that hangs between two or more human beings who otherwise live in a darkened room.'

(Dobyns 1997)

Poetry and midwifery have an ancient connection, in long ago times when the voices of women were strong. Brigid, the ancient Celtic goddess of midwifery and birth, was also the goddess of poetry and all creative acts. Brigid means 'one who exalts herself' and she is a Celtic threefold goddess, her three aspects being:

- Fire of Inspiration as patroness of poetry
- Fire of the Hearth, as patroness of healing, childbirth, midwifery and fertility
- Fire of the Forge, as patroness of smithcraft and martial arts.

Because of her third aspect, she is thought by some to be the Lady of the Lake who forged Arthur's sword Excalibur. Ceridwen, another Celtic goddess of fertility and poetry, was believed to be the mother of Taliesin the Bard. The act of creation – whether it be birthing a child or writing a poem – was a source of wonder and respect. Aesculapius, son of Apollo in the Greek tradition, was the god of poetry, medicine and the arts and demonstrates that this historical intertwining of arts and health was crosscultural.

But the voice of women became silenced over the generations, for reasons too complex to go into here (although they are discussed briefly in the introduction). The truth of their lives, centred around maintaining a home and raising children, became marginalised in favour of the more important 'public' world of men, politics, business and war. Women became muses, inspirations for male creativity and glorified unattainable objects of courtly love. In the Western, almost exclusively male, poetry tradition, subjects deemed 'suitable' for verse were nature, beauty, poetic love and the glorification of God.

Until recently there was little creative literature about motherhood and childbirth. There is some private journalling in diaries by women in the 16th and 17th centuries, but nothing for public consumption or praise. There are a few noteworthy exceptions: Mina Loy's poem entitled *Parturition* published in 1923 (from Bernikow 1979) is a graphic account of labour which echoes Toi Derricote's much later *Natural Birth*, for example. But 'in our century, as in the last, almost all distinguished (literary) achievement has come from childless women' (Olsen 1980). Much has been written about the incompatibility of the creative artist and the daily responsibilities of motherhood (e.g. Olsen 1980). It is no wonder that many well-known female artists chose not to have children, and perhaps it is worth noting the tension and torment that runs through much of the work of many female artists who were also mothers (Bernikow 1979). Often women writers who were mothers chose to focus their poetry on other aspects of life in order not to be pigeon-holed as 'merely women who wrote'. Childbirth was not considered a suitable subject for public audiences and male-dominated publishing houses. 'In the past, women writers often shied away from the subject of pregnancy and birth, possibly aware that men might find it too limited' (Chester 1989, p.2). Even in an anthology of poems specifically on birth and birthdays compiled as recently as 1983, there is only a tiny proportion of poems by women writers (Graziani 1983). Palmeira writes that:

'Talking about birth in our society has largely been seen as distasteful and motherhood as mundane; something private, not public, belonging to women's spheres, unclean even. I have been given the distinct impression in literary circles that writing about it is a stage you go through before returning to "more important things".'

(Palmeira 1990, p.xvii)

But after the Second World War, women were:

'...freed by that cataclysm from their cliched roles as goddesses of hearth and bedroom ... women began to write openly out of their own experiences. Before there was a Woman's Movement, the underground river was already flowing, carrying such diverse cargoes as the poems of Bogan, Levertov, Rukeyser, Swenson, Plath, Rich and Sexton.'

(Kumin, in Sexton 1981, p.xxxiii)

The confessional poetry movement of the 1960s made intimate poetry both acceptable and fashionable – up to a point. Anne Sexton, a confessional American woman poet writing in the 1960s, genuinely shocked the literary world with her poem *In Celebration of my Uterus* written in 1969. 'Not only did she write what was considered by many (especially men) an outrageous poem on an unseemly subject, but she went on the poetry circuit and read this poem to mixed audiences. Men in audiences were heard to say "I wish she'd stop talking about her... "... and they choked on "uterus"!' (Otten 1993, p.xxi). Sexton followed with equally powerful poems on abortion, unwanted pregnancy and adoption, not all to critical acclaim; these topics were still largely taboo. For one critic writing in *Harpers'* magazine, Sexton's poem on *Menstruation at Forty* was 'the straw that broke this camel's back'! This distaste can be heard in the poet Robert Lowell's eulogy to her: 'Many of her most embarrassing poems would have been fascinating if someone had put them in quotes, as the presentation of some character, not the author' (in Sexton 1981). Sexton struggled with mental illness, was hospitalised with postnatal depression after the birth of each of her children and tragically committed suicide in 1974.

The famous British poet Sylvia Plath's long poem written for radio entitled *Three Women,* set in a maternity ward, was written in 1962. It remains perhaps the most powerful piece on women's experience of childbirth. The voices of three women alternate in telling of their experiences on the maternity ward: one who is happy to be having a baby, one who is miscarrying a much-wanted baby and one who is giving up her child for adoption. Plath also gave us some of the most well-known childbirth and mothering poems: *You're* (1960), *Morning Song* (1961) and *Heavy Women* (1961) (Plath 1981). Like Anne Sexton, Plath also struggled with mental illness and postnatal depression and committed suicide in 1963, just 6 months after the radio broadcast of *Three Women.* Two women, both of their time and ahead of their time.

The second wave of feminism in the late 1960s and 1970s gave a new legitimacy to women writing the truth about their own lives. Women's creative writing groups began to appear in towns and cities, successful women-only publishing houses such as Onlywoman Press, The Women's Press and Virago Press provided a vehicle for wide-scale distribution and slowly the body of women's poetry about the reality of women's lives grew. There was a sense of exploring new territory. Adrienne Rich wrote of this exciting time:

'For women writers in particular, there is the challenge and promise of a whole new psychic geography to be explored. But there is also a difficult and dangerous walking on the ice, as we try to find language and images for a consciousness we are just coming into, and with little in the past to support us.'

(Rich 1980)

In its aim to liberate women, feminism remained uncomfortable about motherhood and childbirth, however. There was a central tension; feminists were, and remain, divided and unsure whether the path to emancipation is to be liberated from 'the chains of reproduction and motherhood' or rather to embrace and celebrate the 'womanliness' of these acts. In an anthology of British feminist poetry 1969–79 edited by Mohin (1979), what little there is about childbirth is very negative. Caroline Halliday, for example, writes about 'birth as affliction' in her poem *Reading of Women Born by Adrienne Rich.* In her poem about a D&C, Kathryn Gabriella writes of how 'We have avoided the hyperplastic cancerous leviathan. We have gone beyond the narrow straits of progeny'. Motherhood was an oppression: 'I am in control of my life she said meaning I own a child and can control her to make up for the fact I am not free' (Diana Scott, *Of the Children of Other People*). In this worldview the road to emancipation was clear: easy access to birth control and abortion rights for all women.

Poetry about childbirth itself, barring a few notable exceptions, is thus quite a recent phenomenon. When searching for poems about birth prior to compiling *In the Gold of Flesh* in 1990, Palmeira wrote that she had difficulty finding many. Yet put 'birth poetry' into an Internet search engine nowadays and you will get an overwhelming number of 'hits'. The last 20 years have seen an explosion of childbirth poetry in which women have been liberated to write about their experiences, good and bad, of giving birth and becoming mothers. In this new poetry, giving birth, rather than being seen as an affliction, is more often now celebrated as an opportunity for personal transcendence. Chester writes that:

'Once you become a mother, you are more keenly aware of the fragility of life and therefore of potential tragedy ... Mothering actually gives us direct access to the greatest themes in literature – birth, death, loss, love ... we are opened up as at no other time.'

(Chester 1989, p.4)

Giving birth can open women's eyes to matters beyond the everyday, the ordinary.

'Birth is, and represents, the principle of life, that all things have a source, a moment of creation and taking on of being; that birth resonates throughout life in many different forms – it is a metaphor for all changes that generate new states.'

(Palmeira 1990, p.xvii)

As women discover their power in giving birth, they are increasingly using poetry as a vehicle to share their discovery with others. Childbirth and mothering are now sexy! The Internet revolution has altered publishing beyond all recognition; slim vanity volumes published at poets' own expense have been replaced by everyone's own website, where their birth poems can be freely read by anyone. Many international childbirth websites have 'poetry corners' and poems that touch a chord are often circulated in the e-mail lists and Internet chatrooms of mothers and midwives.

Why poetry?

This new rich resource provides a unique, emotionally heightened, direct way of empathising with and learning about the infinite variety of women's childbirth experiences, and of life itself. Women often struggle to find the words to describe their experiences (just how do you explain what a contraction feels like?). Swedish researchers Lundgren & Dahlberg (1998), exploring women's experience of pain during childbirth, found that women found the pain of labour to be contradictory and impossible to describe. But poets – whose craft is capturing the precise image and whose tools are words – are expert wordsmiths who excel in expressing the essence of an experience in a few stanzas.

Poetry is hard to define and much has been written on what it is and what it is not. Bolton suggests this definition: 'Poetry is an exploration of the deepest and most intimate experiences, thoughts, feelings, ideas: distilled, pared to succinctness, and made music to the ear by lyricism' (Bolton 1999). What a poem does is to 'give enduring and universal life to what was merely transitory and particular' (from www.poetrymagic. co.uk). As John Keats wrote in his letters (1958, vol 1, p.238): 'Poetry should ... strike the reader as a wording of his own highest thoughts, and appear almost a remembrance'. A good poem will strike the reader with a chime of familiarity, a contented sigh of 'aah yes, that's *just* how it is'. 'Poetry humanises because it links the individual by its distilled experience, its rhythms, its words to another in a way which no other form of communication can. Poetry also helps to ease the aloneness which we all share in common' (Myra Cohn Livingston, in Lerner 1994). For example, for a woman experiencing grief after a miscarriage, what a relief to read a poem that encapsulates emotions that she cannot yet articulate herself.

So poetry can communicate emotions and make them universal, and in this it humanises us. Robert Frost (2001) wrote that 'Poetry is when an emotion has found its thought and the thought has found words'. But there is more to it than that.

'We don't read and write poetry because it's cute. We read and write poetry because we are members of the human race. And the human race is filled with passion. And medicine, law, business, engineering, these are noble pursuits and necessary to sustain life. But poetry, beauty, romance, love, these are what we stay alive for.'

Many readers will recognise Robin Williams' impassioned call to his students from the 1989 film *Dead Poets' Society*, directed by Peter Weir.

Poetry in midwifery

There are many ways in which poetry can be used in midwifery: in education, in professional reflective writing and in research. Poetry can be used with women in antenatal classes and in hospital clinics, and as a therapeutic tool in support groups.

Poetry in midwifery education

Educational theory

Reading and discussing poetry is one useful way to revisit the familiar and make it strange, seeing familiar events from the client's perspective (in this case, mother or baby) and thus gaining a heightened awareness of both ourselves and others. Grant (1998), a pioneer in this work who is leading its development at South Bank University in London, suggests that the main purpose of studying the humanities is to enable healthcare professionals to take better care of their patients and better care of themselves. Discussion of the emotional world of the poems can promote ethical reflection, and Grant also suggests that 'as we become more sensitive to the words others use to express their feelings, our communication as health professionals may become enhanced. We may become more inclined to listen'.

Learning takes place in both the affective (emotional) and the cognitive (intellectual) domains. Bloom (1965), a cognitive theorist, draws a clear distinction between the two, both of which need to develop in a parallel pattern of growth to facilitate the highest possible level of genuine learning. Too often in institutionalised education, the emphasis remains firmly on the cognitive. Bloom's famous educational taxonomy incorporates in the affective domain at its base level the notion of 'receiving' – paying attention to stimuli, observing and developing awareness. This is followed by 'responding' in which students are encouraged to formulate a response to the stimuli. Reading poetry can help students develop this skill of first observing and then articulating a personalised response, based on an interpretation of the poet's experience and choice of words integrated with their own clinical experience.

Schon (1987) talks about professional practice being a high ground overlooking a swamp. 'On the high ground, manageable problems lend themselves to solutions through the application of research-based theory and technique. In the swampy lowland, messy, confusing problems defy technical solutions.' Most of the real-world problems encountered by the professional are in 'the swamp', where human situations do not neatly correspond to the academic theories learnt in school and are characterised by uncertainty, uniqueness and value conflict. This is certainly true in midwifery, where Page (1997) estimates that research evidence only currently exists to help answer 12% of clinical dilemmas. The remaining 88% need to be solved by what Schon describes as 'professional artistry', whereby skilled practitioners deal with individual situations by a kind of improvisation, constantly inventing and testing strategies of their own creation. He defines artistry as 'an exercise of intelligence, a kind of knowing, though different in crucial respects from our standard model of professional knowledge'. Calman, a pioneer of this approach in medical education, explains how reading poetry and litera-ture may teach healthcare professionals to tolerate ambiguity and enable them to come to conclusions even when the information is incomplete or when alternative interpreta-tions are possible (Calman & Downie 1996). It encourages them to construct meaning after a period of reflection, and this facilitates deeper learning. This is in contrast to surface learning, in which students aim to memorise as much factual information as they can but pay little heed to understanding it.

Observation is a skill of perceptive watching, an informed way of looking that raises awareness and sharpens understanding. In their professional role, midwives are required to work in situations involving complex human relationships, where actions can have far-reaching consequences. Developing the skill of focused observation while suspending judgement is an essential midwifery skill, and being asked to describe 'what they see' is the first step in this process.

Rogers (1983) talks about the concept of 'whole-person' learning, in which both hemispheres of the brain engage. The left hemisphere is logical and linear and deals in ideas that are clear-cut and defined. The right hemisphere functions in a different way, grasping the essence before it understands the details, and can make creative leaps. It operates in metaphors and can take in what Rogers called the 'whole gestalt', the total configuration. To help students become skilled reflective practitioners able to use professional artistry in their decision making, the right hemisphere needs to be stimu-lated as much as the left. Poetry is one route into this approach; the use of metaphors can broaden thinking, stimulate deeper learning and help students make connections. Students are encouraged not simply to memorise but to articulate 'what it is *like*'. 'If it is like "x" in one way, is it like "x" in other ways, or does it differ', and so on. Synectics is a method of creative problem solving used by Harvard University which follows the process: paradox – analogue – unique activity – equivalent (Bligh 1986). The central process within this is the application of analogies and metaphors to make new connections between familiar phenomena, and it is here that poetry excels.

The aim of teaching is to let students learn (Rogers 1983). Learning can be seen as a process of change, the development of new perceptions and formulation of responses to new material (Rogers 1986). The very nature of poetry, wrote Ezra Pound (1960), is that it is language charged with meaning to the utmost degree and as students 'unpack' that meaning, which has resonance both to them as individuals and with their clinical experiences, they develop new perceptions and sensitivities to that which was familiar.

To summarise, the key elements of the rationale for using poetry as part of midwifery education are to:

* stimulate the development of empathy and compassion
* develop communication skills, especially careful, non-judgemental and deep listening
* develop skills of observation and accurate description, in the face of repetitive occurrences that may dull the senses
* develop decision-making skills, especially in ambiguous or uncertain situations
* begin to make the paradigm shift required for the provision of woman-centred care by seeing and feeling events from the client's perspective.

Practical methods of using poetry in midwifery education

There are many different ways to use this rich resource of poetry in midwifery education, from pre-registration students to Master's level postregistration studies. Start compiling a file of poetry and gather them up wherever you find them; then be brave and use them in the classroom. I personally recommend just leaping in: perhaps a few words about how important it is to understand women's perspectives and experiences but otherwise no big build-up or 'theory of poetry and why poetry is good for you' that will probably put students off!

You could:

- use an existing poem as a 'trigger' for introducing a new topic in enquiry-based learning
- start (or end) each lecture with a poem on the woman's perspective of the topic (students will often remember a poem whereas they have a tendency to forget much of the rest of the lecture!)
- work on individual poems in more depth
- encourage students to write their own poems, perhaps as part of personal reflective portfolios (see *Blackberry stained lips* by Lucy Brown, Box 6.1)
- encourage students to share their poetry in group sessions
- perhaps inaugurate a birth poetry club, like the popular book clubs where each month students gather to discuss their favourite childbirth poems
- launch a birth poetry noticeboard/website and invite contributions (either in real or in cyberspace)
- encourage student readings/performances of Plath's *Three Women* and other poetry, perhaps as part of student-led study days, and invite women and midwives to attend.

Box 6.1

Poetry for reflection

I wrote this poem after being involved with a family who experienced a neonatal death at 35 weeks. The episode had a profound effect on me, particularly witnessing the close physical bond the family had with the dead baby, who they kept with them for several days. I had never seen a dead baby before and the image of the purplish lips impacted on me and gave me the starting point to reflect on the experience through a poem. I find that writing poems about midwifery experiences helps me recognise and acknowledge the mixture of feelings, images and ideas that go through me. When I am ready to write a poem it just flows out. I do not worry about poetic correctness, but am guided by the desire to genuinely express my sense of the event (by Lucy Brown, studying midwifery).

Blackberry Stained Lips
Baby with the blackberry stained lips
Not for this world
The life force stopped too soon for you
No hedgerow rambles to colour your fingertips
You lie still
Perfectly formed
We can almost imagine a faint breath

Box 6.1 (Continued)

A shifting chest
A fluttering eyelid
But look again at the stillness
That has no end
Wrapped – To keep you warm?
Held with loving hands
Kissed and embraced
By those who anticipated you with hopefulness
Now gone
Gazing at you
They try to discover who you were
Their baby
Searching your face for what might have been
And cannot be
A birth
A death
Most unnaturally combined

Box 6.2

Poetry for self-esteem

Hands
These are my hands.
Through these hands I have come to see the world.
These hands have measured the growth of life
and documented the stalling of time.
They guide my ears to places where I hear
the watch-like beating of tiny hearts.
My hands have felt
the hard bony framework of passages
and the softness of muscles
which will bulge like petals of a rose.
My hands have opened windows to the energy
of the souls of those I have touched.
They have held the frigid rigidity
of steel instruments and the softness of a friend.
There are stories in these hands,
read from the pages of the work of women.
With my hands I have felt the power
of the strength it takes to grow
and release new spirit.
My hands were born with the knowing of touch.
The journey has added how and when
and the time to ask for help.

Box 6.2 (Continued)

Teaching hands engulfed mine
until they were ready to fly.
My hands are joined in a circle which is
unbroken through time.
Sometimes my hands do nothing.
Their most important work
to be still with fingers laced
and witness.
'The art of doing nothing well' has been passed
from one generation to the next.
Mine have been taught by some of
the most powerful hands
to watch and wait.
This is perhaps the hardest for
hands born to touch.
If I have nothing else to give you, let me
teach you how to see with your hands.
How to open the windows of life, and close
the door softly when it is time. In the darkness,
it is your hands that will light the way.
These are my hands.
These are the hands of a midwife.
(Jan Weingrad Smith)

Working on individual poems in more depth

To illustrate how poetry can be used as a resource in midwifery education, what follows is a short commentary and discussion based on real-life classroom discussions with pre-registration student midwives of Penelope Shuttle's powerful poem *Giving Birth* – a deeply powerful poem which seems to encompass virtually the whole of the midwifery curriculum! Sections of the poem are followed by an amalgam of the students' comments and discussions. Each stanza clearly articulates the phenomena associated with traumatic hospital birth, postnatal adaptation and new motherhood and provides a depth of emotional insight that no textbook or individual anecdote can match. In classroom discussions, the tutor can provide supporting evidence and linkages with contemporary research on women's experiences of birth, motherhood, posttraumatic stress disorder and so on.

You don't need to be a literary expert to run sessions such as this. Read the poem out first (aural) and accompany it with a visual version on overhead/computer as individual students may have a preference for visual or aural learning.

Prompts that might be useful when working on a poem like this include the following.

- Why do you think the poet chose this (a certain) word or phrase?
- What other resonance or meaning does this word have for you? (Remember that poets 'play' with the multiple dimensions, different contexts and parallel meanings of a single word, such as '*bout*' below.)

- What emotion(s) do you feel on reading this poem?
- What words (nouns/adjectives/verbs) come into your mind when you think of an instrumental birth? Perhaps direct your focus onto one aspect or perspective, e.g. the woman (or the partner, the baby, the midwife, the doctor, the room). Call them out/write them up on a brainstorming board. You could divide the group up: ask each subgroup to work on a different perspective (the mother, the baby, the doctor, etc.) as above.
- Using the brainstorming exercise as a starting point, could you write a few lines or more that capture the essence of an instrumental birth you have seen?
- Would you like to share them with the group (optional, of course) and talk about what you have written and why?
- How might insight into this poem/experience alter your midwifery practice?

Giving Birth

Delivering this gift
requires blood,
a remote room,
the presence of overseers.
They tug a child
out of the ruins of your flesh.

A remote room. Distant. The woman is far away from everything she knows and holds dear, perhaps almost out of ordinary time and space. Or is there something more sinister in that remote room, a torture chamber far away down long corridors, far away from listening ears or any hope of rescue? It requires blood, which echoes perhaps a ritual sacrifice. Who is being sacrificed?

Shuttle chooses the word 'overseers' to describe the midwives and doctors in the room. It implies the power differential and clearly denotes who is in control of what is happening there. What does the image of an overseer conjure up for you? A hard, brutal person, usually overseeing slaves or a chain gang, using whips, shouting, cold, heartless, inflicting pain without caring? These faceless overseers – a cold, impersonal 'They' tug the child out of the ruins of the woman's flesh. Is this an instrumental birth or could it be a 'normal' but 'hands-on' birth? The woman is passive, unmoving, a body, a corpse. The most delicate, private parts of her lie cut, ripped and bloody – ruined, perhaps forever. The episiotomy leaves you in tatters. There is nothing soft, nothing caring, nothing loving here.

Birth is not given.
It is what is taken from you;
not a gift you give
but a tax levied on you.
Not a gift but a bout
that ages both the contestants.

At the time of birth, something is taken from you. What is taken from this woman in this remote room? Dignity, humanity, control, pride, hope? She feels as though she has been in a fight, a bout that ages both the contestants. Why a 'bout'? What images does that word contain? It's a term used in the boxing ring; two people fighting surrounded by a crowd jeering and cheering on the violence. Mother and baby are not working in harmony but are contestants in a bout. Boxers usually end up bloodied, bruised and battered – like a baby after a forceps delivery and a mother after an episiotomy. Both she and the baby are aged by the process. She is not the same woman she was when she started; to get her baby, she has been forced to pay a tax of violation, levied on her by faceless others, a high price for her and her baby. Taxes are not optional; she has no choice and she must pay.

> Birthshocks hold on tight, for years,
> like hooked bristles of goosegrass,
> cleavers clinging to your coat skirt and sleeves.
> The raw mime of labour
> is never healed,
> in giving birth
> the woman's innocence goes,
> loss you can't brush away,
> it stains all your new clothes.

Why a 'mime'? Is the play-acting centred around the fact that she is the one supposed to be giving birth and yet the reality – the shock, the betrayal – is that she is not important at all? And she will never forget or recover, never be healed. Giving birth is a shock; no-one prepares you for what will happen in that remote room. The shock of the birth holds on for years and even if you try to forget it and move on, try to forget what happened, it will not leave you. Like a burr on your coat, you cannot brush it away. The more you try, the more it sticks. Women remember their birth experiences forever. Her innocence and youth are gone, her trust in the world and in others around her shattered. However she tries to move on, the mark of the birth stays with her. It is a stain; she is dirty, unclean, violated. She is changed forever.

> No longer can you be half-woman, half-bird.
> Now you are all woman,
> you are all given away,
> your child has the wings,
> can resist the pull of earth.
> You watch her rush up,
> clowning her way through the cloud.
> And you applaud.

And now as a new mother, you have responsibilities and ties. Your freedom and youth must be left behind. You are all given away. You are empty, drained and exhausted. You are heavy, laden down with gravity. There is nothing left of the 'you' you thought you were. That carefree young woman is gone forever. Now your child is the one who has the freedom to be careless and free, to resist the pull of responsibilities, to play. And you are no longer centre-stage but relegated to audience, as you passively watch her as she grows and clowns around. And you applaud her – but how: joyously or slowly and heavily? What emotions do you feel? Was she worth the price you paid?

D.H. Lawrence wrote in 1936 that 'the essential quality of poetry is that it makes a new effort of attention and discovers a new world within a known world'. Experienced midwives can perhaps particularly benefit from this kind of 're-seeing' their familiar world from a multitude of different perspectives.

Poetry for professional development

In a slightly different context, creative writing is now being encouraged as a means of professional reflection. Bolton, a research fellow in the growing field of medical humanities at Sheffield University, explains how 'through writing stories and poems about their work ... professionals discover areas about which they need to think and reflect more deeply, on their own through further writing and in discussion with others in carefully facilitated groups' (Bolton 1999). She explains how the therapeutic value of writing poetry about an experience is far more than the initial outpouring; the working and reworking bring further insight and crystallisation as the writer tries to capture the emotions with clarity and succinctness; as she explains, 'poetry can create order out of mental turmoil'. There is also the finished product, which can enhance satisfaction and self-esteem. She runs courses for doctors and nurses which combine creative writing with professional reflection, in which group members write creative pieces (poetry or prose) exploring aspects of their work and then share and discuss them in small, closed groups. This creates 'a dynamic and vivid professional development process' (Bolton 1999).

Box 6.3

Poetry for professional development

This poem was written by Jenny Green when studying midwifery in 1999. She wrote it as part of an assessment for a module called Images of Women at the Anglia Polytechnic University.

With Woman
Will you be with me?
No I mean 'really' with me?
I can feel this power rising up within, sweeping along
on huge waves, I need someone, you see, because I am frightened.
I am also exhilarated to be on such an exciting journey.
I am tired to tears of people who will not listen and I
barely have the strength to protest at the formulaic
phrases and litanies of self-comfort. I cannot bear
now to be reduced to a product of tunnel vision.
Not now, not when I am at my most powerful, my most
dangerous, my most beautiful.
I am incredibly sensitive. Your body does not lie and
When you touch me I will know if you are really 'with me'
If you do not respect me. Do not insult me with platitudes or
Falseness for convention's sake. I would rather be alone.
Sanctify me. We are equal. Do not collude with those misguided, or more sinister still
those who would emasculate me.
You are powerful and so am I. Touch me gently.
Share the power of life with me honestly, let me be me.

Poetry in research

Midwifery is developing a rich body of research literature in the qualitative paradigm that uses words, not numbers, to communicate the lived experience of women during pregnancy, birth and motherhood. Sara Wickham (2003) writes of the importance of 'seeing the women in the numbers'; it is imperative that we hear their voices and understand their experiences.

There are many different types of qualitative research methods, most commonly based on in-depth interviews, which aim to represent the reality of individual lives. Transcripts are analysed in detail, looking for shared common themes and unique differences. The challenge is then how to represent those data in a way that is faithful to the voice of the interviewee(s) and yet communicates their essence to an audience. One way of presentation is to shape the narratives into poems.

The researcher, having interviewed the participants, works with the tape and transcript of their narrative to find key phrases that seem to highlight their perspective. She works carefully with the words, putting them into stanzas, recreating the pauses, pace and tone, using the participants' own words and the order in which they told their story.

Poindexter (2002) gives details of how she used this methodology in her work with a couple experiencing the shock of an HIV-positive diagnosis, and presented the data as two powerful poems from each partner's perspective. 'The intent of the research poem is both aesthetic and empathic. It can communicate the respondent's emotional world effectively and efficiently' (Richardson 1993). There is a methodological issue that remains unresolved of how this medium can be evaluated for validity and so on, but Poindexter argues that the most applicable standard is simply if the poetry increases empathy and understanding within the audience. Poindexter explains how she uses her research poems often at the beginning or end of a presentation, to further empathy and understanding. It is the economy of words and the direct impact that make this such a powerful medium. Others to follow up are Gee (1991), Richardson (1992) and Becker (1999) who have pioneered this approach in differing fields of healthcare. It has yet to be tried in midwifery research.

Poetry in antenatal education

Poems can be a rich trigger for discussion and reflection in antenatal group sessions. They can engage the heart and mind in a way that a factual discussion of pain and pain relief will never do. One of the challenges, for example, is to describe what a contraction or giving birth feels like. In her poem *Oxytocin*, Susan Taylor talks of natural contractions as 'fierce arched rainbows' or the pain that rises and falls 'like breath' (in Palmeira 1990). Sharon Olds, in her poem *The Moment the Two Worlds Meet*, viscerally describes the process of the baby emerging 'when the slick whole body comes out of me ...' (in Donnelly & Bernstein 1996).

People are most often moved to write poetry during life's intense events: the giddy 'falling in love' of a new relationship or the break-up of an old one; the death of a loved one or a time of despair and unhappiness. Giving birth is surely such an event. Midwives can suggest that women try their hand at writing about their experiences – celebratory or otherwise. Some of the most moving poems have been written about grief: for a loss of a baby or for the loss of a normal childbirth experience. Consider that Bolton (1999) believes there is a 'right' time to write poetry: too soon after the event and everything is too raw and jumbled (although an outpouring onto paper may be cathartic), too late and events can become grey and indistinct.

The tradition of the celebratory birthday poem is an ancient one. Poems were written to celebrate the birth and birthdays of rulers and other important people as far back as Roman times, then by poets to their patrons and gradually extending to ordinary friends and family members in the 19th and 20th centuries. As childbirth and parenthood has now become an acceptable topic for male and female contemporary poets, there is a growth of male writers writing about their experiences during their partner's pregnancy, in the birth room and as new fathers. There is a section of the *Virago Book of Birth Poetry* entitled 'Male Participation' which gives a small selection (Otten 1993). Fathers-to-be may like to read some of the contemporary poems to be found there written from father to new child, such as *Hello* by John Berryman, *To a Child Before Birth* by Norman Nicholson or the well-known *Prayer Before Birth* by Louis MacNeice. Parents may even like to consider writing a poem to their own child and encourage others such as godparents to do the same. They can be read at the christening/baby naming ceremony, kept in a keepsake box and read at each birthday thereafter. You can start them off with a simple 'All the things I wish for you …' or the more provocative 'The things I've learnt so you won't have to …!'.

Poetry as therapy

The word 'therapy' comes from the Greek *therapeia*, meaning to heal through dance, song, poem and drama, i.e. the expressive arts. Using poetry for healing has a long history, from the whispering spells, chants and incantations of priestesses across

---

Box 6.4

Poetry for inspiration

Being born is important
Being born is important.
You who have stood at the bedposts
and seen a mother on her high harvest day,
the day of the most golden of harvest moons for her.
You who have seen the new wet child
dried behind the ears,
swaddled in soft fresh garments,
pursing its lips and sending a groping mouth
toward the nipples where white milk is ready –
You who have seen this love's payday
of wild toil and sweet agonising –
You know being born is important.
You know nothing else was ever so important to you.
You understand the payday of love is so old,
So involved, so traced with circles of the moon,
So cunning with the secrets of the salts of the blood –
It must be older than the moon, older than salt.
(Carl Sandburg)

---

continents to the actual eating of words! In Egyptian times, words were written onto papyrus and then dissolved into a solution so the words could be physically ingested by the patient. The Roman physician Soranus prescribed tragedy for his manic patients and comedy for the depressed ones. The first hospital in the United States, founded by Benjamin Franklin in 1751, used reading, writing and publishing of their writings for treatment of mentally ill patients. They published their creative work in their own paper, *The Illuminator*.

The term 'bibliotherapy' was coined by Samuel Crowthers in 1916, whereby psychiatric patients were given books to read that might 'draw them out'. The hospital librarian and doctors worked closely together to find suitable literature to inform and stimulate. This took on a new dimension in the 1960s when group therapy became popular; patients were encouraged to share their responses to existing literature and express their own experiences through their own creative writing. 'Poetry therapy' or 'psychopoetry' began to be recognised as a form of healing within mental healthcare, focusing on two aspects: an emphasis on the evocative value of poetry and the beneficial potential of patients writing their own responses to poems or creating their own, based on their own experiences and emotions. The Association for Poetry Therapy was formed in the United States in 1969, to attend to what poet Joy Shieman, a pioneer in this field in the 1960s, called 'a realignment of the soul'. Poets-in-residence and poetry therapists began to appear in some psychiatric hospitals. At the same time, others were using poetry to 'draw out' different groups: young people, children, victims of abuse, those addicted to drugs, as part of counselling and so on. Anne Sexton's work, for example, was being recommended by psychiatrists for other mentally ill patients to read. In the 1970s other institutes were founded, such as the Poetry Therapy Institute on the West Coast and the American Academy of Poetry Therapy in Texas. A corresponding body of literature began to appear and in 1980 the Association for Poetry Therapy became the National Association for Poetry Therapy (NAPT). The *Journal of Poetry Therapy* was launched in 1987. The NAPT began to set national standards for training and now offers two designations: as a Certified Poetry Therapist (CPT) or a Registered Poetry Therapist (RPT). The NAPT is the official membership organisation for poetry therapists within the United States, supporting a wide range of educational and research activities.

There is no similar national organisation within the UK at present, but on the Poetry Society website you can find details of many fascinating projects using poetry in a healthcare context. 'Poems for the Waiting Rooms', for example, is an Arts Council/King's Fund project which has commissioned poems on the subject of 'waiting' to be displayed (or, in a separate project, given out as pamphlets) in outpatient and surgery waiting areas. Why not 'poster poems' in postnatal wards or in antenatal clinics where 'waiting' has a double resonance?!

'Poets-in-residence' is another scheme where poets have worked alongside GP surgeries, children's hospitals, community drug teams and all manner of healthcare settings to offer patients and staff the opportunity to give voice to their feelings, either by writing their own poetry or the poet-in-residence writing poetry to capture their experiences. Again, why not in a maternity or neonatal setting? Marilyn Krysl (1989) produced some beautiful poetry when she was poet-in-residence at the Center for Human Caring of the University of Colorado School of Nursing in 1987–88, such as *The Womb is the Body's Most Powerful Muscle*.

Bolton (1999) has used creative writing in many different healthcare settings. Here she describes her work with women in the postnatal period while attached to a GP practice.

Box 6.5

Poetry for strength

To My Daughters
I'll tell you about power:
We are born with the potential
for every daughter we will ever have
embedded like pearls in the dark flesh of our ovaries.
You were already there, in me,
while I was yet curled within my mother, as she was, inside my great-grandmother;
each mother birthing her grandchildren, through her pelvis,
ivory cradles protecting secret worlds within our own seas,
worlds of fierce hearts and minds beyond knowing.
Is there a greater power than holding the entire
universe in your belly?
All of Creation? What about our own galaxies pouring forth?
The summoning of all that is love
and alive into our very breasts, our marrow,
our coursing blood, a luminous milky way
so bright it blinds, with all the power and force of life,
heaven meeting earth, giving to those worlds we hold,
that we see in the irises of our daughters' eyes.
(Corey Alicks 2002)

'A couple of workshops in a GP surgery for new mums was part of this project. Six or eight mothers, their babies and some toddlers attended the hour-long workshop, along with the GP, the practice nurse and the health visitor (all women). One of the mothers wrote a graphic poem about her father dying very close to the birth of her baby. It was read to the group, and received with a great deal of feeling and support; my later feedback from the GP was that the mother had found it extremely helpful. Two of the mothers later published their writings: one about her child having meningitis and the other about having a Down's syndrome baby. The latter (written after the session, as I encouraged the group to continue writing) describes the heartaches and joys of parenting such a baby. It is not a poem, but there are certainly poetic passages in it: "I didn't want people to say *I'm sorry.* If you met Lucy, you'd know why there's no need to be sorry".

This opens the way for poetry – both reading and writing – to be used therapeutically for women experiencing miscarriage, antenatal or postnatal depression, posttraumatic stress disorder or just simple disappointment with their experience of birth and mothering. This can be done in support groups or one to one. As Longo (2004), a practising poetry therapist, writes: 'One of the benefits of poetry reading and writing is not only that it helps to define the "I" but strengthens it ... and when we feel ourselves as not alone in the world, but a part of and integrated with all that exists, self-esteem grows'. There are now many books and articles that provide more information on the application of poetry as therapy which you can find in the reference list below. There is an important ethical dimension not to be forgotten: clearly any therapeutic work such as writing poetry may cause some individuals distress, although Bolton (1999) argues that it is likely to be temporary and, if handled with skill and sensitivity, can lead to personal growth and resolution. Skilful group facilitation is needed, with appropriate back-up, supervision and support.

Conclusion

'What would happen if one woman told the truth about her life? The world would split open.'

(Rukeyser, in Bernikow 1979)

Why does a woman write a poem? Adrienne Rich has an answer: 'Every poem breaks a silence that had to be overcome' (Rich 1995).

Poetry is not an option; it is an imperative. Women continue to suffer unnecessarily every day on the labour wards of the world and midwives have become complicit in their suffering. Too many have hardened their hearts and closed their eyes so they no longer see other women's shocked and horrified faces. Writing a poem may be the only way that a woman can truly tell her story; we have an obligation to listen. It may be, after all is said and done, poetry that finally wakes us up.

'Because this race of women, the women poets, have opened a music in their lives, that out of a mixture of strength and weakness, sex and protest, visibility and invisibility, offers us a glimpse of possibility that we may be on the edge of claiming.'

(Rukeyser, in Bernikow 1979)

We hear the terrible, sad and negative stories and weep silently but birth poetry also gives us a glimpse of another possible universe, one where giving birth is a glory, a triumph and a celebration. We are indeed *just on the edge* of claiming this as a woman's birthright. As we slowly move from being two-dimensional birth technicians, we too reclaim our own heritage as midwives.

Giving a woman a chance to be heard is important. Giving women a collective voice is potentially world-changing. 'It is time that these experiences are shared in poetic form. It is time for women's voice to be heard collectively: collectively they make a powerful sound' (Otten 1993). In this, I include the experiences of women who attend other women; thus the voices of midwives need to speak and be heard too. Midwifery and childbirth is still wearily lost in the world of separation; poetry gives us one way to overcome our silence, to connect with ourselves and each other, and to remind the world that 'Being born is important' (Sandburg, in Graziani 1983).

When you read a beautiful or moving poem about childbirth, perhaps just remember for a moment that you are 'standing on the shoulders' of the generations of women before you who have made it possible for us to give voice to this aspect of the truth of women's lives. It was not always so.

References

Becker B 1999 Narratives of pain in later life and conventions of story telling. Journal of Aging Studies 13(1): 73–87

Bernikow L 1979 The world split open. Women poets 1552–1950. The Women's Press, London

Bligh D (ed) 1986 Teach thinking by discussion. SRHE and NFER Nelson, Guildford

Bloom B S 1965 Taxonomy of educational objectives. Longman, London

Bolton G 1999 'Every poem breaks a silence that had to be overcome': the therapeutic power of poetry writing. Feminist Review 62: 118–132

Calman K, Downie R 1996 Why arts courses for medical curricula? Lancet 347: 1499–1450

Chester L (ed) 1989 Cradle and all. Women writers on pregnancy and birth. Faber and Faber, London

Dobyns S 1997 Best words, best order. Essays on poetry. St Martin's Griffin, New York

Donnelly K J, Bernstein J B (eds) 1996 Our mothers, our selves. Writers and poets celebrating motherhood. Bergin and Garvey, Westport, CT

Eliot T S 2004 Complete poems and plays. Faber and Faber, London

Frost R 2001 The poetry of Robert Frost. Vintage, New York

Gee J 1991 A linguistic approach to narrative. Journal of Narrative and Life History 1(1): 15–39

Grant J 1998 Different ways of knowing. Practising Midwife 1(11): 41

Graziani R (ed) 1983 The naked astronaut. Poems on birth and birthdays. Faber and Faber, London

Hazlitt W 1818 On poetry in general. Oxford World Classics, Oxford (reprinted 1991)

Keats J 1958 The Letters of John Keats: 1814–1821, 2 vols. Harvard University Press, Cambridge, MA

Krysl M 1989 Midwife, and other poems on caring. National League for Nursing, New York

Lawrence D H 1936 Preface to Chariot of the Sun. In: McDonald E (ed) Phoenix: the posthumous papers (1968). Viking, New York

Lerner A (ed) 1994 Poetry in the therapeutic experience, 2nd edn. MMB Music, St Louis, MO

Longo P 2004 Poetry therapist. Available online at: www.poetrytherapy.org

Lundgren I, Dahlberg K 1998 Women's experience of pain during childbirth. Midwifery 14: 105–110

Mohin L 1979 One foot on the mountain. An anthology of British feminist poetry 1969–1979. OnlyWomen Press, London

Olsen T 1980 Silences. Virago Press, London

Otten C (ed) 1993 The Virago book of birth poetry. Virago Press, London

Page L 1997 Evidence-based midwifery practice. British Journal of Midwifery 5(2): 18–22

Palmeira R (ed) 1990 In the gold of flesh. Poems of birth and motherhood. The Women's Press, London

Plath S 1981 Collected poems. Faber and Faber, London

Poindexter C C 2002 Research as poetry: a couple experiences HIV. Qualitative Inquiry 8(6): 707–714

Pound E 1960 ABC of reading. WW Norton, New York

Rich A 1980 On lies, secrets and silence: selected prose 1966–1978. Virago Press, London

Rich A 1995 What is found there: notebooks on poetry and politics. Virago Press, London

Richardson L 1992 The consequences of poetic representation: writing the other, re-writing the self. In: Ellis C, Flaherty M G (eds) Investigating subjectivity: research on lived experience. Sage Publications, Newbury Park, CA

Richardson L 1993 Poetics, dramatics and transgressive validity: the case of the skipped line. Sociological Quarterly 34(4): 695–710

Rogers A 1986 Teaching adults. Open University Press, Milton Keynes

Rogers C 1983 Freedom to learn for the 80s. Charles E Merrill Publishing Co, Bell and Howell, Colombus, OH

Schon D A 1987 Educating the reflective practitioner. Jossey-Bass, San Francisco, CA

Sexton A 1981 The complete poems. Houghton Mifflin, Boston

Wickham S 2003 Seeing women in the numbers. MIDIRS Midwifery Digest 13(4): 439–444

Further reading

Note: I have chosen not to reproduce well-known poetry that is accessible elsewhere; it saved me from that heart-wrenching, Desert Island Disc trauma of having to choose only a small number out of my many favourites! Instead, I have provided references to where you can begin your search for your favourite birth poetry, and have chosen to give public voice to some women who may not otherwise be heard.

Chester L (ed) 1989 Cradle and all. Women writers on pregnancy and birth. Faber and Faber, London

Couzyn J 1999 A time to be born. Firelizard, London

Derricote T 2000 Natural birth. Firebrand Books, Ann Arbor, CT

Donnelly K J, Bernstein J B (eds) 1996 Our mothers, our selves. Writers and poets celebrating motherhood. Bergin and Garvey, Westport, CT

Ferguson G K 2001 Baby: poems on pregnancy, birth and babies. Canongate Books, Edinburgh

Graziani R (ed) 1983 The naked astronaut. Poems on birth and birthdays. Faber and Faber, London

Krysl M 1989 Midwife, and other poems on caring. National League for Nursing, New York

Otten C (ed) 1993 The Virago book of birth poetry. Virago Press, London

Palmeira R (ed) 1990 In the gold of flesh. Poems of birth and motherhood. The Women's Press, London

These books go in and out of print but you should be able to source them via secondhand booksellers on the Internet.

Useful websites

www.lapidus.org.uk An Arts Council-funded UK organisation founded in 1996 to promote the use of literary arts in personal development and health.

www.poetrytherapy.org The website for the US-based National Association of Poetry Therapy, with details of the Poetry Therapy Journal.

www.poetrymagic.co.uk The largest resource for learning about poetry on the web.

www.poetrysociety.org.uk The website for the UK Poetry Society, which has a dedicated section on poetry and health.

www.endeavor.med.nyu/lit-med A website from the New York School of Medicine which offers a useful searchable database of art and literature resources for those interested in using the humanities in healthcare.

CHAPTER SEVEN

How Do They See Us? Portrayals of Childbirth and the Role of the Midwife in Literature

—————————(•)—————————

TERRI COATES

This chapter started as an exploration of how midwives are described in literature but because of a dearth of material, the research was broadened to look at how childbirth and the attendants at the birth are described. I undertook a short review of midwives as they have been portrayed in fictional literature (Coates 1998) and this was used as a starting point.

Sheila Kitzinger (1991, p.1) wrote:

'In childbirth today the obstetrician usually stands centre-stage. The midwife is invisible. Yet historically, ever since the first recorded accounts of birth midwives have had the main responsibility for giving care before, during and after the baby is born, and in many societies today the health of most mothers and newborn babies still depends on midwives.'

There are references in novels that give some insight into who practised midwifery and how it was practised at the time. The novels and other sources that have been examined are presented in chronological order and grouped together as small collections in context.

The process of birth has been experienced by every member of our species and the process of becoming a mother has for most women been in the company of a midwife, at least in the broadest sense. So it would seem reasonable to search for the midwife in literature, as she, or he, touches most lives, even if rather briefly. Over the centuries authors have touched on every job imaginable and doctors, nurses, vets, barristers, police and criminals have all become household names through fictional portrayals of their profession. A well-researched portrayal of a profession can give an overview of the day-to-day requirements of a job and often mirrors that profession's current standing in the community. So looking for midwives in literature may seem narcissistic but an interest in fictional portrayal of a profession, particularly one's own, did not seem unreasonable.

In literature the birth narrative has largely been a feature of the 20th century. Whilst this makes the available narratives contemporary, it does not guarantee the presence of a midwife.

Many midwives use birth stories as practical work tools and the stories can become an important part of our work of teaching at all levels. Some midwives become skilled story tellers. The use of case histories to describe our own or vicarious experience is an everyday occurrence. Kirkham & Perkins (1997) suggest that the use of birth narrative can be a way of improving the care we deliver by looking at ourselves from someone else's point of view.

Childbirth in literature

Birth narratives evolving from the 18th or 19th century are all written by male authors, even when written from the female perspective. Examples are rare but those that are still in print or available include Laurence Sterne's *The Life and Opinions of Tristram Shandy* (1759), Tolstoy's *Anna Karenin* written in 1873 and Chekhov's (1888) description of premature labour and birth in *The Party*.

Tristram Shandy (Sterne 1759) is the fictional author whose conception, birth, christening and circumcision form a major narrative. The story is around 250 years old but the themes are unnervingly relevant to practice today. Tristram relates his own birth and family history, drawing upon stories and hearsay and adding an abundance of his own opinions. Tristram's father, Mr Shandy, is well read and criticises medical opinion as he believes that it could not be superior to his own. Shandy spends much time deliberating the new caesarean operation for extracting the child as he believes that it would be a more desirable method of giving birth, and becomes convinced that the normal method of childbirth is wrong. He is dissuaded from this course of thought but decides that the baby should be turned to breech and the head protected from the crushing shock of birth by forceps. Doctor Slop is the local male midwife and scientifick (sic) operator who has a pair of the recently invented delivery forceps. In the end, Tristram's mother, Elizabeth, insists on having a midwife to attend her rather than Doctor Slop, out of resentment at not being allowed to deliver her child in London. Doctor Slop has written a book expressing his distain for the practice of midwifery. He is only interested in surgical and medical advances and opts to simply keep Tristram's father company during Elizabeth's labour. Elizabeth births with the local midwife in attendance and the child is named Tristram. Sterne's view of childbirth is rather chaotic and neither the midwife nor the doctor emerge particularly well.

Two births described by famous Russian authors can be used to compare and contrast two different views of midwifery skills. Both were written contemporaneously. The birth of Kitty's baby in *Anna Karenin* was inspired by Tolstoy's own reactions to the birth of his first child. During a 22-hour labour, Kitty is attended by Lizvaveta Petrovna, one of the few midwives in literature to be given a name. Lizvaveta Petrovna is also worthy of note as she remains a calm and resolute presence throughout Kitty's arduous labour, delivers and resuscitates the baby with 'skilful hands' whilst the doctor keeps company with Kitty's distraught husband. The midwife here is known, trusted, respected and appreciated.

Chekhov (1888) was a doctor, so he wrote with professional insight when describing a premature labour on a humid day. The midwife is not a source of help or comfort whilst sitting with Olga through her labour and is a figure of ridicule as she pulls out drawers to speed labour. Here the doctor's view of midwifery practice is that it is ignorant and superstitious, though he shows his own profession in a positive light as the doctor relieves Olga's pain and suffering.

Female novelists of the 19th century were affected by the sensibilities if their age and direct references to pregnancy or childbirth were rare and oblique.

Jane Austen wrote domestic novels about the lives of women, though as a spinster she was perhaps not the best informed about the processes of pregnancy and childbirth. Births are only described in four of her books and they all take place off stage. Whilst the delivery of an infant is never described, Austen does refer obliquely to the events, using the terms 'lying in' and 'delivery'.

In *Jayne Eyre* (1848), Charlotte Bronte omits any account of a pregnancy or birth. The baby is introduced to the reader when he is described as closely resembling his father, having been placed into his father's arms. The other Bronte sisters are equally circumspect about recording the appearance of a new generation and avoid the use of the words 'birth' or 'born', which was the norm for that generation of authors. Any reference to the appearance of a new baby is described with the utmost delicacy so the inclusion of a character that is as blatantly connected with childbirth as a midwife is wholly unlikely. In fact, any young woman expecting to gain any information regarding marriage and the production of heirs from these novels would remain mystified by the whole process.

At the time Dickens was writing *Martin Chuzzlewit* (1844), midwives in England were hardly considered to be respectable. Dickens describes the character of Mrs Sara Gamp as a monthly nurse and almost apologises for her brazen sign which proclaimed her a Midwife. The garrulous gin-swigging Mrs Gamp was distinctly unprofessional but perhaps not as bad as other midwives of the era known as Mother Midnight (Carter & Duriez 1986). Unfortunately, the fictitious Mrs Gamp 'established a stereotype for the midwife in history' (Donnison 1988).

Dickens' portrayal of Sara Gamp did little for the midwife's standing and recent fictional portrayals written in a historical context have done little more.

Garfield's (1994) short story about a midwife called Moss and her apprentice, Blister, form part of a collection of short stories about apprentices in 18th-century London. Moss and Blister helped to perpetuate the image of the midwife as 'pig ignorant' (p.57) but they could deliver a baby 'as safely as kiss your hand' (p.58). Moss and her apprentice Blister attend a woman in labour and ask for the mirrors to be covered so the child would not be born blind and instruct that all knots be untied and drawers opened to hasten delivery. This tale does little to impress upon children and young people the role of the midwife and makes the midwife look like a historical curiosity similar to other characters in the book, such as the lamplighters and pawnbrokers (Coates 1998).

A more positive portrayal of the midwife for a young audience is *The Midwife's Apprentice* (Cushman 1997) set in 14th-century England. The story is a skilful weaving of fact and fiction that offers a wise and sensitive portrayal of the midwife in medieval England. The woman's knowledge is considered valuable and the book includes some information written by Jane Sharp, a real midwife who practised in the 17th century and who is believed to have been the first woman to produce a manual for midwives. A version of her book is still in print (Sharp 1671) and is documented well by Donnison (1988) and others.

Laurel Thatcher Ulrich (1991) has used her skill as a historian to bring the diary (1785–1812) of Martha Ballard, a midwife and healer, to modern readers. The diary is a record of her work (undertaking 816 deliveries) and domestic life.

From the start of the 20th century there was a reversal in the way birth is viewed. Until the 20th century, births that were described were usually recalled from the audience's point of view. Subsequently births have usually been written about either in the first person or specifically from the woman's point of view (Atwood 1986a,b, Byatt 1986, Drabble 1968, Hansford Johnson 1955, Lessing 1964, Lette 1993, McCroy 1989, Weldon 1980). Births in these books are without exception viewed from the heroine's point of view, with the midwife portrayed as a cold and distant character, a source of irritation rather than comfort (Coates 1998). The persona of the midwife in these novels is that of a universally nameless character, peripheral to the birth, moving in and out of the text, undertaking tasks and giving off an air of brisk untouchable efficiency. The labour and birth are usually written without using professional jargon, telling the reader only what the heroine would have known or felt at the time. The omission of midwifery and medical jargon gives the descriptions of labour and birth an air of authenticity but whilst this gives women a strong voice in contemporary literature, it hides the midwife's role in supporting labour and birth.

The Squire by Edith Bagnold (1938) is a notably rare exception, giving a midwife a role and character which lasts more than a paragraph. The 'Squire' is mistress of the house and whilst her husband is away, she takes on his title (Squire) in his absence. The book was first published in 1938 and is a sensuous exploration of late pregnancy. As the household waits restlessly for the birth, the Squire contemplates the woman she was and the birth to come. She is distracted from her deep contemplations by her friend and companion Caroline, the day-to-day running of the household and her four children. The midwife arrives to await the onset of labour and senses a change in the Squire that has been put down to an overindulgence in fruit that day. Like Chekhov's (1888) description of labour, there is an element of heat and an impending storm brewing on the horizon. The night passes with the distractions and discomforts bound up with early labour. The doctor and midwife keep a quiet watchfulness whilst the Squire paces the garden regarding the pair as a monk and nun. The processes and progress of the labour are couched in metaphors.

> 'The monk and nun were about her bed, acutely directed on her, tuned to her every manifestation. With eyes fast shut she lent herself to their quiet directions, clinging to the memory of her resolve that when the river began to pull she would swim down with it, clutching at no banks.' (p.144)

Bagnold (1938) said that it is hard to gauge the pain of labour and describes the process of labouring as hallucinated swimming. The Squire delivers under an anaesthetic administered by the doctor and so the delivery itself is not described. The description of labour goes from the Squire experiencing corkscrew contractions to the shocked cry of the newborn, already dressed, with smiling faces looking on. The doctor leaves having administered morphine to keep the Squire calm and to prevent her from wanting to get out of bed, whilst the midwife makes tea and folds baby clothes. Through the weeks after the birth the midwife stays and sorts small troubles then leaves the household established with the new baby and disappears, 'leaving not a ripple'.

In *Cold Comfort Farm* (Gibbons 1932), Flora believes that women who have had no experience of childbirth will derive information from novels. She then makes fun of the different styles of description, such as those where many dots follow staccato phrases and those that are dismissive of childbirth with cheerful brightness. Best of all, she believes, is the lazy old-fashioned description.

Women of the era may well have been gathering information from the novels they read, but they would be no wiser about the birth of a baby unless they could disentangle metaphor from flowery description that actually avoided any indelicate facts. For its time, Bagnold's 1938 novel is remarkably frank. More usually, authors who did include a pregnancy in their novel used announcements in *The Times* or phrases such as Gibbons (1932) suggests, 'She was brought to bed of a fine boy', to cover the indelicate matter of labour and birth.

In *The Pursuit of Love* (Mitford 1945), the Radlett girls are fascinated by childbirth and are compelled to uncover all the facts they can. They find lurid descriptions of labour and birth which are all screams from behind the bedroom door and running for the doctor. As they surmise that this fate will one day be theirs, they ask Aunt Sadie

who has just had her seventh. Their aunt is far from reassuring; she tells the girls that labour is the worst pain imaginable but 9 months too late to put a stop to the whole process. This rather confirms the descriptions they have found. The Radlett girls do discover the facts regarding the physical process of childbirth but they don't seem to be much wiser for the knowledge. This sort of apprehension regarding childbirth, where misinformation is obtained from the pages of the novel, was what Dick Read (1942) worked so hard to dispel. He believed that novelists were keen to gain the attention of the reader by describing childbirth with drama and associated horrors, producing a fear of childbirth, and concluded that young women were very unlikely to approach mother-hood cheerfully if their only information was gathered from books or newspapers where straightforward births were not considered to be good copy.

Doris Lessing was one of the early protagonists in the groundswell of feminist writers, who by the 1950s and 1960s were writing novels of stark domestic real-ism describing the forgotten lives of women. Lessing was one of the first women to offer a realistic account of childbirth from the participant's point of view. In *A Proper Marriage* (1964), she described Martha's labour in a South African hospital in a manner that reads like a documentary script. This was a huge departure from what had become a traditional silence regarding the processes of birth in works of fiction. Lessing does not attempt to romanticise pregnancy and birth and the novel could not be construed as an escapist read for any but those of a stout constitution. When Martha realises that she is in labour she is 'lifted on a wave of excitement' and cries out 'Hurray, this is it!'. As the labour progresses, she describes very graphically the changes in the intensity of the con-tractions, the pain and agony and the exasperation at not being able to remember the agony in the painless moments between contractions. Despite the careful description of the labour, the nurses (midwives) attending Martha remain out of sight for most of the time, appearing only occasionally to examine her progress. The delivery itself is quite shocking. It is performed under chloroform after a nurse has 'plunged her pink rubber sealed hands' into Martha's body and declared Martha to be 'ripe'. Martha regains con-sciousness to hear that she has a baby girl and shrieks, at which the nurse says 'Oh, drat it' and Martha is once again anaesthetised with chloroform. Here is an objective view of labour and delivery with the heroine observing the process of labour with interest and detachment. The description of the birth is bleak and attendants are not a source of comfort or support and lack empathy. They appear only to undertake procedures that are seen as degrading and depart with brisk disapproving comments.

Margaret Drabble (1968) introduces Rosamund who is academically brilliant but finds herself pregnant after one sexual encounter. Arriving at the hospital in labour, Rosamund describes with incredulity the porter who insists that she is not allowed to walk so she allows herself to be wheeled to the labour ward. The descriptions of the staff continue in the same vein, with midwives referred to as 'them' or 'they'. Rosamund describes her labour in a detached way, but she remains in control of her labour within her own mind. She expresses irritation with the staff, whom she overhears discussing their social lives, and when she asks them to '...pack it in, can't you?', the staff think she is calling for help. She does not maintain her irritation but responds the way she thinks that the staff would expect, saying that she believes her drugs have worn off. They respond by telling her that she can't have anything else until later and leave her alone again. Rosamund describes her contractions as violent sensations that promise pleasure rather than pain. Towards the end of her labour she describes hearing herself moan violently, the sound of which makes the staff quickly reappear. The delivery is described succinctly by Rosamund as 'within five minutes my child was born' but she goes on to

describe the midwives arguing among themselves up to and beyond the delivery. The midwife who had taken on the 'task' as the calmer and soother of nerves sounded more panicked than soothing to Rosamund. Even after the delivery, the midwife, who shows no warmth or kindness, is described as 'all smiles and starch'.

In *The Waterfall*, Drabble (1969) describes birth in very different circumstances. The heroine, Jane, waits alone in a cold house for labour to start; her husband has left her and her first child has been sent to visit grandparents until after the birth. Jane is so used to silence and isolation, the cold house and the snow that she is surprised that she manages to call the midwife when her labour begins. The reader is told that the cold and Jane's isolation concern the midwife who can only concentrate all the sources of heat available within the bedroom. The delivery is not described but the arrival of the baby is announced by informing the reader that the doctor was too late to assist but arrived to put in some stitches. The midwife makes tea and baths the baby. She waits quietly with Jane until a cousin arrives to stay overnight, and then does get a couple of lines of dialogue: 'I'll be off then' and 'I'll be back in the morning, nine o'clock'. This is a brief but believable portrayal of a midwife seen through a mother's eyes.

Fay Weldon writes prolifically about the lives of women. The realism that she uses to portray pregnancy in *Puffball* (1980) is a tribute to sound research and is a departure from other novels of the same era that stick to the heroine's viewpoint, telling only what they could have known of the pregnancy or labour. *Puffball* describes Liffey's pregnancy and development of her fetus in a way that separates her from her life and emotions. The only appearance that the midwife makes is at an antenatal clinic, as Liffey has a placenta previa and undergoes an emergency caesarean section.

The Handmaid's Tale (Atwood 1986b) is a bleak story of America some time in the 21st century. The country is so polluted that birth is a rare occurrence. Families are split up and women are expected to have sex for the purpose of reproduction only. Birth is a rare event and is a time for a joyful gathering and celebration of women. Birth is celebrated by women and seen as crucially important for the continuation of the human race. The birth is attended by many women but the role of a midwife is not described.

Looking back to London of the early 1950s, Worboyes (2004) describes a close-knit family life and the pregnancy of Maggie, a 15-year-old girl, in *Time will Tell*. The supportive extended family keep Maggie hidden and pretend that the girl's mother is pregnant, hoping eventually that the baby will be brought up as Maggie's brother or sister.

Midwives are mentioned several times throughout the book. Worboyes introduces the local convent where midwives are trained and there are memories of another birth within the family when the midwife had to shout for help and wait for a sixpence for the meter before she could see to help a woman deliver. When Maggie goes into labour, a midwife arrives on a bicycle; she calms the household, examines Maggie and leaves instructions for the labour. The midwife's instructions are followed carefully and Maggie is well supported by several generations of female relatives. The midwife returns promptly when summoned and is kind and compassionate.

The unusual aspect of this fictional delivery is that the midwife has been given a voice; she has several pages of dialogue with Maggie and her relatives. She has also been given a background, arriving from the local convent maternity home. As a midwife she is credible; she carries with her the tools of her trade, equipment that you would expect a midwife to carry such as a stethoscope, cord clamps, scissors, bowls and gauze, which are spread out on a chest of drawers near the bed ready for delivery. The birth itself is unusual as it is the only fictional birth that I have found that accurately and realistically describes the processes of a vaginal delivery which was gleaned from

research and watching a few births (Worboyes, personal communication, 2005). This is a birth from an observer's point of view, not completely detached but without really describing any of the physical sensations associated with a birth.

Birth as portrayed in the romantic comedy novel

In recent years several authors have written romantic comedy novels with gritty descriptions of pregnancy, labour and birth as observed from their heroine's point of view. They lack the jargon of the midwifery and medical profession and therefore confer an air of authenticity to their birth stories.

In *Fetal Attraction*, Kathy Lette (1993) describes Maddy giving birth. The labour description starts when Maddy is already in the second stage. Maddy's midwife is unusual as she has lines of dialogue: ' "Bear down, bear down!" the midwife enthuses.' Then after application of the Ventouse cup, she instructs Maddy to pant as the baby's head is delivered. This is a short but realistic portrayal of a midwife as a kind, tolerant and competent professional working as part of a team.

The Wives of Bath (Holden 2005) chronicles the lives and unlikely friendships of two fictional couples, their experiences of pregnancy and early parenthood. The labours and deliveries are given scant coverage. The nearest that a midwife gets to making an appearance is when Alice goes into labour and calls the local NHS maternity unit. She discovers that there are not enough midwives available to attend a home birth that night so she chooses to go to the local private maternity unit instead and is delivered by emergency caesarean section. Her friend Amanda, who had chosen an elective caesarean section in the private maternity unit, has a normal vaginal delivery in the NHS maternity unit. The delivery is referred to only in retrospect, so the midwife is omitted again.

Second Prize (Manby 1997) introduces Julie who labours quickly at home, is helped into a very small car and is then rushed to hospital but she delivers her baby on the back seat.

In *Life Isn't All Ha Ha Hee Hee* (1999), Syal describes Chila's labour in a series of words strung together, such as *OHMYGODOHMYGODOHMUMSHANTIOMY-GOD*, that leave the reader in no doubt that labour is less than comfortable but without mention of attendants, midwife or otherwise. Green (2001) uses similar series of words and letters to describe Maeve's feelings during labour: *NNNNNNNnnnnnnnnnnnnnnnnnnnnn nnnn, NOOOOOOOOOooooooooooooo* and *NNNNNNNNNNNNNRRRRRRRRRH-HHHHHHHHHHH*. A midwife makes an appearance, saying 'Come on, Maeve love' (p.305). The delivery is not described but the baby does appear later in the book, rather similar to the style of novels written before the 1940s.

One father's view of the midwife can be found in *The Family Way*, by Tony Parsons (2005). The midwives are seen as eye candy for the consultant obstetrician as they loiter around him, 'giggling and blushing, hoping that he would notice them'. The birth described is premature, complicated by preeclampsia and a caesarean section which is well described. It is a pity the midwives didn't feature in an equally positive way.

American authors' views of birth

American authors have been writing in a similar genre to contemporary British writers. In *Small Changes*, Piercy (1972) describes Miriam's 17 hours of labour. She is supported by Neil but appears to be alone with her thoughts. She describes being robbed of dignity

in a tiny gown and experiencing contractions that don't hurt any less for not being called pain. She is delivered by Doctor Forman. In a way that seems fairly typical in American novels describing birth, the doctor is given a name whereas a nurse assists but is a very peripheral character.

Maternity Leave (Camp et al 2000) is a collection of three novels with the same theme of impending motherhood. The stories are hopelessly romantic and the births are all rather improbable. Needless to say, as in most American tales of hospital birth, there are no midwives and all the babies are delivered by dashing doctors.

In *The Diary of a Mad Mother to Be* (Woolf 2003), the softly spoken obstetrician is rather charmingly described as the Crotch Whisperer. He makes various appearances through the novel as the heroine attends her antenatal visits and then when she is in labour. The first really audible thing uttered by the Crotch Whisperer is 'Good lord, this woman is a pain in the ass!' because Amy wants to delay the birth until after midnight so her baby will not arrive on April Fool's Day.

What is striking about the American fiction compared to British fiction is how many of the care providers who conducted the deliveries had names and a rapport with the labouring woman. These American doctors would have been chosen by the pregnant woman and paid by her for all the visits. The obstetric nurses who provided care in labour call the doctor for the delivery so that he can appear like the cavalry at the last moment and deliver the baby with a flourish.

Stories of fictional midwives

Fictional midwives who turn to murder really give the profession the ultimate in bad press. *Whitechapel Mary* (Worboyes 2001) is set in London 1888, the time of Jack the Ripper. The main character is Mary who is lured into becoming a courtesan. Her friend and neighbour is a hard-working midwife called Jacqueline Turner. Jacqueline turns to murdering prostitutes.

An American tale of midwifery (Moran Laskas 2003) that starts in 1913 portrays a fourth-generation midwife, Elizabeth, learning the art of midwifery from her mother. Knowledge and skills passed down from mother to daughter would seem like a positive reinforcement of the midwife's art but even here there is a dark side. The generations of midwives have recorded births they have attended in black ledgers whilst the secret contents of a small red ledger reveal an unpalatable record of illegitimate babies killed at birth. Elizabeth is uncomfortable with the knowledge of the red book, loses faith in her vocation and feels that she has to cease to practise. The births and deaths described are alarmingly accurate but described without professional jargon. The accuracy of Moran Laskas' writing is explained by her acknowledgements which include a long list of midwifery texts both modern and historical.

The town of Trinity is the fictional setting for a midwife practising in 1830s Pennsylvania (Parr 2003) This American story about a midwife is written in a much lighter and more optimistic vein. The midwife is very much part of the community and the attendance at birth an important aspect of the novel. However, the descriptions of midwifery skills and births are superficial and lack authenticity.

Chris Bohjalian (1997) wrote a fictional story of an American midwife that reads like a factual account of events. The central story, narrated by the midwife's daughter, is of a difficult labour in an isolated house during an ice storm. The labour goes badly and the midwife, her apprentice, the labouring mother and her husband are cut off from the community, trapped by the weather. The mother dies and the midwife does a post

mortem caesarean section, saving the baby, but is then accused of killing the mother. The events leading up to the night, the labour, birth, the court case and the trial are gripping and chilling. The clinical detail is so well written that it is difficult to believe that it is fiction. The courtroom drama and death are harrowing but the midwife and her supporters are portrayed in a kindly fashion. The tale does little to inspire public trust in midwives and would put many off ever contemplating a home birth, no matter what the weather.

Non-fictional midwives

There are few portrayals of the midwife in literature but my call for midwives to write (Coates 1998) about their work and give a realistic literary image of it did at least produce one response. *Call the Midwife* (Worth 2002) is a description of one midwife's working life in the East End of London during the late 1950s and early 1960s. Worth's reminiscences offer us a vivid piece of social history and a unique insight into midwifery practices within this period. She also describes the pleasure of working within midwifery, weaving in friendships she formed with the women and their families whilst working in the poorer areas in the East End of London. Worth's descriptions of midwifery are evocative of a bygone era, but many of the practices she describes are current or would be recognised by midwives today.

There is a sharp contrast between the drab existence of many of the women's lives in 1950s London and the world where Peggy Vincent (2002), an American licensed midwife, practised. Vincent's memories are of more recent practice, working as an independent nurse midwife in California. In *Baby Catcher: Chronicles of a Modern Midwife*, Vincent describes the American way of home birth. Each birth is skilfully portrayed and the descriptions of supporting women and their families through the birth process are written with sound professional insight. Both books are fascinating and give a privileged glimpse into the day-to-day practice of other midwives and add a significant contribution to the tradition of oral history. Other notable resources that can be added here are the collection of interviews tracing the oral history from handy woman to professional midwife (Leap & Hunter 1993), the biography of the Middlesbrough midwife (Cleveland Biographies 1999) and Allison's (1996) study of district midwives working around Nottingham between 1948 and 1972.

Non-fictional birth narratives

A collection of letters from working women who were members of The Women's Co-operative were edited and published as *Maternity* by Margaret Llewelyn Davies (1915). The letters are autobiographical portraits of what motherhood was like in the late 19th and early 20th century. Like the fiction of the time, pregnancy and the birth itself are only mentioned obliquely. The women must have endured a great deal, as there was an almost universal lack of antenatal care and no maternity benefit. The letters frequently detail a lack of food and hard physical work right up to the confinement. For most women there was an almost immediate return to household chores or work. The overall impression from the letters is one of resignation, despair and endurance.

In an attempt to balance the apparent shortfall in midwifery presence in fiction, a search for some non-fictional birth narratives was undertaken. Birth narratives themselves are numerous. Collections of narratives include Oakley (1986), Attallah (1987) and Kitzinger (1987). More recent birth stories can be found on the Internet where a search will bring up hundreds of birth stories on dozens of sites. Again, it is interesting to see how seldom the midwife appears, especially in the British birth stories. Around 50% of the American women who posted birth stories that I read on various websites named their obstetrician and heaped praise on him (all men), usually for just getting to the birth on time. In the same cases the nurse midwives who cared for the women in labour are rarely mentioned or are just referred to as 'the nurse'.

Oakley's (1986) book consists of transcripts of interviews with a group of women who were questioned about their experiences of pregnancy, childbirth and motherhood before and after the birth of their first children. The selection of accounts for the book clearly serves to contribute to a specific thesis. Oakley points out that although the overall impression of the accounts does seem to emphasise the less than satisfactory experiences of childbirth, it affords the reader a 'realistic idea of parenthood' (p.6). The women being interviewed spoke in general terms about people *doing things* to them. Some of the women appeared to be passive and almost detached from their labour. It was, however, surprisingly difficult to find a midwife mentioned at all in spite of the fact that there is a whole chapter of the women's less than complementary descriptions of their medical care during pregnancy and childbirth.

In contrast, Kitzinger's (1987) collection illustrates the editor's natural approach to childbirth. The stories of birth in this book have a greater coherence than those in Oakley's. This could be accounted for by the fact that they were all written accounts and not transcripts of oral material. As with previously described birth narratives, there is scant evidence of the midwife here either.

Some women who have written their birth narratives (Kitzinger 1987) used medical and obstetric terms and as such were seen to maintain a greater degree of power over their birth as they spoke the same language as the midwives and doctors (Arney 1982).

There are many similarities between the two sets of accounts but it is the differences between the two which seem to be the most interesting. These differences undermine the claim of either to be showing the *real* version of birth. In reality, the selection of accounts serves to demonstrate the spectrum of birth experiences rather than one being more realistic than the other. In both sets of accounts, however, the midwife's presence is rarely discussed.

Another collection of birth narratives can be found in *Women* (Attallah 1987). Attallah (1987) interviewed 289 women on feminism, sexuality, motherhood and relationships. Although not all of these women were mothers, those who had experienced childbirth described their labour and delivery in some detail. In the 200 descriptions of birth, there is not one mention of a midwife; two male doctors and one male gynaecologist are mentioned, and there is one delivery undertaken by a husband, but no midwives. The interviews were done mostly in Britain and it is likely that all the women delivering in this country would have encountered a midwife (Ball 1987).

Accounts of pregnancy and birth written by 'celebrities' have been cropping up for the last few decades. Sue Limb (1986), a writer and broadcaster, wrote *Love Forty*, contrasting the kind, supportive midwives with less than helpful medics who wander in and out of her labour room looking at monitor printouts but forgetting to acknowledge the person attached. This is a rare glimpse of a midwife at work in the believable surroundings of a local general maternity unit. Paula Yates (1990) chose to have her baby in a private hospital and describes the delights of private care. Prelabour preparation includes 'bonding with your obstetrician'. The midwife does make an appearance but only after the birth. The midwife is described as a useful pair of hands to plug in the heated rollers for the hairdresser so that Paula could look her best for the press photographers. Mel Giedroyc (2004) described her pregnancy as 'one mother of a journey'. Her pregnancy diary is written as a countdown to delivery; the number of days left to delivery are used as chapter headings. The midwifery service does not appear to have much input in Ms Giedroyc's pregnancy but otherwise the pregnancy is very detailed. A midwife called Valerie calmly organises an epidural while Ms Giedroyc delivers a series of colourful expletives. The epidural is sited by a pair of anaesthetists but only numbs one leg before the baby is born. The midwife really only serves to perform a series of tasks which are peripheral to Giedroyc's birth narrative.

The stories of the process of birth are told in these narratives and in the telling, women appear to have regained control of the experience by excluding the midwife. It is a sobering thought that the midwife can be rendered invisible by either an author's omission or an editor's pen.

One notable exception to these narratives is written by Rachel Cusk. In *A Life's Work* (Cusk 2001), she describes the process of becoming a mother. In the introduction she explains that she expects childbirth to be painful and remembers a film that she was shown at school where a woman gave birth with little support. The midwife in the film is remembered as a shadowy figure sitting in the corner murmuring support and encouragement. The midwife's presence is described as giving an air of authority to the proceedings but she does not appear to move until there is a baby to catch. Cusk describes her own antenatal care but the midwife is only a source of information leaflets and books. She decides to have a home birth but the presence of the delivery pack in the bedroom gives her nightmares after she has seen the contents. A diagnosis of placenta previa makes this choice of birth impossible for Cusk and her daughter is delivered by caesarean section. The midwives are never personalised or given names and are constantly referred to as them or they. Once again, midwives are seen as part of the system – a group of faceless professionals who do things to you when you are pregnant.

In a frank and open account of pregnancy, birth and early motherhood, Ann Enright (2004) describes her experiences with disarming candour. Transition to motherhood is a rollercoaster of emotions and there are some experiences that Enright describes that strike a chord of truth for anyone who has shared them. Enright explains that she wrote the book because she thought it was important for women to know what having a baby was really like. The descriptions of amniotomy and a short stay on an antenatal ward in early labour, whilst leaking copious amounts of amniotic fluid, is something that should be part of every student midwife's reading list. In all the pages of wonderful eloquent description of early labour and establishing contractions, the midwife gets a couple of passing mentions, 'arranging things on a stand' and later when she hands over to another midwife who then runs ice cubes around Ann's belly to check the level of the epidural analgesia. Then a second midwife takes over and there is a rapport between them, perhaps because Ann feels that she has control of herself and her labour again as her epidural is working and she can see further than just the next contraction. The midwife 'Sally is lovely: sweetness itself. She is the kind of woman who is good all the way through'. Whilst she gains a name she also gains some credibility as a midwife in the eyes of other midwives. Sally catches the baby whilst the obstetrician watches, cheering like a football hooligan. After the delivery the midwife and obstetrician disappear from the text. Ann and Martin examine their new daughter with the intense observation and surprise that is only possible following the birth of a baby.

Twentieth- and 21st-century versions of the old wives' tale

Oakley's (1986) book relies on oral testimony; several women recount their mothers' stories of their own births. These have the ring of folk tales celebrating extraordinary events. However, they cannot be counted as true birth stories as they are answers given in response to a researcher's questions. Mothers' birth stories are traditionally occasioned as advice from a mother to a pregnant woman (Carter & Duriez 1986).

Pregnancy does attract comment in the form of unsolicited advice and birth stories. Not every woman is thankful for this sort of attention. Oakley (1986) includes one woman's experience of receiving just such advice. The woman explains to the interviewer how she is not going to listen to her mother or mother-in-law because they '...just describe how awful it was ... and enjoy telling you about it' (p.79). It is interesting that Oakley tells us that this particular interviewee later wonders if her mother-in-law might have been right all along.

Our own mothers' birth stories are a generation out of date. The birth stories that are told by groups of new mothers will be of births that only happened weeks or months ago. The recency of these experiences may improve the perceived reliability of these tales.

Networks of local groups, for example the National Childbirth Trust (NCT), may have taken over some of the supportive roles from the extended family. The groups provide information and, perhaps more important, a network of like-minded and experienced mothers to support new members. These groups help to perpetuate a type of female oral tradition as a source of information and support.

The equivalent of the stories exchanged by a group of friends was published as *The Fat Ladies Club* (Gardener et al 1999), the indispensable 'real-world' guide to pregnancy. The authors are a group of five women who met at NHS antenatal classes who have written their views of pregnancy and the maternity services. They poke fun at the antenatal class teachers and exercises, their own bodies, maternity bras and other things that came as a bit of a shock with their first pregnancies. The labour stories are told by each author in individual chapters. Each woman approaches labour in a different way but all omit any aspect of care delivered. There are two midwives mentioned; the first author explained that a midwife had patiently passed on messages from one grandmother-to-be who had phoned the labour ward at frequent and regular intervals. The second midwife mentioned would not allow a grandmother into a postnatal ward until the official start of visiting.

A prospective study undertaken by Green et al (1988) looked at women's expectations and experiences of childbirth. They recorded women's views and expectations at 36 weeks of pregnancy, before they had any personal experience of labour ward practice or even much experience of the hospital antenatal clinic as they had most of their antenatal care in the community (Green et al 1994). Women in several hospitals were questioned and were found to have virtually no differences with respect to what they wanted in labour but the women's expectations of the staff varied according to the expected place of delivery (Green et al 1988, 1994).

Green et al (1994) suggested that when questioned before labour, the adjectives used by women having their first baby to describe the midwife's care in labour were the same as those used by multiparous women. It would seem therefore that the primiparous women had heard on 'the mothers' grapevine' (Green et al 1994) all about the midwives and having babies, even if they hadn't attended any antenatal classes. Green et al (1994) conclude that the 'unit ethos' (p.22) exists not only as a researcher's abstraction but also in 'the local beliefs and ideas about hospitals that women pass on by word of mouth' (p.22).

It would seem that until midwives provide a service that mothers want, like and respect then the primary effect of the contemporary 'old wives' tale' is not going to enhance the midwives' reputation. It appears that it is the medicalised system of childbirth and the alien process of being hospitalised (Kent & Dalgleish 1986) that is resented and disliked by many of the women who write birth narratives.

Reading birth narratives, whether real or fictional, is like listening to a woman sharing a birth story or debriefing following childbirth. In all cases midwives can listen and learn.

As the midwife has been missing from birth narratives for decades, it is difficult to guess whether authors' perceptions of the midwife have improved. If we are to reflect upon practice then perhaps as a profession we should read factual and fictional accounts of birth. The use of birth narratives may help midwives reflect upon practice by first becoming impartial witnesses to a written scenario before being required to recall their own practice.

Midwives appear to be part of the medical system. We still (mostly) wear a uniform (Brady 1991, O'Luanaigh 1994) and we often use inappropriate language or professional jargon (Oakley 1980). There are women who do not know a midwife when they see one (Brady 1991). Is it possible that it is the uniform that is seen and only the professional jargon that is heard by labouring women? Or is it the uniform and the jargon that make us blend so successfully into the surroundings that we are not noticed?

Where have we as midwives gone wrong over the centuries to be apparently overlooked by authors? Where we have been mentioned, it is frequently with irritation or the memory of an unpleasant occurrence. But perhaps we have been getting our job right for the most part. Midwives can perform a quite unobtrusive watchful waiting role in many labours, not disturbing the women we care for, not intruding on their focus and control. Perhaps we should be glad that we are not in print more often, as so frequently when authors or mothers seem moved to add us into their birth stories, it is because we have intruded into their birth experience.

Perhaps to understand why the midwife is nigh on invisible in literature we need to look at the difference between the high-profile doctor (Kent & Dalgleish 1986) and the no-profile midwife. An essential difference between doctors and midwives may be in the apparent passivity of a midwife caring for a labouring woman. The doctor, however, may feel compelled to justify her or his presence by doing something (Arney 1982). This was most evident in American birth stories.

The only consistent thing that I have found that has defined every birth in fiction and non-fiction is the stating of the sex of the baby. As midwives we are there to share the moment, but the moment is for celebrating the birth, not the presence of a midwife.

In retrospect, was the search for the midwife in the birth narrative unrealistic? During a labour we often undertake a quiet role, watching, waiting and observing and supporting women. The lack of midwifery presence may be an indication that on the whole we do our job well, rightly enabling women to recall labour as a personal triumph.

Kirkham & Perkins (1997) suggest that reading birth narratives may help midwives 'to develop their capacity to listen to a mother's story without persistent impulses to defend practice, and perhaps give the busy midwife time to reflect and perhaps reassess care given in the past'. Midwives would do well to read a selection of birth narratives, not least to see midwifery practice in a different light.

References

Allison J 1996 Delivered at home. Chapman and Hall, London

Arney W R 1982 Power and the profession of obstetrics. University of Chicago Press, Chicago

Attallah N 1987 Women. Quartet, London

Atwood M 1996a Giving birth. In: Dancing girls. Vintage, London

Atwood M 1996b The handmaid's tale. Vintage, London

Bagnold E 1938 The squire. William Heinemann, London

Ball J 1987 Reactions to motherhood: the role of postnatal care. Cambridge University Press, Cambridge

Bohjalian C 1997 Midwives. Chatto and Windus, London

Brady M 1991 Midwives' uniforms. MIDIRS Midwifery Digest 1(1): 27–28

Byatt AS 1986 Still life. Penguin, Harmondsworth

Camp C, London C, Woods S 2000 Maternity leave. Silhouette, London

Carter J, Duriez T 1986 With child: birth through the ages. Mainstream Publishing, Edinburgh

Chekhov A 1888 The party and other stories (trans. 1985). Penguin, London

Cleveland Biographies 1999 Number 1: a Middlesbrough midwife. Cleveland Historical Biography Group, Cleveland

Coates T 1998 Impressions of the midwife in literature. RCM Journal 1(1): 21–22

Cushman K 1997 The midwife's apprentice. Macmillan, Basingstoke

Cusk R 2001 A life's work: on becoming a mother. Fourth Estate, London

Dick Read G 1942 Childbirth without fear, 2nd edn (reprinted 1958). Heinemann, London

Dickens C 1844 Martin Chuzzlewit. Penguin, Harmondsworth

Donnison J 1988 Midwives and medical men. A history of the struggle for the control of childbirth, 2nd edn. Historical Publications, Hong Kong

Drabble M 1968 The millstone. Penguin, Harmondsworth

Drabble M 1969 The waterfall. Penguin, Harmondsworth

Enright A 2004 Making babies: stumbling into motherhood. Jonathan Cape, London

Gardener H, Betteridge A, Groves S, Jones A, Lawrence L 1999 The fat ladies club. Penguin, Harmondsworth

Garfield L 1994 Moss and Blister. In: The apprentices. Mammoth, London, pp.55–80

Gibbons S 1932 Cold comfort farm (reprinted 1984). Penguin, Harmondsworth

Giedroyc M 2004 From her to maternity. Ebury Press, London

Green J 2001 Babyville. Penguin, London

Green J, Coupland V A, Kitzinger J V 1988 Great expectations: a prospective study of women's experiences of childbirth, vols 1 and 2. Centre for Family Research, Cambridge

Green J, Kitzinger J V, Coupland V A 1994 Midwives' responsibilities, medical staffing structures and women's choice in childbirth. In: Robinson S, Thomson A M (eds) Midwives research and childbirth, vol 3. Chapman and Hall, London, pp.5–29

Hansford Johnson P 1955 An impossible marriage. The Companion Book Club, London

Holden W 2005 The wives of Bath. Headline Books, London

Kent G, Dalgleish M 1986 Psychology and medical care, 2nd edn. Baillière Tindall, London

Kirkham M, Perkins E R 1997 Reflections on midwifery. Baillière Tindall, New York

Kitzinger S (ed) 1987 Giving birth: how it really feels. Gollancz, London

Kitzinger S 1991 The midwife challenge, 2nd edn. Pandora, London

Leap N, Hunter B 1993 The midwife's tale: an oral history from handy woman to professional midwife. Scarlet Press, London

Lessing D 1964 A proper marriage. Flamingo, London

Lette K 1993 Fetal attraction. Picador, Basingstoke

Limb S 1986 Love forty. Corgi, London

Llewelyn Davies M (ed) 1915 Maternity: letters from working women. Virago, London

Manby C 1997 Second prize. Hodder and Stoughton, London

McCroy M 1989 Katie Ellen takes on the world. In: Bleeding sinners. Minerva, London

Mitford N 1945 The pursuit of love. Penguin Books, Harmondsworth

Moran Laskas G 2003 The midwife's tale. Piatkus, London

Oakley A 1980 Women confined: towards a sociology of childbirth. Martin Robertson, Oxford

Oakley A 1986 From here to maternity. Penguin, Harmondsworth

O'Luanaigh P 1994 Uncovering midwives – do we need a uniform? Modern Midwife 4(7): 4

Parr D 2003 Home to Trinity. St Martin's Press, New York

Parsons T 2005 The family way. Harper Collins, London

Piercy M 1972 Small changes. Penguin, Harmondsworth

Sharp J 1671 The midwives book or the whole art of midwifery discovered (ed. Hobby E, 1999). Oxford University Press, Oxford

Sterne L 1759 The life and opinions of Tristram Shandy. Penguin, London

Syal M 1999 Life isn't all ha ha hee hee. Anchor, London

Thatcher Ulrich L 1991 A midwife's tale. The life of Martha Ballard, based on her diary 1785–1812. Vintage Books, New York

Tolstoy L 1873 Anna Karenin. Penguin, Harmondsworth

Vincent P 2002 Baby catcher: chronicles of a modern midwife. Scribner, New York

Weldon F 1980 Puffball. Flamingo, London

Woolf L 2003 Diary of a mad mother to be. Orion, London

Worboyes S 2001 Whitechapel Mary. Hodder and Stoughton, London

Worboyes S 2004 Time will tell. Hodder and Stoughton, London

Worth J 2002 Call the midwife. Merton Books, Twickenham

Yates P 1990 The fun starts here: a practical guide to the bliss of babies. Pan, London

Further reading

Atwood M 2001 The edible woman. Virago, London

de Beauvoir S The second sex. Penguin, Harmondsworth

Carter J, Duriez T 1986 With child: birth through the ages. Mainstream, Edinburgh

Chevalier T 2004 The lady and the unicorn. Harper Collins, London

Curtis P 1990 Midwifery: an historical interpretation. Working Papers in Applied Social Research (19). University of Manchester, Manchester

Department of Health 1993 Changing childbirth part 1: Report of the Expert Maternity Group. Department of Health, London

Diamant A 1997 The red tent. Wyatt Books, New York

Hamilton M 2001 Staircase of a thousand steps. Penguin Putnam, New York

Hunt S, Symonds A 1995 The social meaning of midwifery. Macmillan, Basingstoke

Inch S 1989 Birthrights: a parent's guide to modern childbirth, 2nd edn. Green Print, London

Kitzinger S 1991 The midwife challenge, 2nd edn. Pandora, London

Kohner N 1988 Having a baby. BBC Books, London

Levy A 2004 Notes from a small island. Headline, London

Llewelyn Davies M 1931 Life as we have known it. Virago, London

Mitford J 1992 The American way of birth. Gollancz, London

National Childbirth Trust 1989 Birth reports. NCT Leicester Branch

National Childbirth Trust 1990 Baby annual. Imperial Group, London

National Childbirth Trust 1995 Pregnancy plus, autumn/winter. NCT Publications, Glasgow

Noble E 2003 The reading group. Coronet Books, London

Oakley A 1986 The captured womb: a history of the medical care of pregnant women. Blackwell, Oxford

Oakley A, Houd S 1999 Helpers in childbirth: midwifery today. Hemisphere Publishing (for World Health Organisation), London

Raphael-Leff J 1991 Psychological processes of childbearing. Chapman and Hall, London

Riley M 1968 Brought to bed. Dent, London

Sherr L 1995 The psychology of pregnancy and childbirth. Blackwell, Oxford

Woolf L 2003 Diary of a mad mother to be. Orion, London

CHAPTER EIGHT

Blue Moons and Wise Hands:
Birth Knowledge and Stories of Mindful Midwifery

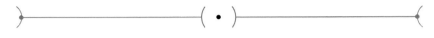

NESSA McHUGH

'Yf they saye the mone is belewe, We must believe that it is true.'

(1528 rimester)

'The body in the woman and the story in the woman are inseparable.'

(Behar 1991, p.270)

Introduction

One of my best, safest memories from my early childhood was curling up on my mother's knee, in front of the fire to 'listen with mother'. Precious time with my mum, the hectic world stood still for that brief time while we listened to the stories on the radio together. Of course, that is how my memory reconstructs those events. We probably didn't have blazing coal fires in June and my mother was probably just relieved to have a time in the day when her youngest child actually managed to sit still and fall asleep for a while. I was, of course, a true child of the 1960s, a signed-up member of the Jackanory generation. I listened to stories on the television, I listened to the chat, gossip and tall tales of my relatives at frequent family gatherings, learning of past exploits and making connections between the past and the present.

So what has any of this got to do with midwifery? The short answer would be nothing and everything. Stories give structure and meaning to information, they aid recall of events and they colour perceptions. Stories put things into a context and as such enable us to shape the meaning of the world around us. Stories can be problematic, they may contain truths – but the tale changes over time and tellers. They are not hard and factual, they contain shifting parameters of meaning and symbolism, which we may find infuriating, upsetting, reassuring, unimportant, all depending on our own sets of values, experiences and beliefs. Most important of all, stories put our senses and emotions into knowledge. They bring to life dry words and phrases, evoking images and emotions that we can recognise and relate to. Beneath every story there is a set of unspoken cultural rules and societal norms that are imparted from tellers to listeners, the means by which social and cultural norms are reinforced. Most of us are familiar with the fable of the boy who cried wolf once too often; we can understand the message explicit in the tale.

Over the past decade there has been an increasing interest in the use of story telling as a legitimate way of informing practice and gaining knowledge. We are recognising the shortcomings of relying upon purely reductionist accounts of truth, fact and meaning. There are many truths, and facts are not fixed givens but are subject to interpretation and relational fluidity. At their best, stories bring to our knowledge base the concept of *metis* or transformational intelligence. They give us the ability to connect and learn in a way that is creative and interconnective. At their worst, stories can be used to frighten and control, ensuring rigid adherence to a system or culture where words have the power to scare, frighten, dismiss, humiliate, ensure ignorance and diminish.

In many ways the story or legend of the ancient Greek goddess Metis stands as an important allegory for contemporary and future midwifery. Metis, the first consort of the ancient Greek god Zeus, was a titaness and goddess of wisdom. She was considered to be the most knowing of all beings. An oracle of Gaea told Zeus that Metis would give birth to a daughter and then to a son, and that the son would overthrow Zeus. Being the archetypal scheming god, Zeus tricked Metis into changing into a fly and promptly swallowed her to prevent the prophesy from coming true. However, Metis was already pregnant with her daughter, the goddess Athena. While still inside Zeus and coming towards the end of her pregnancy; Metis set about hammering out a beautiful helmet for her daughter to wear. Unfortunately for Zeus, this activity gave him apocalyptic headaches, which caused him to roar out in agony (I have to admit to not feeling much sympathy for him). Hephaestus, the blacksmith of the gods, decided to take a wedge to Zeus's skull and split it open, upon which the goddess Athena sprang forth fully grown (and wearing a full set of armour with a very nice helmet). No more is heard of Metis except that she was able to impart wisdom from within Zeus.

As a metaphor for takeover and control, this story clearly shows how wisdom, and especially birth wisdom, were appropriated. The ancient Greeks believed that men were solely responsible for the conception of a child and the woman's only role was to carry the fetus until it was born. Therefore Metis is not given any credit for Athena's birth, but she has become the symbol of transformational intelligence and wisdom beyond the basic premise of *logis* or logic.

The above account could be seen as a distant tale, which could be argued to have little bearing on contemporary life and contemporary midwifery in particular. However, as midwives, our knowledge base is often unrecognised; we inhabit a world where emotion is often disembodied from experience. There are many ways of knowing but few of them are recognised. Within this context I intend to explore how we use stories in our everyday lives, in our growth and our practice of mindful midwifery. Dalmiya & Alcoff (1993) write about epistemic discrimination, which is the process of defining systems of knowledge that have traditionally excluded women's beliefs and sources of knowledge. The expression 'old wives' tales' can be traced back to early midwifery knowledge that was passed on through observation and oral transmission. These early forms of knowledge were for the most part preliterate; that is, knowledge tended to be based in experience, had practical applications and was not written down but passed on orally. They stem from the time when the gossips got together and useful information was passed on alongside socially conforming and controlling information – structuring one generation to the next. This was the knowledge that was seen as subversive and dangerous because it often existed out of the control of men – in the birthing room where women's talk was viewed as a potentially dangerous thing. Kramer & Sprenger (1948, original 1486) stated that no-one does more harm to the church than midwives.

'We are assured that the gossip's bridle was a measure to prevent disorder, but
a nagging suspicion remains that even when men held all the reins of power
they were still apprehensive lest women topple them simply by the use of their
tongues.'

(Burford & Shulman 1992, p.61)

In modern Western midwifery we have large resources to draw upon. Journals and textbooks are widely available. Practice is dictated by a plethora of written guidelines, policies
and national dictates. Amidst all this array of information it is very easy to underestimate
the impact and importance of stories as a legitimate source of knowledge.

This exploratory journey will start with the stories of becoming; how we learn to be
and where we get our identity. I then intend to look at the stories that heal; those stories
that highlight how we relate with each other and with the women and families we come
into contact with. The journey then will lead onto the stories of crisis and identity;
our political stories looking at the politics of control, how others see us, and where we
place ourselves. Finally I intend to look at mindful midwifery; the stories that frame our
connected consciousness and encapsulate a way of being that we may aspire to.

Stories of becoming

Midwives pride themselves on belonging to one of the oldest professions in the world.
Through time and across many cultures, wherever babies are born there is likely to be
someone who is known as the birth attendant or midwife. The stories of becoming are
the accounts of deciding to become midwives – the experiences and inspirations that
lead to the decision to becoming a student or apprentice midwife. They are also the
stories that then shape the student or apprentice into the future midwife.

There are many different paths into midwifery across many different cultures;
sometimes the calling may be considered to be in the blood, inherited through another
family member.

'Grandmother taught Jesusita other lessons, too – patience, how to take care
of herself, and the fact that all people are different. Most important she taught
her granddaughter how to touch. "I touch the people as soft as I can, like my
grandmother showed me," says Jesusita softly, showing tribute to instructions
issued many, many years ago.'

(Perrone et al 1989, p.116)

Sometimes the call to midwifery comes in through more subconscious channels; the
traditional Mayan *comadrona* or *iyom* comes to midwifery through a supernatural calling. The future midwife receives various birth signs, omens and dreams that signify her
destiny or *mandado* (Cosminsky 1982). In Britain the decision to become a midwife is
usually based on different criteria. Between the mid 1930s and early 1990s the majority
of midwives (but not all) trained as nurses first and it was common to view midwifery
as an addition to nurse training. Now the majority of student midwives are on direct-
entry midwifery courses. For some, a personal experience of birth or a passionate desire
to work with women during a huge life-changing event may act as the trigger and take
the individual down the route of gaining the right qualifications, entering the lottery of
gaining a precious place on a course and then the pressures of constant practical skill

acquisition and academic assessment. Although the British call to midwifery may be through structured routes, the first step is always made by the aspiring midwife, who often shows a strong passion to be part of something important and special.

'I saw an advert in the feminist magazine *Spare Rib* for a VSO midwife in Peru and knew that that was what I wanted to do.'

(Allison Ewing, independent midwife, personal correspondence, 2005)

Becoming a midwife is not always the first choice that people make or else they harbour an interest that may manifest itself at a later point.

'I did not find university a very positive experience the first time and wanted to do something practical. Having applied for a number of jobs and done some voluntary work I needed to find something meaningful to do. It occurred to me out of the blue, that I wanted to be a midwife. I didn't really know much about it – but the more I found out the more I really wanted to become a midwife and look after women having babies, it remains a passion within me.'

(Research participant, 2005)

Reading accounts of different midwives' experiences of entering into midwifery gives us a global perspective of not just different cultures but also the different types of midwife. The fact that within Britain and Europe midwifery is a legislated and professionalised occupation but that elsewhere across the world this is often not the case helps us to see the politics and history of such a woman-focused profession, something that should be but is not always apparent in the everyday working lives of midwives. When we read or hear other midwives' stories of becoming, we can see many similarities and of course many differences. The similarities would appear to focus on the desire to be with women at a crucial time in their lives. This connection or ability to reflect and see ourselves as part of a wider picture is a crucial part of becoming a midwife. The understanding generated takes us outside our immediate sphere of experience and helps to expand our knowledge and understanding of both the vocation we have been called to and the context of our contemporary experience.

Learning to be: just who do you think you are?

The period of training, education or apprenticeship teaches the skills required to become a midwife but there is also another type of learning taking place. Within Britain the hidden curriculum plays an important part in teaching student midwives how to fit in and how to behave in what is a highly structured and regulated working environment.

The expectations may come from within ourselves and what we bring with us to our midwifery. If the impetus to become a midwife wells up from our own unresolved negative birthing experiences then being thrown back into a similar environment where feeling helpless as a student can trigger the memories of feeling helplessness as a mother, we can find ourselves in an unbearably painful position. I have observed that among the students I work with, there will be individuals whose experiences as mothers and as women will act as a catalyst to self healing and also as a challenge to their personal sense of self. I believe that an important part of our learning to be is to discover just who we think we are and what we went through to become that person.

Sometimes the most difficult stories to tell are our own personal narratives. Lea Gaydos (2005) observed that personal narratives are a form of autobiographical story telling that give structure to individual experiences. In opening ourselves up to others, we also lay bare our vulnerabilities, but as midwives we are often privy to the vulnerabilities and difficulties of our clients as they journey through their pregnancies and births towards parenthood. In midwifery we frequently talk about the importance of trust and working with women in partnership. Student midwives are also subject to the expectations of other students, midwives, professional groups and the clients we interact with.

> 'Our first clinical placement was on the community. The first day you walk out of the house wearing a uniform confirms that this is for real. It is surprising how wearing a uniform can make you feel part of a profession. The uniform also makes others see you as someone who knows the answers to their questions, this is a scary but nice feeling.'
>
> (Set Six Student Midwives 1998, p.13)

This process of learning to be can be at best a bumpy ride and at worst an ordeal that is so overwhelming that the only way to deal with it is to leave the profession before the conflicts become too great. The decision to leave is usually made at great individual cost, where the process of becoming a midwife becomes incompatible with personal beliefs and situations.

> 'The decision to leave the course was difficult. I had been so keen to become a midwife and had hoped that knowing I did not have to practise within the constraints of NHS hospitals when qualified would maintain my motivation. However, the whole situation was far more depressing than I ever expected.'
>
> (Westmacott 1997, p.35)

I started my own student training in 1988 and I can still clearly remember my first shift on a postnatal ward. Having completed my nurse training, I clung to the rituals that I was already familiar with – doing 'the obs', making beds and trying hard to fit in. I was amazed that seemingly healthy women were having more routine observations taken than the patients recovering from heart attacks on the medical ward I had just left. One of the midwives asked me to take a new mother upstairs to the neonatal unit, as it would be good experience for me. The woman had just given birth to her first baby who had been diagnosed with a diaphragmatic hernia and the baby was losing the fight to hold onto life. I had become accustomed to death and dying in adults but I had never seen a seriously ill baby in my life. I had no idea what a diaphragmatic hernia was and although I could hazard a guess, a guess was no basis to presume any understanding. I was terrified, I didn't know what I would see, I had never been on a neonatal unit before and I was unable to answer any of the desperate questions that this new mother was anxiously asking me. When we arrived on the neonatal unit the baby was rapidly baptised before she died in her mother's arms. I felt totally helpless, scared to say anything in case I made it worse for the mother. In the end we sat and sobbed together while she held her dead baby close to her chest. The fact that someone thought this would be a good experience for me on my first day as a student midwife still amazes me, but my socialisation to that working environment had begun.

There is a process of socialisation that has to be undergone and endured. Bosanquet (2002) writes that in order for student midwives to qualify, they have to learn their place within the NHS culture, accepting medicalised values and modifying their behaviour to fit in. Listening to students relating their practice experiences in reflection groups, it would appear that this shaping starts very early on. Student reflections are full of stories of control and often humiliation.

'I can still remember the midwives who made my life miserable when I was
a student. The awful experience of standing on labour ward after report
waiting while mentors were allocated for the shift, and praying that I wouldn't
be allocated to the bitch troll that was on the same shift as me. Then the flood
of guilty relief as some other poor student was the sacrifice for the shift and
not me!'

(Research participant, 2005)

The above account forms part of a more complex story that becomes part of an
individual's personal mythology. It remains embedded in their experiences and colours
how they are shaped as a midwife and how they in turn relate to other midwives and
students. Someone once raised the question of why midwives are so aggressive towards
their students. Maybe this should be rephrased as why some midwives are bent on
aggression towards their students. I think that perhaps Hadikin & O'Driscoll (2000, p.7)
may provide an answer when they state:

'It is a feature of the human condition that the majority of people in new
surroundings or with a new cohort first observe the accepted behaviour, dress,
mannerisms and speech patterns and hierarchy of the group whilst on the fringe
of the group. To be accepted by the group the newcomer has to quickly prove
that she understands the culture and accepts it.'

Stories of the wicked and the wise

So part of our learning to be is imbibing the culture around us and stories can serve to
reinforce this culture by the disclosure of negative learning environments and experiences.
The skill that students then have to learn is how to take hold of something negative and
use the story as a medium for courage, healing and for change. Reflection on practice is
an integral part of student development, where experiences are looked at from a number
of perspectives to see what can be learnt from the stories we have to tell.

McDrury & Alterio (2000) maintain that there are two important reasons for telling
stories about our practice experiences: firstly, to enable emotional release and secondly,
to make sense of a series of events. McDrury & Alterio go on to state that often the
strongest motivating force behind the telling of a story is the cathartic effect of releasing an affective response to a situation which the story teller has been actively involved
in. Hopefully, when a degree of catharsis is achieved the story teller should be able to
move forward and look at the story to gain insight and achieve a state of learning and
some degree of resolution. If the midwife who told the 'bitch troll' story had been able to
reflect and pull apart the story, she might have gained ways of dealing with the
situation or taken strength from other students who had had more positive experiences.
It would also have been possible to look at the underlying structures that supported an
environment that let such bullying relationships flourish. In the case of the 'bitch troll'
story, there was no opportunity to reflect but what did happen was that the student
midwives learnt a lesson of humiliation and fear. Catharsis was not achieved and the
affective response of fear and anxiety was subsequently learnt and passed on to other students. Everyone knew which were the midwives to avoid and when the student midwives
qualified they were already part of a destructive cycle.

The 'bitch troll' story is one that I recognise very clearly from my own student
experiences and would appear to be very much alive and kicking in midwifery in the

21st century. In many respects it would appear that part of the experience of being a student midwife is learning about the pecking order and just which part of that order you occupy. Begley (2002) observed that student midwives in Ireland were very much aware of the hierarchy of the hospital system. In exploring the experiences of Irish student midwives, she found that students felt that the sometimes difficult relationships they had with qualified staff were related to the hierarchical nature of the healthcare system.

As we progress towards midwife status and go through the rites of passage that are part of being a student, our stories are not just of bitch trolls and ogres. They are also of people with amazing skills and strengths, women who are awe inspiring as they give birth, midwives and other professionals who are outstanding in their enthusiasm, compassion, skill and determination.

> 'The best thing about going to ARM meetings is being inspired by the other
> midwives there, so that when I go back I feel like a bit of their wisdom might
> have rubbed off on me. You know what it's like in the coffee room – all
> bitchiness and complaining … It just drags you down after a while. I need
> my ARM fix just to keep going sometimes.'
>
> (Research participant, 2003)

When midwives talk about their experiences, whether as students or as qualified professionals, they often include accounts of people who have been a source of support, strength or inspiration. These are the stories of the people who help us to keep going, the people who inspire us to develop and change our practice. They are the stories of the women we work with and the colleagues we work alongside.

> 'I always feel blessed when I am at the birth of someone I know. These are
> for me just the best of births. They take on a whole life of their own and
> the connection between the woman, her loved ones and the midwives is very
> special. Time shifts as the birth unfurls. The change in the woman becomes
> mesmerising as she connects with her baby during labour. The ability of the
> midwives to synchronize their thoughts and actions in support and care of the
> woman is something that I have mostly seen in this context. Where the woman
> is unknown it is very rare for that connection to exist even with the most
> intuitive midwives and connected women.'
>
> (Research participant, 2004)

The ability to learn from such positive experiences shapes the knowledge base of a student and extends the skills of the midwife. Sharing these stories where connections are identified and the strength of the labouring woman is acknowledged is a critical part of reflective practice. McDrury & Alterio (2000) write that when we tell and retell stories that are significant to us, new learning can occur. This is especially true when stories are retold as in these situations the story teller makes deliberate choices about which part of the story to tell and how to tell it.

Nicky Leap (2004) clearly identifies the key people who inspired her in her growth into midwifery: the inspirational community midwives she met when she had her own babies.

> 'They exuded wisdom during my contact with them for antenatal care, during
> their daily postnatal visits to my home and later during the baby clinic visits.'
>
> (Leap 2004, p.190)

Most of the midwives and student midwives I know have someone that they consider to be a source of support and inspiration. Like a number of the student midwives I trained with, I waited with bated breath to discover which community midwife I would be placed with for part of my training. There were certain midwives that I definitely wanted to avoid; one disliked having a student so much that we went to visits in separate cars for most of the placement (which was actually a huge relief). However, there were others that I was desperate to be placed with because I knew they liked having students and they were kind to their clients. They actually listened to women and supported them – what a revelation! There were some glorious midwives on labour ward who made turning up for work pleasurable, and a couple of obstetricians who showed patience with and respect for the women who were booked there. As student midwives, we learnt very quickly who was approachable and who wasn't – developing a list of people that we could go to with any query and not be immediately belittled or humiliated. One midwife in particular was so calm and serene that when she came into a room everybody was actually considerate of each other, at least for as long as she was there.

Working with the glorious midwives means not just learning from the current experiences of the day but also listening to accounts of their previous experiences. By listening, we learn through other people's experiences as well as our own. Sitting with experienced midwives when it was quiet, with a pot of tea and talking midwifery. The pot of tea disappeared a few years ago when it was decreed that the midwives didn't look busy enough and that hot teapots were a health and safety hazard. The bitch trolls teach us to be cautious, to keep our heads down and the glorious midwives teach us how to be midwives with positive stories full of inspiring and useful information and, best of all, with attitude.

Stories that heal

'Stories are medicine. I have been taken with stories since I heard my first. They have such power; they do not require that we do, be, act anything – we need only listen. The remedies for repair or reclamation of any lost psychic drive are contained in stories. Stories engender the excitement, sadness, questions, longings, and understanding.'

(Pinkola Estés 1992, p.14)

How can telling a story heal anything? Stories are just anecdotes, little tales or subjective accounts of life's events. They are not objective purveyors of facts and sometimes the finer details can become blurred or misinterpreted.

Being able to tell your story can be part of a healing process. Telling your story means that you are voicing and framing your own experience. What is written in a set of notes will give a type of story about someone's pregnancy or birth but it is rarely written from the perspective of the woman undergoing that experience. There will be a lot of information about the pregnancy or birth but very little about how the woman felt, what her views are.

Personal reaffirmation

Being able to tell your story means you have an opportunity to reaffirm your identity and sense of who you are. When we are put under a lot of pressure or experience prolonged stress as a result of difficult events, then our sense of self can rapidly dissolve and the boundaries of our identity can become blurred. When story telling is part of a healing process, the reaffirmation of self is not just centred on the individual's perception but also on the recognition of that reaffirmation by those who are listening. The fact that someone is listening to the story teller can be perceived as a measure of worth. It brings another dimension and the recognition of worth, something that rapidly vanishes when our experiences are ignored or suppressed.

Kilty (2000), when writing about illness stories, states that the telling of the story is therapeutic for the teller, giving them an opportunity to be heard but also to hear themselves. Again, when silence and repression are part of your lived experience, the ability to frame your own words becomes a significant part of the healing process.

'Telling their story has given them the opportunity to step outside of themselves and witness who they are. This dis-identification allows new possibilities to emerge.'

(Kilty 2000, p.1)

Frank (2000) writes that stories, as acts of telling, are relationships themselves; the act of telling therefore can redirect the relationship within which the story is told. This becomes clearer when we consider the importance placed on listening skills and the impact of debriefing on the healing of traumatic experience.

'At first it was too much to say, the words hurt and got stuck in my throat like I was choking. I felt I was going to explode but I couldn't speak. Then I got words out, jumbled and all mixed up. I felt the strength of my own feelings and anger. I began to use the anger and I started to relish telling what happened to me – watching for the reactions I got as I told what had happened. Too shocking to be true? But also flashes of recognition, unspoken, but there in the eyes and faces of others. I was not alone.'

(Research participant, 2005)

Women who have been traumatised by their birth experiences feel further brutalised when their perspectives are discounted by the people in the service they assumed were going to care for them and keep them safe.

Part of the impact of hearing stories is the recognition of experiences similar to your own. The realisation that you are not the only one who has experienced something distressing or undergone difficulties can decrease feelings of isolation. Again, the sense of depersonalisation is often increased by isolation; the feeling of being the only person to whom this has happened can turn inwards on an individual and perspectives can encompass distortion of self-worth and increase perceptions of guilt. We appear to have a strong need to identify with others, perhaps demonstrated in the plethora of women's magazines which specialise in readers' 'true stories'. We need to listen to other people, read about them and through the Internet we make more connections with other people's stories than ever before. The Internet is full of websites which focus on women's experiences and stories of their births, bring women together in sharing their stories and hopefully create change through the process of strength through group activity.

Healing connections

Another dimension is the impact of a story on the people who hear it. Sometimes it is hard to hear that someone interprets your actions in a way that is completely at odds with your intention. However, sometimes that feeling of dissonance can be channelled sensitively and lead to self-growth on the part of the listener. Watson (1985) maintains that in the shared moment of connection between the client and carer, changes take place as the phenomenal fields of both interact and intersect.

When women as service users are asked back to talk to health professionals and students about their experiences, it can make for difficult listening. It can be very hard to hear how women view their experiences of the health service and the quality of support or care that they received, especially when the health professional feels that they have done their best or have provided a good service. It can also reinforce how significant small actions can be and that although we may feel too overwhelmed to make big changes, we can start making a difference in our personal practice and these actions will make a difference to the individual women that we encounter. When we hear someone else's story, we make sense of it through our own sense of perspective and that process of interpretation leaves us with the indent of someone else's experience. For better or worse, we are forever altered by it.

In 1999 the postnatal care and support subgroup of the Leicestershire Maternity Services Liaison Committee (MSLC) arranged a series of meetings with women from health service user groups representing a range of ethnic minority communities in Leicestershire. This was probably the first time that midwives, health visitors, community workers and community mental health workers had all met together with some of the women who had experienced the maternity service provision of Leicestershire. Listening to women's experiences of being pregnant, giving birth and the prejudices that they encountered was very depressing. However, listening to how both health professionals and women misinterpreted each other's actions was a revelation. The stories brought insight into how uninformed some of the maternity service providers were of the range of women's needs. Fairbairn (2002) recognises that story telling has a therapeutic value not just for individuals but also for communities, where the telling and retelling of stories of disturbing or difficult events serve as a way of remembering, coming to terms and regaining control. The stories also showed how women sometimes misinterpreted the actions and responses of some of the health professionals they met because of previous negative experiences they had with other service providers. When the different groups met and talked to each other as people rather than stereotypes, real connections could take place and understanding could start to develop.

Listening to and engaging in other people's stories is a way of developing empathic understanding, a connection to the personal rather than maintaining an emotionally safe distance. Of course, as every good (and closet) feminist knows, the personal is always political.

> 'There is a story going around our area that a midwife at one of the local units discharged a refugee woman who had nowhere to go and was made to get on a bus to go over a hundred miles to another part of the country. This poor woman was four days following a caesarean section, she had no money, no friends and no clothes for her baby. How could that midwife have been so cruel? I'm not really interested in politics but that's got to be wrong! What's happened to us that anyone would find that okay?'
>
> (Research participant, 2003)

An objective discussion of maternity provision for disadvantaged groups can sometimes bring a backlash of forgetting the majority and their needs but a story of someone's personal experience is more likely to resonate with our empathic natures – though obviously not with the midwife in the story.

Identity and crisis: political stories

'Narratives that explore certain individuals and groups self-identified by gender, race, sexuality, class or ethnicity tend to validate the tellings not only in terms of their specificity, credibility, dynamism, and the cultural or political work they perform but also in terms of how they can be seen to respond to the dominant tales of social identity and power within and against which they are produced.'

(Kreiswirth 2000, p.310)

Yoder-Wise & Kowalski (2003) state that stories serve to give us insight into our selves, our roles and visions or goals but also how these fit into the broader structures within which we function. Midwifery in the UK is in varying degrees of crisis and at the time of writing this, midwives are an endangered species. There are not enough midwives in parts of the UK to provide a safe service, let alone a quality service. The 'One Mother, One Midwife' campaign is gaining momentum in an attempt to turn the tide of maternity care. Many midwives work in environments that stifle innovation and destroy motivation; our identity is being slowly eroded and our bleakest fears are of a future of automatons, not autonomous practitioners.

'I have been a midwife for over eighteen years and during that time every single midwife who was a manager of our local labour ward had a nervous break-down. At the last unit meeting the head of midwifery actually stated that if the midwives wanted to be autonomous practitioners then they should go and be independent because we didn't want them here! Well that's probably just what she needs, if not what she wants. If I could afford to leave, I would.'

(Research participant, 2002)

When we are immersed in our own difficulties and lives, it can be hard to take a step back and regain perspective or the strength to find a different solution.

How do we maintain our sense of identity when we feel overwhelmed by crisis and it's just enough to go to work without having to do politics as well? Stories can be so powerful that they can bring about action in ways that we cannot always envisage. Ochberg (1988) believes that the stories people tell are important because they offer a window into subjective experience, but also because stories are part of the image people have of themselves. When we become political, we change the agenda and we start to create stories of empowerment and resistance. The opportunity to protect our identities as midwives is challenging but we are strengthened by the stories of resistance.

'In the tidal wave of debate about childbirth – home versus hospital, natural versus drug assisted – one vital figure, the midwife, has kept silent. But silence hides anger. Indeed some midwives have become so frustrated that they have formed themselves into a group called the Association of Radical Midwives, ARMS for short. It is not merely self interest which motivates them. Doctors, they claim, are turning childbirth into an illness which needs medical intervention unless proven otherwise. The midwives say childbirth should be a normal process until proved otherwise. They are also angry that obstetricians have taken control, leaving midwives, often as not (no) more than assistants.'

(Excerpt from a letter published in the SUNDAY TIMES, July 1977)

This represents the public starting point of the Association of Radical Midwives, something that had been brewing for some time. It could be argued that midwifery has always had a small but strong tradition of radical resistance and political grassroots activity. Midwives marched with the suffragettes and they were ready to defend their identity and women against the ongoing crises within childbirth. By meeting together and sharing experiences, knowledge and stories, the aim was to gain mutual support and bring about change.

> 'Women make up the majority of people working in the health service. It is
> crucial that we women health workers support each other. We must give each
> other the confidence to use our strengths as women, rather than becoming
> divided by the insecurity and alienation of working within a large, male
> dominated bureaucratic system.'
>
> (MacKeith et al 1979, p.4)

Looking back to the letter published in the *Sunday Times*, we might be forgiven for thinking that nothing has changed, that we are still in the same place except there are even fewer of us now than there were then. Well, without our stories of political activity and resistance then that might be the depressing conclusion. The intervening years of stories and strengthening identity have seen changes in practice. We know from listening to the stories of those midwives who have been around through all these changes that we no longer have to 'accidentally drop' the scissors to avoid episiotomies. We have the evidence base to hand, thanks to the brilliant idea of the ARM to form a research data base for midwives which went on to become MIDIRS. The Vision for Education radically changed midwifery education and while we may still struggle to have professional control over our education, we are not in immediate danger of becoming another branch of nursing (although there are still those who despair of direct-entry midwifery and hark back to the good old days – whatever they were). In the technologically driven age of laptops and the Internet, I am so impressed by the stories of midwives who were so motivated that although they feared being identified as troublemakers at first, they learnt how to set up printing presses to make a newsletter that would print birth stories and provide information for midwives.

> 'I had been a member of the ARM since I was a student but I'd never been to a
> national meeting. Midwifery Matters was a lifeline throughout the isolation of
> my training, and I still read it cover to cover when I get it. I was qualified when
> I went to my first national meeting – where I was, there was no chance of a
> local meeting – and was dead worried that I'd be a bit intimidated by all these
> right-on women – maybe it'd be a bit much, you know?
>
> At first it seemed there was a debate about who would make the tea and
> whether it was time for a cake or not. Then there was another debate about
> something else and then yet another lengthy discussion. Hell's buttocks,
> does nobody ever make a decision around here? Just as I was beginning to
> wonder why on earth I was there – although the cakes were very good –
> someone mentioned the recent case of two midwives who had been suspended
> for attending a woman for a home birth, in East Herts, I think. Well it must
> have been something in the cakes! Decisions were made, letters written and
> a list of MPs was drawn up and a plan of action including a protest march
> was organised – in less time than it had taken to decide the agenda for
> the day.'
>
> (Research participant, 2003)

The strongest political stories bring women and midwives together, but often the politics of control bring them into direct conflict with each other. Wilkins (2000) rightly identifies that the professionalisation of midwifery has placed women as mothers and women as midwives in different spheres of being. Wilkins points out that the professional paradigm, through the concepts of professional knowledge and control, subliminally encourages the midwife to see the woman as client in an object orientated way.

This ties in very clearly with the hegemony of gendered control, where the midwife is not in control and the woman has to be controlled. The object orientation is a cultural artefact that many midwives would struggle to admit to or recognise. However, the sharing of women's stories discourages objectification and helps to dismantle the professional barriers that have evolved within the current healthcare climate.

The most recent midwifery study days I attended were to update myself, but mainly to meet up with midwives and pick up new tips. What I got was my latest political story; the two days were full of useful information and sharing of ideas and some depressing accounts of the demise of midwifery in parts of the UK. In one part of England, a popular birth centre was set to close 'temporarily' – and let's face it, would it ever open again, we cynically ask ourselves? But the best story was the plan for midwives and pregnant women to stage a sit-in on the beds. At the time of writing, I don't know whether it will happen but the planning just showed how politically powerful women and midwives are together. The power of a good story and the transformational knowledge it generates should never be underestimated.

Mindful midwifery

'It is in these precious moments that we begin to see life is a timeless and eternal process of birthing. We give birth to new understandings, new hopes and dreams, heightened awareness, and new undertakings. We birth new challenges and new ways of being in the world, as well as giving birth to new life. We each come to midwife ourselves in these processes and we learn to midwife each other as we support, encourage and love those close to us.'

(Shatar 2002, p.1)

Mindful midwifery evolves through the seeds of transformational knowledge that we all carry within us. Sometimes it takes a good story to germinate those seeds. Stories have been for a long time a type of folk knowledge, usually seen as something quaint and nice to look back at, but not really the gold standard of the knowledge circuit. Davies (1999) has suggested that although women/midwives produced a body of knowledge based upon observation and experience that was transmitted via non-literary means, this knowledge was in effect confiscated once it was written down and recorded with the name of the (usually) male author attached to it.

'In the field of midwifery the confiscation of women's knowledge was evident in the way in which barber surgeons and physicians gained knowledge of childbirth first through the observations of midwives' practices, then confiscated this knowledge as their own.'

(Davies 1999, p.7)

Davidoff (1998) recognises that midwifery is undergoing a conflict between the so-called rationality of scientific procedure and the continued influence of orally transmitted knowledge in the form of stories or what was once known as old wives' tales. What the contemporary interpretation of this epistemological dichotomy within midwifery points to is the weaving of hearts and minds – the transformational knowledge that allows mindful midwifery to flourish even in the bleak places of modern maternity care where postnatal care is a telephone call away but women are unlikely to have the support of an experienced community midwife.

Maher & Souter (2002), in their study on the making of midwifery narrative, suggest that we have to allow for a combination of several sorts of narrative. It could be argued that the skilled midwife takes the different discourses and narratives of birth and creates stories of connection. A prime example of this would be where midwives have combined an ability to utilise objective knowledge, such as anatomy, and combine it with experiential knowledge to create new theories for midwifery practice. When an experienced midwife such as Jane Evans teaches ways of supporting a breech birth, she is combining her midwifery knowledge, the stories of the women she has worked with and her application of science to evolve a more accurate theory of the mechanism of breech than that currently described in the majority of midwifery and obstetric textbooks.

Ulrich (2004) recognises the rich value of stories in developing professional affective socialisation for midwives. Ulrich analysed the 'lost my hat' stories posted on the bulletin board of the Frontier School of Midwifery and Family Nursing. Tradition has it that historically, student midwives were given a hat to be placed on the heads of all babies born into the hands of nurses of the Frontier Nursing Service. At a student's first birth she gives the parents a hat and tells them the story of the frontier nursing service. To lose your hat means you have been at that crucial first birth that marks your path towards becoming a midwife. Ulrich found a number of themes emerging from the lost hat stories, not least being the importance of good preceptors and the implicit woman-centred approach to care. However, embedded deep within these stories was a huge pride in their profession, the sense of rite of passage as each student recognised the symbolism and significance of this traditional action.

Stories keep us mindful, they help us learn in ways that are connective and cooperative. The title of this chapter was chosen because I believe that a good midwife has wise hands and a strong heart but that these are rare qualities – as rare as a blue moon. However, in the process of writing this chapter I discovered that blue moons are not as rare as you would believe. A blue moon is the name for the second full moon that sometimes occurs in a calendar month and as I picked through the rich sources of stories that midwives have told me, I remembered that we are a profession of many wise hands – it's just that sometimes we need our stories to remind us.

References

Begley C M 2002 'Great fleas have little fleas': Irish student midwives' views of the hierarchy of midwifery. Journal of Advanced Nursing 38(3): 310–317

Behar R 1991 The body in the woman, the story in the woman: In: Goldstein L, Arbor A (eds) The female body: figures, styles, speculations. University of Michigan Press, Michigan

Bosanquet A 2002 'Stones can make people docile': reflections of a student midwife on how the hospital environment makes 'good girls'. MIDIRS Midwifery Digest 12(3): 301–305

Burford E J, Shulman S 1992 Of bridles and burnings: the punishment of women. Hale, London

Cosminsky S 1982 Childbirth and change: a Guatemalan study. In: MacCormack C (ed) Ethnography of fertility and birth. Academic Press, London

Dalmiya V, Alcoff L 1993 Are 'old wives tales' justified? In: Alcoff L, Potter E (eds) Feminist epistemologies. Routledge, London

Davidoff L 1998 Regarding some 'old husbands' tales': public and private in feminist history. In: Landis J B (ed) Feminism, the public and the private. Oxford University Press, Oxford

Davies D 1999 Embracing the past, understanding the present, creating the future: feminism and midwifery. New Zealand College of Midwives Journal 20: 5–10

Fairbairn G J 2002 Ethics, empathy and storytelling in professional development. Learning in Health and Social Care 1(1): 22–32

Frank A W 2000 The standpoint of storyteller. Qualitative Health Research, 10(3): 353–365

Hadikin R, O'Driscoll M 2000 The bullying culture in midwifery. Butterworth Heinemann, Oxford

Kilty S 2000 Telling the illness story. Patient's Network Magazine 5(3): 1–3

Kramer H, Sprenger J (1948; original 1486) Malleus maleficarum. Pushkin Press, London

Kreiswirth M 2000 Merely telling stories? Narrative and knowledge in human sciences. Poetics Today 21(2): 293–318

Lea Gaydos H 2005 Understanding personal narratives: an approach to practice. Journal of Advanced Nursing 49(3): 254–259

Leap N 2004 Journey to midwifery through feminism: a personal account. In: Stewart M (ed) Pregnancy, birth and maternity care: feminist perspectives. Elsevier, London

MacKeith C, Spinks J, Kirkham M, Cudby H 1979 Editorial. ARM Newsletter February: 4

Maher J M, Souter K T 2002 Midwifery work and the making of narrative. Nursing Inquiry 9(1): 37–42

McDrury J, Alterio M 2000 Achieving reflective learning using story telling pathways. Innovations in Education and Teaching International 38(1): 63–73

Ochberg R L 1988 Life stories and the psychosocial construction of careers. Journal of Personality 56: 173–204

Perrone B, Stockel H, Krueger V 1989 Medicine women, curanderas and women doctors. University of Oklahoma Press, Oklahoma

Pinkola Estés C 1992 Women who run with the wolves: contacting the power of the wild woman. Rider, London

Set Six Student Midwives 1998 Reflecting on seven months. Midwifery Matters 78: 13

Shatar K M 2002 Sacred path of midwifery. Llumina Press, Florida

Ulrich S 2004 First birth stories of student midwives: keys to professional affective socialization. Journal of Midwifery and Women's Health 49(5): 390–397

Watson J 1985 Nursing: human science and human care: a theory of nursing. Appleton Century Crofts, Norwalk, CT

Westmacott J 1997 An educational tragedy. Midwifery Matters 74: 35

Wilkins R 2000 Poor relations: the paucity of the professional paradigm. In: Kirkham M (ed) The mother–midwife relationship. Macmillan, Basingstoke

Yoder-Wise P S, Kowalski K 2003 The power of storytelling. Nursing Outlook 51(1): 37–42

CHAPTER NINE

Looking at Ourselves:
Using Theatre to Examine Structures Around Birth

) |————————————(•)————————————((

KIRSTEN BAKER

Giving birth to ourselves

There is a moment in birth – any birth – where a woman delivers something that had been a part of herself into another, outside space. This moment is often and in many cultures shared with a midwife, a presence to help her make the process of transition from one to more-than-one, and who observes the first watchful gaze of the new parents as this other-being begins to fill its own space and time.

This chapter is an exploration of some overlaps between notions of birth, notions of theatre, and the structures and praxis of both. It describes some ways in which theatre can be used to analyse and reflect on the role of the midwife, and in particular the work of Progress Theatre, who use theatre to work with midwives and their stories of clinical life. This work is based on the notion that there are some damaged and dysfunctional structures around birth, oppressive to midwives and women. The work generates some broader questions about the nature of theatre and the nature of being, and the connections and contributions these can make to one another. This is related to birth as well as to the role of midwifery, and has at its heart the notion of connectedness and the healing of fractured and divided entities.

Watching a part of oneself in its own space and time is, in essence, what theatre is. Augusto Boal, a South American dramaturge, relates the following birth parable in his book *Games for Actors and Non Actors* to describe theatre.

> *'Xua-Xua was a prehuman woman who lived contentedly with her mate,*
> *sharing all the good things in life: food, fun, sex. Over a period of time,*
> *Xua-Xua became aware that her body was changing: her belly grew, and grew:*
> *she felt it move, and one extraordinary day it moved and she moaned and*
> *the experience took her quite out of her body as she became engulfed by its*
> *sensations. Then her baby was born, and Xua-Xua knew that now she had two*
> *parts to her body. Sometimes the two rejoined as the baby attached itself to*
> *her, and even when separate they were always close. Time passed, and one day,*
> *as she slept, her mate who had observed the one-body-becoming-two from a*
> *distance, became curious. He approached the sleeping figure, and took the small*
> *child with him to wander, and to teach him to hunt and fish.*
>
> *It was some days before Xua-Xua saw the other part of her body again.*
> *When she saw him, and saw his difference, something took the place of her*
> *grief at losing part of herself. She saw that he was her and also not-her.*
> *This recognition made her look at herself: who was she? ... In this moment,*
> *theatre was discovered.'*

(paraphrased from Boal 1992)

Watching in another space and time

In this parable, Xua-Xua is drawn into observation of what she thinks of as a part of herself. She sees her child's actions and reactions, with his environment and with others, and as she watches, Xua-Xua wonders about herself. She seems to feel simultaneously close and separate from what she is watching. This quality, of watching a part of oneself, is a key element in theatre. Theatre, perhaps uniquely, can portray life in its minute-by-minute, breath-by-breath detail: people within their context. Nothing is static; there are layers of human interactions as characters, contexts and spectators collide and jostle with each other. Those watching can sometimes barely feel the separation between themselves and what they are watching; at other times the space allows for a critical distance and appraisal of what is on the stage.

The tension between this closeness and separation, and the different uses to which they can be put, has been debated for many years in writings about theatre. There are a number of mainstream traditions. Greek dramatists classically used stories to evoke grief, pity, sorrow, anger, desire; moving the audience through the feelings with the actions and through identification with the characters so they, in effect, do their emotional work as the action on stage evolves. This kind of theatre, sometimes called Aristotelian theatre after the playwright and writer Aristotle, aimed to engage people in order to generate a sense of catharsis: a feeling of release through identifying with the movements and feelings portrayed on the stage. Following the spectacle, the spectators are able to leave the theatre purged, cleansed of their own powerful and potentially destructive emotional responses.

In response to this, Bertold Brecht, a 20th-century German Marxist, saw this form of theatre as a tool of the ruling classes, designed to curtail any desire in the audience to challenge the conditions of their lives. He developed a form of theatre where identification with characters was discouraged; he wanted the audience to see aspects of life with a critical distance in order to generate a desire to act against the unjust conditions portrayed.

Augusto Boal (1992) coined a word which, in a sense, *contains* the tension between identification and separation. He describes 'spectactors' – those who are drawn into watching a scene in which they could themselves be acting – and he expands this notion by actually drawing the spectators into the scene and asking them if they would like to act out a different set of events and experiences. This is because the stories he uses are drawn from unsatisfactory and unsatisfying situations: individuals oppressed by each other and by their context.

Access to complex structures and interactions can, through theatre, be made enjoyable, safe and provocative. As *spectactors*, we can watch our own familiar environments and reactions take shape in their own space and time. This can provide a powerful trigger for the emotions that the same situations evoke in real life, whilst also maintaining the possibility of observation and analysis. Fervour for change, at an individual and collective level, can be invoked. The spectators are drawn into their own story and, seeing themselves, can live through – or perhaps change – the ending.

Theatre allows for this scrutiny and review of reality, and for rehearsal of change. It can offer a means of challenging how things are and a safe space for exploring how it could be; showing life as it is and as capable of transformation.

Progress Theatre

The work of Augusto Boal is used as a basis for the work of Progress Theatre, a midwifery theatre group who have worked with midwives in workshops across the UK since 1999. As a founder member of Progress Theatre, much of what is described below is the accumulation of my personal experience of using theatre to explore midwifery culture. This work is premised on the belief that midwives will be unable to care better for women unless we access more honestly our own processes, those processes which touch us and our relationships with them.

'Swimming in Concrete' is a show performed by Progress Theatre. It consists of a series of scenes and images which depict midwives at work. These scenes were devised by the midwives who form the theatre company and draw on their own experiences as well as that of many other midwives whose views and experiences were elicited. Within these accounts there is an enormous richness of material and of course, the stories contradict as well as overlap with one another. There are also many layers to the telling, with much being revealed as well as being stated about the experiences of midwives and student midwives in the UK.

Brenda, Sarah and Louise are characters who appear in 'Swimming in Concrete' and who are based on the midwives' tales.

Brenda is having a particularly hard day at work. It is the usual story: as coordinator on delivery suite, she is yet again desperately plugging the gaps for midwives who have phoned in sick. And the staff she has for this particular late shift are the wrong skill mix. She is finding one of them, Louise, particularly irritating; apparently she has a first-class degree but she seems to have no common sense at all. What is more, she still needs to be supernumerary – to have a preceptor to hold her hand – and is of little benefit to the unit.

Louise, meanwhile, is having trouble with a piece of equipment and gravitates towards her preceptor, Sarah, for help. She is looking after 'an induction' and the drip doesn't seem to be working. Sarah is at the desk – the legendary desk on delivery suite where many of the midwives whose faces fit seem to gravitate – and Louise dreads having to announce publicly that she can't quite manage to fix things up.

Sarah is waiting for an emergency; that is to say, she is waiting for a '28-weeker with twins' to be brought in by ambulance. She is enjoying sharing a moment at the desk with Brenda and is also enjoying sitting with Brian who is the new SHO and who, like Sarah, is on the organising committee for the staff ball. The interruption by Louise makes Sarah feel uncomfortable. She is torn between her desire to fit in, with her relatively new position at the desk, but she can also remember the feelings of isolation and embarrassment that she, like Louise, experienced when she was newly qualified.

Recognition

The characters and their stories in this and other work by Progress are deliberately heavily laden with unexplained references to aspects of maternity hospital culture. This dense familiarity allows for a close sense of identification from those who recognise themselves and their own situations in parts of the material. Midwives watch midwives and are astonished to see themselves: they laugh, gasp, cover their eyes with their hands, barely able to watch. *Watching* how they are is different to *being* how they are; suddenly all the strange rituals and jargon of everyday life seem to be just that.

This watching is complicated. The point of showing this material is not to reinforce such behaviour but to encourage people to see it as problematic. The range of reactions can be wide; in their responses and where different people identify their own sense of dissatisfaction and frustration. The reactions are, of course, a reflection of their own experiences and values. The sketching of the characters of Brenda, Sarah and Louise is also fairly minimal, allowing for each spectator to impose their own finishing touches. We are also left to imagine how each of them would relate to a woman in their care; in the scene she, who should be at the centre of care, simply does not appear. Indeed, it seems as if the staff are so embroiled in their relationships with each other and with the system of care that the woman is somewhat marginal. In fact, it may even be, for some of the characters in the scene, the labouring woman who is the cause of frustrations at work; the ward would run so much more smoothly if it weren't for her …

Using this material as a springboard, we can then unpick some of the behaviours which have been observed and recognised. The scene has been constructed around midwives' stories, after researching and listening to how they experience their clinical lives. After showing the piece to midwives, the first question we ask is whether they recognise what they have seen. For this theatre to work, recognition is important because without recognition, there can be no sense of ownership. The following story, told in *Theatre of the Oppressed* (Boal 1979), is about recognition and ownership, and flags up some important issues for learning, for theatre and for midwifery. Embedded in this is the crucial question of agency; of who is the prime agent in how this experience is developed and the structures around it are built.

As part of a literacy project in Peru, students were asked what they understood by exploitation and were given cameras to produce images which epitomised this. Some returned with pictures of government offices, landlords or the police whilst one of the children brought along a picture of a nail hammered into a wall. The first images were resonant for many as emblems of oppression. The nail, however, caused much bemusement amongst the adults but for many of the other children, it clearly reverberated strongly. The boy explained: from the age of 5 or 6, boys work in the city shining shoes, making the daily journey in from the barrios where they live. Their equipment is cumbersome and to avoid carrying it back and forth, they rent a nail on the wall of some business on which to hang their shine boxes. This rent takes a chunk out of their meagre earnings; the image, therefore, represents oppression in a direct, highly recognisable way. Boal points out that a picture of Nixon or Uncle Sam would not.

Like the nail, the characters and behaviours shown in 'Swimming in Concrete' are deeply resonant to those who find themselves caught up in this culture, whatever their level of consciousness or collusion. This *showing it how it is* can of course be tailored; Progress Theatre's show 'I Don't Know How She Got Pregnant' focuses on the maternity care of survivors of sexual abuse, for example, and highlights the midwifery care pertinent to that. Working with students, or supervisors, or those involved in different care environments may make different material pertinent as a starting point.

Theatre to explore context

Theatre, of course, portrays people in their context and we can use it to try to analyse the relationship between context and self.

The theatre of Augusto Boal is called Theatre of the Oppressed and using this with midwives is based on a premise that midwives are an oppressed group. This analysis is not simply an observation about the behaviours of individuals within this culture; it is a recognition that there are structural pressures which make such behaviour likely. Unwillingly placed on the fault line between the nurturing and the technical demands of medicalised childbirth, there is a huge strain within and around the role of midwifing. The reproduction of oppressive behaviour – for those who are oppressed are likely to turn into oppressors themselves – can even be seen as a survival mechanism, an adaptive response to tensions inherent in the construction and organisation of maternity care. It is as a result of these dysfunctional and unhealthy 'norms' that the labouring woman in 'Swimming in Concrete' has been forgotten. An important part of remembering her and of connecting with her is to enable the midwives involved to explore their own sense of alienation.

It appears that this alienation represents a crisis currently facing the profession; there is evidence that, for the many midwives who leave the profession, an inability to practise midwifery in the way they want is the most significant factor (Ball et al 2002). For many of those who stay, however, this disaffection becomes the daily reality and mechanisms of self-protection develop. These mechanisms can include a replication of the disloca-tion: a clinging on to systemic ritualisation and a parallel process of disempowering colleagues and clients. This is what the midwives who watch Brenda, Sarah and Louise are observing.

There are a number of ways in which theatre can work with this. What is important is not to use theatre to humiliate or to impose a hierarchy of correctness. This can be difficult. There are parallels here with what we offer as midwives; in working with women and by enabling each individual to draw down and work with her own experi-ences and desires, we sometimes have to consciously let go of what we think is a 'better' or 'worse' experience of birth. So it is with theatre. The *spectactors* are not empty ves-sels into which we pour our analysis and solutions. A form of theatre called 'agitprop' – agitational propaganda – which proliferated in the UK in the 1970s can sometimes be criticised for doing this. At its worst, groups of well-meaning actors devised and toured shows about the follies of the workers – their audience. The intent was to demonstrate how wrong their situation and, by implication, they were. This was theatre from the outside in and indeed, it was this sort of theatre which Augusto Boal moved away from as he began to work with the idea of the *spectactor*. His theatre troupe had initially been involved in showing landless peasants the importance of taking up arms against their oppressors, the landowners. In developing Theatre of the Oppressed, however, he was looking to find a way of using theatre from the *inside* of people's stories, so they could bring *their own* critical gaze to it. This was fundamentally different from using the theatre itself to criticise what was being portrayed.

When working with midwives, Progress Theatre uses a form of theatre which is simple, accessible and readily adaptable to a range of circumstances and environments. The starting point is a dramatic exposition of *what it is like in real life*. In other work-shop situations, the starting point could be stories midwives or student midwives tell, and a willingness to delve a little. Ideally, the sense of *what it is like* will be a shared one with the group or, at least, similarities will be identified. Then, an individual who is prepared to be a blank sheet is placed in the space. The facilitator asks what is the thing that is having the biggest impact on her, on this individual, at this moment. The spoken responses from the group can then be placed in the space and related to the central individual in a way that evokes the experience. This could equally be set up as a set of hurdles between the individual and their ideal experience. What kind of hurdles are there which impede us working as we would wish? What might a hurdle look like and how near or far from the individual is it? As each of these thoughts – hurdles, pressures, factors which affect us in any way – are suggested, they can be placed in the space. How and where they should be in the space can generate discussion and debate, ostensibly about the position of an arm or leg but on another level about the nature of what is being portrayed. In terms of the midwives' experience, and very sadly, they often select the labouring woman as one of the key pressures and she is duly placed in the 'scene'. As the implicit feelings are given an explicit and visible form, she might pull at the arm of the midwife or press down on her shoulders – the group can decide. This picture can be built and built, and a small tableau is formed. In a development of this static picture, the different components can then be given some movement or a voice; 'paperwork', for example, might bleat 'I'm still here' as she flutters about the picture. Poignantly, the midwife and the labouring woman in the structure are given the same line, often 'Help me'. Even with its fractured heart, there can be a complete aural mirroring of the midwife and the woman.

Creating a safe space

Portraying and playing with the relationships between individuals and contexts can enable a critical review and a degree of analysis of the intersection of structures and behaviour. Because of the nature of this work, people often seem to be working at quite a deep level of their own consciousness. It is often the case that when we invoke artistic expression in learning, we are inviting learners to reveal more of themselves than if we simply used didacticism.

For people to engage readily with this sort of exercise, the space within which the issues are addressed needs to feel safe. When what is being discussed is a *lack* of safety, where people are drawn to describe their experiences of feeling overpowered by what is happening around them, this can be tricky. Initially what trickles out in this sort of exercise is a reproduction of the values being described; there are unkindnesses and judgements among midwives, and between midwives and women, which take shape as the picture builds. Sometimes this passes without question but sometimes as the exercise develops people do begin to make different sorts of observations. This new sense of seeing can also enable people to take responsibility for their own behaviour. 'I can see,' said one participant in a Progress Theatre workshop, 'that I have to think about how I behave – and decide if I want to change – and not just wait for everyone else to change.'

In asking people to engage with and absorb new ways of seeing themselves and their world, they are being asked to go beyond what they already know. To leave familiar territory needs the accompaniment of an enabling and safe-making practitioner. Being alongside learners, knowing when to intervene and when to leave alone, is in some respects like being a midwife. The 'midwife-equivalent' here can be called a number of things: director, teacher, joker (this is a word Augusto Boal uses – a kind of wild card), facilitator, counsellor – and the key to the job is the maintenance of a safe space without judgement. This can be harder than it sounds, and requires trust in the process and in the individuals engaged in it to do it in the way they choose. If what people express is to be seen to have value, it is important that they are not met with a response of 'right' or 'wrong'.

Theatre: choosing our story

The choices people make and the values that guide these choices are nowhere more apparent than in their stories. Gather together any group of midwives, student midwives, new or expectant mothers and the likelihood is that they will begin to talk, to regale each other with stories about how it was when such a thing happened, what happened then and who it was who did it. Story telling is a part of life and serves an important purpose as we live and incorporate our own stories. We use stories to reveal or conceal parts of the lived experience; a translation takes place, as Nessa McHugh discusses in Chapter 8.

Sexing up: the art of spin

As part of a research project at the inception of Progress Theatre, we asked student midwives to talk about their clinical experiences. The stories they told were spellbinding. They were heard very differently by the two of us who pored over the transcripts. For Bill, not a midwife, he was astonished at the accounts of courage and assertiveness in the face of precipices of clinical risk, unresponsive colleagues and complex clinical tasks. For me, as a midwife, the hyperbole was familiar; the stories of heroism were part of a recognisable canon of student culture.

In all the stories the women for whom they were caring had virtually disappeared. They appeared fleetingly as a clinical procedure – a vaginal examination or recordings of a fetal heart – but the women themselves were not there, not present in the stories. What seemed to be revealed in these accounts was a separation of the carer and the cared for. This is a deeply uneasy polarisation, based on an intrinsically unhealthy relationship, lacking in mutuality or respect. In fact, on closer examination, it causes not one but both parties to disappear. The student midwives, although ostensibly central to the stories, described themselves too as a series of medical procedures. There was little sense of ontological engagement within their descriptions of practice. It was as if they were attempting to make themselves visible by framing their input in terms of the dominant medical model, and casting themselves as high-status players within that.

As they told their stories, however, the student midwives were living the moments in a different way. Gestures and animations filled the room, voices were raised and lowered to invoke the chosen version of what happened. In selecting and (re) presenting the material, it has been translated; material is selected, discarded and tweaked to convey what the teller chooses to reveal. When we formalise stories into pieces of theatre, the finished product is shaped by the purpose to which it will be put. From quaking in our boots as the ogre appears, to being unbearably moved at a moment of great tenderness, there is an alchemy that takes place between the story, its chosen presentation and ourselves.

Theatre can also enable us to make some choices about our own stories. In a sense this happens each time we recount something that has happened, as the student midwives were doing. They were selecting and refining how they described their experiences – and indeed how those experiences would then be framed in their memory in a way that fitted the purpose.

These choices and the potential for different meanings within stories can be mobilised to bring a further level of scrutiny to our behaviour. Starting with a seemingly straightforward reenactment of a story, for example, the action can be frozen and other meanings added in. In psychodrama this technique is used in different ways to develop this telling. This usually takes place in a therapeutic group where the story of one member – the protagonist – is central. Members of the group are allocated roles within the story and the scene is acted out. The director of the drama works with the protagonist and the scene to explore meanings and to incorporate new ways of seeing. Past and present experiences can be mobilised; these can be animated and placed within the scene using other members of the group. Careful attention to context, and to the connection between memory, body and experience, enables the director to facilitate a difficult process for the central character. Once again, the role is similar to that of a midwife: holding, intervening, enabling people to do difficult and painful things. The process can be a healing, a significant move within a process of self-actualisation. The director *midwifes* the transition.

Work at this level and with this explicitly therapeutic aim requires a strong mandate from group members. However, we have used a similar technique at an accessible and engaging level in Progress Theatre workshops, and this can be adapted to a range of circumstances. It can be a way of adding layers and exploring meaning at a number of levels. Using the starting point of a tableau, for example, or a frozen moment in a scene, spectators can be asked what they think the thoughts and feelings of the characters are. By coming into the scene – by becoming *spectactors* – and standing alongside the character for whom they speak, they can give voice to their *own* perceptions and thoughts. This can provoke much discussion about what is contained within and beneath the obvious presentation of stories and behaviours.

Reflection on and in action

Moving between being and the telling-and-showing of being is, in essence, a process of reflection. The values mobilised by this process are a construct of the *lived experience* of the individual and the *context* in which the reflective process takes place. As it is for childbearing women, the semiotics (or embedded meaning) of the space provide a powerful determinant for this mind and body incorporation. Much will depend on how much the expectations and values of the participants are held in common. In a consciously therapeutic group there are rules, rituals and expected norms; so it is with any group who share their moments, their stories.

This reflection can also become a form of theatre. Using a trigger such as the tableau described above or an enacted scene, participants can reflect actively on what they see. They can, for example, be invited to stand within the scene and give voice to what they see. They can enter into a dialogue, using other participants to reflect on different and possibly contradictory aspects. Inconsistencies, tensions, different interpretations and agendas can take shape, form and voice. Layers can be added as new participants, perhaps stopping the action with a handclap, can enter the 'scene' and add their version. Using theatre like this can mobilise feelings between the watcher and the watched; each is engaged in a form of exploration of self, of being. Sameness and difference between people and perspectives can be explored. The therapeutic enactment and reenactment of parts of one's own story can reincorporate painful and difficult parts of oneself.

Minds and bodies

What makes this different from talking is that people are engaging with their bodies as well as their minds. This is a joining together of what are usually held to be separate and polarised concepts, a separation which is particularly unhelpful in midwifery and childbearing. Not only do we learn about life in our bodies as well as our minds; we also *store* our lives in our bodies and minds. As a series of moments involving sight, sound and touch, theatre can stimulate an intensity of emotion; engaging physically with a story can evoke unforeseen responses as a body memory is dislodged. Theatre will be affected by the space and the context in which it occurs. Response at a visceral level can be unexpected, however much planning has gone into it. The enactment of a moment can connect with a lived experience which has been carefully and sometimes consciously buried away only to be reawakened in its rawness by the sight, sound and sensation of the new moment.

In this, it is like birth. Bringing an awareness of the connectedness of minds and bodies is a part of midwifery. Paradoxically, in becoming a 'professional' midwife, we can collude in a cultural fragmentation of mind and body. There is sometimes a false dichotomy between learning 'theory' and 'practice'. Within a professional model, greater value can be placed on theoretical learning compared with the acquisition of the more lowly 'skills'. Conversely, childbearing can in some models of thought be reduced to a physical event, as opposed to one where there is a complex interplay between mind, spirit and body. This is a particularly knotty issue for midwives. The polarisation can be seen as an attempt to limit the points of connection between the carer and the cared for. If we are to be fully and effectively alongside women whose physical and metaphysical experience is particularly intense, we also have to engage ourselves holistically, honestly and at many levels.

Professionalisation, as we know it, is very culturally specific; in many cultures, past and present, the midwife's status within a community is not that of a 'professional', with its connotation of being part of another, removed community. In essence, though, however *theoretically* knowledge and learning are transmitted, part of becoming professional, or adopting a new role, very often means *physical* learning. There are overt and covert questions as to how much we need to physically reproduce. In the learning of a midwifery skill, for example, as the teacher 'acts' the skill for the apprentice to begin learning, the learner picks up how to move her body appropriately. Looking at this through a theatrical paradigm, how much of the body language, the thinking and the feeling of the 'performance' needs to be absorbed by the watcher, the learner? Is the 'delivery suite bustle' a skill? Or is it simply part of the performance of the role? In learning about vaginal examinations, many of us learnt a 'technique', a clinical, de-personalised 'procedure' where lack of eye contact further dehumanises those involved. Quite apart from the debate about when or whether to 'perform' vaginal examinations, how accurately does this behaviour need to be replicated for the skill to be acquired? How much does the apprentice need to reproduce to be deemed competent?

Equally, in trying to unravel aspects of the role, we can use some of the reflective techniques discussed to separate out component parts. As well as using the tableau or frozen image idea, people can adopt or mould each other into different work postures to look at them afresh. Thoughts becoming movements or postures, and postures evoking thoughts and feelings, all of these perceptions and framings can be drawn back into an awareness of how it is for women. Giving birth is the apotheosis of connectedness of mind and body, and so it should be for midwives.

This connection – or disconnection – can work on another and very simple level. In the classroom, for example, active listening can quickly turn to passive listening in inert bodies. Skilled teachers can spot this; a simple break-up of the format of the class can reengage the learner. Turning to share with a neighbour or breaking into small groups allows several new stimuli to occur. There is change of delivery in voice and pace, and the simple act of moving the head, body and limbs can reawaken a response. This can, of course, be done consciously: whole rows of learners can be invited to stand, shake out, tap out a rhythm on their bodies before resuming their sitting-and-listening position.

Role play and the 'magic if'

Blame for the resistance to 'using drama' can often be laid at the door of role play. Much of what has been discussed here is, of course, role play: playing with roles, turning them over and over to unpick their component parts, having the freedom of play to explore roles and being. Much of what children do when they play is 'role play' but asking adults to do it is to almost guarantee toe-curling resistance. The potential to feel exposed, embarrassed and foolish is huge. The gap between the aim of the exercise and the experience of the participants can be equally vast. Done well and in safety, however, role play has the potential to offer a magical reality, where insight into one's own and others' experience can be powerful.

One of the critical questions here is who is in role, and why. 'Playing' our own roles is an important part of adopting them. It can also pull at the edges of these, and can entail a loss of certainty. In play, as Dorothy Heathcote, a leading practitioner in drama in education, explains, we can move between the world as it is and the world as it could be – the 'as if' world. Engagement in the 'as if' world, though, may also entail some loss of control; play is at the edge of where 'I am making it happen' meets 'it is happening to me' (Heathcote, cited in Johnson & O'Neill 1984).

This sense of danger can be a pit into which people's experience of role play can nose dive. The setting up of role play can often fail participants too; asking people to expose themselves can often lead to a degree of hilarity but with little insight gained. Feeling uncomfortable will almost certainly block any potential for insight and learning and behind the hilarity, there can sometimes be an undermining of any potentially serious point. Setting up scenes where midwives or women are just silly and laughable might make for a lively session, but what point is being made?

One of the keys here is to be clear about who is in role. If a midwife and a woman are meeting, for example, is the midwife 'playing' herself or pretending to be someone else? And in the 'playing' of the woman, there is potential to represent her in ways that reinforce cultural stereotypes about how women behave and are experienced by midwives. Equally the same exercise could be set up to feel with her: to empathise. Empathy – feeling with – is an essential prerequisite for actors who portray characters with detail and realism.

Konstantin Stanislavski was a Russian dramaturge who was a contemporary of the playwright Anton Chekhov. Their collaboration hinged around densely realistic texts and the development of an acting technique which reproduced very accurately and naturalistically the characters and actions of the play. Stanislavski (1937) wrote about the training that actors required to truly understand and empathise with the characters they were playing. Strange as it might seem, there is much in what he wrote which is relevant to midwifery.

One of the most important things he expected of his actors was that they should have, and be aware of, an 'emotion memory'. This consists of a detailed log of their life experiences to which they should bring a sharp and refined self-awareness. This forms an important part of the skills of an actor.

In playing a character, however, there is little likelihood that the experiences of the character and the experiences of the actor would be absolutely the same. Stanislavski introduces the idea of a 'magic if' to *apply* material from the emotion memory in ways that are relevant to the character. This 'magic if' can, in the imagination of the actor, transform the experience they have had and inform the experience of their character.

This emotion memory and the 'magic if' can also be harnessed in role play but perhaps more importantly, they can be harnessed in seeking to empathise with someone else. Using imagination to mobilise the 'magic if' ('*if* I had just walked into this room for the first time, how might it feel?') is not the same as saying 'I know exactly how you feel'. Nobody can say that. But the 'magic if' can dislodge our certainties. It can cause a moment or two of wondering what it might be like to experience a different set of circumstances. Empathy, therefore, moves beyond a professional skill ministered by one to another; it becomes a key connection between the human experiences of two people.

This can also inform how case scenarios, often used as a trigger for learning, are written. When a woman's situation is offered to students, is she silenced by the way in which she is written? Instructions such as 'what would you [the midwife] say to her?' can convey the impression that women are empty vessels waiting for professional input. Written differently, the scenario could invite the learner to think themselves into the position of another, much as Stanislavski urged his actors to do. It can provide a trigger not simply for a set of professional instructions but for putting oneself in the shoes of another. Building on this empathy, the midwife can imaginatively join with the woman in her concerns. She can also be more in touch with her own feelings and experiences rather than being a set of functions and a dispenser of information. Indeed, the feelings and experiences accessed may be of *not* knowing more than of knowing.

Theatre to help *un*know

Theatre is not an event that needs buildings or specialists or a 'how to' manual. Learning to use theatre is firstly to recognise how much of theatre we use already, and what purpose it can serve. Theatre in its broadest and most commonly owned sense can move between fragments of experience, can reunite or separate minds and bodies, can expose dissonance and give form to fractured and unarticulated experiences. It can humble rather than aggrandise, expand and pressurise certainties, implode familiarity and professional presumption.

Theatre happens every time a story teller animates their words with gestures, demonstrating how who said what to whom. As we watch and listen to each other, observing something take shape in time and space, absorbing through our bodies and our minds, theatre is born. So what is true for theatre in its traditional sense – a place of rules, rituals and expectations – is true for the interactions of individuals recounting what happened yesterday, and equally for those consciously and therapeutically engaged in their own drama.

The theatricality of ritual in religion, in healing, in teaching all aim to touch the very core of being, to enrich and deepen the experience. Theatre can be used to enhance knowing and to imbue a sense of *un*knowing. Theatre can be a way of moving beyond words into a telling and a being which incorporates the lived and stored experiences. There is also much that is shared with childbearing women.

Like other art forms, theatre can show humanity aspects of itself, evoking a pre-lingual, visceral response of recognition, joy and despair. The engagement of the senses can be a conduit to the soul.

For those of us involved in childbearing, we fragment our minds and bodies at our peril. In this sense theatre is not a physical building or a set of techniques; it is a framework we can choose to bring to ourselves and to others to enrich the experience of birth. When we are fully and openly engaged, the distinction between spectator and actor dissolves, for in life we are *spectactors*, constantly engaged in a dance of watching and acting ourselves.

References

Ball L, Curtis P, Kirkham M 2002 Why do midwives leave? Royal College of Midwives, London
Boal A 1979 Theatre of the oppressed. Pluto Press, London

Boal A 1992 Games for actors and non actors. Routledge, London

Brecht B 1978 Brecht on theatre. Methuen, London

Johnson L, O'Neill C (eds) 1984 Dorothy Heathcote: collected writings on drama and education. Hutchinson, London

Stanislavski C 1937 An actor prepares. Geoffrey Bles Publishers, London

Further reading

Itzin C 1980 Stages in the revolution. Eyre Methuen, London

Schutzman M, Cohen-Cruz J (eds) 1993 Playing Boal: theatre, therapy and activism. Routledge, London

www.simplyprogress.co.uk

CHAPTER TEN

The Rhythm of Life:
Music and Childbirth

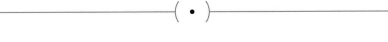

JANICE MARSH-PRELESNIK AND LORNA DAVIES

'I can only think of music as something inherent in every human being – a birthright. Music coordinates mind, body and spirit.'

(Yehudi Menuhin, 1916–99)

Introduction

Music plays a significant part in most of our lives, regardless of who we are, where we are or what we do. Music gives us pleasure, provides a distraction, helps us to concentrate, allows us to make meaning, acts as a conduit for our emotions and our spirituality, and facilitates our healing. Within a cultural and social context, music helps us, amongst other things, to create ritual, to celebrate, to commiserate, to greet, to mourn, to serenade and to create a sense of identity.

Within this chapter, we intend to explore the value of music within the sphere of maternity care from both theoretical and experiential perspectives. We will begin, however, by exploring concepts around music more generally and then apply the principles to the period around childbirth.

Before we begin, it may be useful to acknowledge that, musically speaking, we come from very different backgrounds. Janice is a classically trained musician who studied clarinet, voice and music education in college. Lorna, on the other hand, has had no formal musical training, plays no musical instruments, cannot read music but loves to sing and has what she feels to be a primal understanding of music, its power, its mystery and its therapeutic qualities. The dialogues contained within boxes throughout the chapter are the thoughts and observations of Janice as a musician and midwife. The quotes were transcribed verbatim from taped discussions that we had during the preparation of the chapter. We felt that these experiential 'asides' added a perspective of immediacy to the discourse.

Physiological benefits of music

The discipline of music therapy is gaining increasing authority within healthcare as a result of its now widely disseminated track record of success. Clinicians in the fields of oncology, paediatrics, psychiatry, care of the elderly, and some pioneering practitioners in maternity care, now extol the value of the use of music in the therapeutic context. Music therapy has provided us with a sound body of research-based knowledge that enabled the profession to catalogue the advantages of music therapy over other perhaps more invasive therapies in medicine.

Music indisputably has the power to alter our physical state of being by eliciting a physiological response, and there is a good deal of evidence to suggest that music has healing potential (Davis 1992, Fried 1990, Gaynor 1999, Hanser & Thompson 1994, Lane & Wilkins 1994, Rider 1985).

Gaynor (1999) has listed the major effects of music on a variety of physiological functions and parameters.

- Reduced anxiety
- Decrease in respiratory rates
- Lowered blood pressure
- Reduced heart rate
- Increased immune cell messengers
- Lower levels of catecholamines
- Boost in natural opiates

Emoto (2004) uses a unique approach in order to demonstrate how music affects the physical state. Using high-speed photography, Dr Emoto discovered that frozen water crystals exposed to gentle words and soothing music changed into lovely symmetrical, colourful crystals. In contrast, water crystals that were exposed to negative words and angry music became asymmetrical, chaotic and dull. When we consider that our bodies are composed of approximately 70% water (Meyerowitz 2001), it logically follows that the music we sing, play through an instrument or listen to does change the frequency within us. If music has the ability to alter the arrangement of water molecules, then it has the ability to alter our physical state because it can transmute the arrangement of the fluid that bathes every cell of our body. This theory has astonishing implications because it means, to all intents and purposes, that we can choose whether we want our lifeblood – water – to be beautiful or chaotic.

In his book The Hidden Messages of Water, Dr Emoto writes:

'The music from various cultures of the world has similarly various rhythms and melodies. Water captures these characteristics and reveals them to us through crystals.'

(Emoto 2004, p.112)

This groundbreaking text contains many photographs of water crystals that have been exposed to various types of music. Each photo appears to take on its own life and does indeed seem to represent, through its shape, the type of music it was exposed to, at an emotional level.

Metaphysical benefits of music

Emoto's experiments may be seen as rather esoteric in some scientific circles but others firmly believe that they may prove to be the best demonstration that we have about how the physical effect of music can move us into the realm of the metaphysical.

Sounds and vibrations are all around us and in us, and are the essence of the human soul and of all life. Music is an expression of emotion and in the words of philosopher Suzanne Langer, 'Music sounds the way feelings feel' (Langer 1942, p.6).

Music wakens the soul life, the emotional and intuitive life within a person. Music bypasses the cortical or thinking part of the brain, moving directly to the limbic brain which is the emotional brain centre. While actively engaged with sound, whether listening, singing, drumming or playing an instrument, that person enters into the creative, intuitive realm of their inner being.

Music and being

Music therapy is probably the discipline that is best able to shed light on the complexity of the association between the physical and metaphysical properties of music. It also provides a language that verbalises the holistic value of music.

In his book *Music and Therapy in Healthcare*, Gary Andsell writes:

'We make and experience music because we have bodies which have pulses and tone, tensions and resolutions, phrasing of actions, bursts of intensity, repetitions and developments. Music gives us, in short, access to a whole world of experience, bodily, emotionally, intellectually and socially.'

(Andsell 1995, p.8)

To paraphrase Andsell, music is part of the fabric of our very being and we cannot look at the impact on our physiology without considering the emotional, social and, we would include, spiritual elements of being and vice versa.

During a discussion in the presence of 13-year-old Helen some years ago, we were commenting on how compartmentalised the national curriculum made learning and teaching and commending the value of a more integrated approach to curriculum development. Helen suddenly interjected by commenting that you had to look at the individual subjects in order to make sense of them. 'Take music,' she said 'You can't read music in a mathematical way, although rhythms can be phrased in numbers 1-2-3 1-2-3, and music can't be seen scientifically, the only scientific thing is where the note strikes the air and travels as sound waves until it hits the ear.' The 13-year-old logic had shot itself in the foot, by articulating the individual subject components that construct music in a physical sense. Although music can be broken down into scientific, mathematical and biological function, it is, as we have already ascertained, so much more than that.

It would be a pointless exercise looking at the subject of music in a fragmented way without first acknowledging the all-embracing quality of music that touches the physical, emotional, cognitive, social and spiritual cores of our very being, our humanity. When we consider the words and phrases that we use to describe our physiology – rhythms of speech, tone of voice, circadian rhythms, beating heart, pulsing veins, muscle tone and so on – we are music personified (Andsell 1995).

Speech as a musical origin

One linguistic school of theory believes that music is a fundamental part of our psyche because in the rudimentary stages of verbal communication, we used song rather than speech.

'Our language has more in common with the singing and calling of birds, than with the vocal signals of apes.'

(Aitchison, 1997)

This school of theory hypothesises that language is musical in origin and that our ancestors learned to communicate by using vocalisations based on song rather than speech (Vaneechoutte & Skoyles 1998). Tomatis (in Whitwell 2005), a French linguist, pointed out that songbirds hatched by silent foster mothers never learn to sing. Likewise, babies born of deaf mothers appear to miss the important first lessons in language development. There are still tribes in evidence who do use a song-based language with which to communicate (Vaneechoutte & Skoyles 1998). There are also a number of studies that strongly indicate that children actually learn language this way by utilising a melody-based recognition of intonation, pitch and melody sequencing and phrasing (Sansavini et al 1997). This theory will be revisited later in the chapter and will be examined more specifically in relation to the maternal–child relationship in the early days, weeks and months following birth.

Music in the childbearing period

Music has a specific significance in the domain of birth. In cultures across the globe, women connect with their unborn child with the help of music. In New Zealand, a female choir traditionally charts the progress of the pregnancy of Maori women in song. The Galla of Ethiopia are expected to choose an accomplished singer to act as one of their birth companions (Kitzinger 2000). In Western antenatal exercise classes, women are encouraged to use rhythm to help them to cope with the demands of labour. In childbirth education, they are asked to consider their choice of music for birth. Physiotherapists advise pregnant clients to relax to music in order to connect with their baby and to rest. In societies as far apart as Afghanistan and Zaire, babies are welcomed into the world with song, ululation and instrumental music. In many cultures, lullabies, a seemingly universal phenomenon, have been sung to babies since time immemorial.

It is not altogether straightforward to assemble the manifold uses and, one would presume therefore, the benefits of music during this important rite of passage in our lives. Although there are many studies into very specific areas of benefit, such as neurological benefit in the preterm neonate or the value of music in relieving pain, the information is fragmented and usually 'borrowed' from other fields. What we hope to do is to build up a holistic perspective on the use of music during pregnancy, birth and the postpartum period.

Antenatal benefits

Fetal hearing

Let us for a moment stop to consider what the world of the unborn must be like. Although it is known that the fetus can open his or her eyes from 24 weeks' gestation and can probably therefore distinguish daytime from night, the world of the uterus is likely to be a shadowy place with limited exposure to vision. The primary sensory response of the fetus is therefore auditory.

We know that the ability to hear develops in the fetus at a much earlier stage of gestation than we previously credited and the brain is learning to hear speech from long before birth. In the work carried out by Shahidullah & Hepper (1992), as early as 20 weeks, when a broadband stimuli was changed from a single sound to a series of 2-second pulses, an increased number of fetal movements was observed. Equally, the unborn baby is responsive to music long before birth. It is believed that the fetus perceives the human voice as a melodic medium (Vaneechoutte & Skoyles 1998) and therefore the most frequent external sounds that are heard in utero are quite literally music to the ears of the unborn.

It has been hypothesised that musicality is structured by an ensemble of protorhythms of biological inheritance (Friedman 1993). The sounds that are most prominent to the developing fetus are internal in origin. What the baby is primarily subjected to in utero are sounds such as its mother's heartbeat, her gurgling digestive system and the flow of blood through arteries. Friedman (1993) further speculates that this prenatal exposure may explain some universally significant cross-cultural musical features that are comparable to the rhythmic elements in utero such as the maternal heart beat. Is this the reason why we find the sound of a rhythmical drum beat so compelling? Perhaps this phenomenon could explain the human affinity with the sound of water, which offers many of us inexplicable comfort. Could this be a primal response relating to time spent within the safety and warmth of amniotic fluid? The current trend for companies to provide employees with a 'meditation room' enshrines this theory by offering a safe, quiet, darkened room complete with the sounds of water. Add the beat of a human heart and perhaps meditation 'womb' would be a more fitting description!

We know that the uterus acts as an acoustic filter that introduces the fetus to sounds that represent the outside world. Fifer & Moon (1994) claim that the most prominent of these is the voice of the mother. Although the voice of the father is clearly recognised by many newborn babies, the mother's voice communicated either by speech or song stimulates greater recognition because it is transferred to the uterus via bone conduction internally and by airborne sound waves. The father's voice is known only by the airwave resonance (Fifer & Moon 1994). It may be useful to explain this to parents-to-be during pregnancy and suggest that if the father wants to speak to the baby, the closer he gets to the mother's abdomen, the more likely the baby is to become familiar with his voice which may lead to more immediate recognition of the father's voice after birth.

Studies which have played specific selections of music in the presence of pregnant women have demonstrated unequivocally that very young babies recognise and respond to music that they heard in utero. Hepper (1991) studied the effect of prenatal music exposure on infants of 2–4 days, using a television soap opera that their mothers had watched during pregnancy. The TV learning group experienced a decrease in heart rate and movements and a change to a more alert state while listening to the same melody 2–4 days following birth. No reaction was observed in the control group of mothers who had not watched the programme. The rapt attention observed led the researcher to conclude that the babies had a long-term memory of exposure to sound in utero.

In 1977, Clements (cited in Whitwell 2005) discovered that the fetus of 4–5 months' gestation appeared to be soothed by Vivaldi and Mozart, but was disturbed by loud passages from Beethoven and rock music. Likewise, Federico & Whitwell (2001) list a number of types of music which they would not recommend during pregnancy. These include rock, opera and jazz. They claim that the loud sounds of rock and drama of opera may disturb babies and cite anecdotal evidence of mothers having to leave rock and opera concerts because the noise appeared to disturb the baby. Jazz, they say, is not advisable because of the rhythmic displacements known as syncopation.

It would appear that the unborn child shows a preference for slow music that bears a resemblance to a normal adult heart rate, as does the classical lullaby, and that as early as 4 months into development, they prefer consonance to dissonance (Zentner & Kagan 1998).

Interestingly, a recent research study carried out in New Zealand claimed that trying to stimulate the fetus with music during pregnancy was actually a waste of time because human babies and other animals are locked in a deep sleep until they are born and gain little from such experiences (Mellor 2005). The research conflicts with the current idea that fetuses become sentient and conscious while still in utero.

The research on which physiologist Mellor based his findings was carried out on animals, mainly sheep, because it would have been unacceptable and too risky to experiment on humans. He pointed out that similar experiments on goat, horse, cattle and monkey fetuses have produced much the same results, suggesting it is a feature of all mammalian pregnancies that fetuses stay deeply unconscious until after they are born.

When this information was shared on the UK Midwifery List (a bulletin board for midwives and mothers: http://health.groups.yahoo.com/group/ukmidwifery/) many of the correspondents responded indignantly, countering such claims with stories of their experiences of the effects of using music during pregnancy on their own babies.

Mellor is writing a second paper about sentience and consciousness in the human fetus, which we await with interest.

Relaxation

'Music alone has been shown to diminish stress-induced increases in stress hormones.'

(Spintage & Droh 1987, p.88)

Box 10.2

When I was at college and pregnant with my first baby, I was a music major, studying voice and clarinet. I was working on a specific vocal piece and my baby from about 7 months on kicked strongly whenever I sang a high F. When I realised this, it became a fun game that she and I played. For the remaining $2\frac{1}{2}$ months, whenever I would sing a high F she would kick. I thought that it probably resonated in her body, maybe tickled her or maybe she kicked because she thought 'that really sucks' because I wasn't really any good! This time really added to our relationship. When she was born, maybe within the first hour or so, I had to see how she reacted when I sang that tone. When I sang the F there was no reaction, so I sang some other notes and it was the C below the high F that was the one that she reacted to. She shivered and started kicking and squirming. Twenty years later, my daughter was also a vocal major in college. She came home one day and said 'I've started this new song and it seems as though I already know it'. It was that song. It was the same song I had worked on when I was pregnant with her. I told her, 'Of course you know it. That's the song that I was working on when I was pregnant'. It was a song that every vocal major learns. I hadn't heard that song since she was born. I just put it out of my life.

This story is just so amazing to me. Why did her preference for the F change to the C? Well, my thinking is that the amniotic fluid muffled the sound, so that the pitch didn't change but the water may have changed the overtones. An example would be how sound changes when you have your head underwater.

We know, at an emotional level, that music can lift us up and invigorate us but also can leave us sad and contemplative. This emotional response will be reflected in our physical state and as we have already established, we know that music can have a profound effect on the body's systems by increasing or decreasing heart rate, blood pressure and ventilation. Who can say what effect music has on the neurohormonal state of a pregnant woman and how that may affect her mood and state of being and, consequently, what effect this may have on her developing baby? In a musical environment imbued with such qualities as beauty, calm and joy, the endorphin levels of the mother are more likely to increase and affect her baby positively.

In an article called 'Using Music in Childbirth', Caryl Ann Browning, a music therapist and doula, discusses a study in which the effect of using music for relaxation in pregnancy and subsequently during labour was monitored (Browning 2000). She stresses that the choice of music should be identified and used for relaxation purposes during pregnancy, in preparation for use in labour. The mother should be the guide, but she does identify that certain types of music are more anxiolytic (which means reducing levels of anxiety) and the mother may appreciate some advice based on the experience of other women.

Federico & Whitwell (2001) claim to have created a technique known as Relaxation Through Movement (RTM), which they describe as the awareness of hearing music and reflecting the music in the air by moving the arms. RTM is an attempt to achieve an active musical meditation directed towards the different sensations within the uterus. They separate the pregnancy into three sections:

Box 10.3

When vibrations of different wavelengths meet one another, they begin to resonate together, which is called entrainment. Basically one vibration goes through another and soon they have the same wavelength. Entrainment of vibrations also happens in our bodies. That is why it is very important prenatally to be really careful about what is coming into your body and what you are letting yourself be bombarded with, not only music but any kind of sound. Sounds like yelling affect our make-up. They change the energy of the body and how it is moving. The goal is for the energy circuits and meridians to be free flowing like an electrical circuit; you don't want a kink in it. Fear puts a kink in it, which is often why when people have stress in their neck and they hold tension there, it blocks vibrations or energy from moving through. It's like a kink in a hose; you turn the water on and the water won't get through. The energy of the water is still moving but it is really chaotic and what is moving forward has to move back. Then if you let the kink out, the water rushes forward. This is how I visualise energy moving through the body. How that relates to pregnancy is that it is one of the most important times, and why primitive cultures wanted to protect their pregnant women from being scared or nervous. I believe that they intuitively knew that connection. I believe that it is hard in Western culture to avoid being bombarded by unwanted energy; we harden ourselves to it, just so we can survive. As a midwife, I recommend to women that they shield themselves as much as possible, and explain why it is important. It is important for pregnant women to pay attention to how different sounds and words affect their whole body. One of the partner's jobs is to protect the woman from noise pollution, sounds or music that adversely affect her.

- conception to $4\frac{1}{2}$ months
- $4\frac{1}{2}$–7 months
- seventh month to birth.

Each section has its own specific themes, with music that corresponds with the ongoing transformation of mother and fetus, according to the therapists. As the gestation increases, the intensity of the delivery of the music concurrently increases. The music of preference is that produced by string instruments because it has good conduction qualities that may be transmitted more effectively by the amniotic fluid.

In the first period, the activity is designed to focus on bonding and establishing a connection with the growing baby, exploring the qualities of beauty, love and creativity.

In the second period, the intention is to enhance awareness and to encourage the mother to believe in her ability to give birth successfully.

The connection of mind, body and emotion is a continuing theme but one that features most strongly in the final period before birth. The researchers stress that the purpose of the exercise is not to elicit a fetal response but simply to provide a pleasant experience for the baby by means of the mother's response.

Interestingly, the exercises are specifically used to bring about an understanding that relaxation is not achieved through passive conditioning but is rather active and self-initiated. It can also be used in any number of positions, which makes it a valuable tool for discussing the use of mobility and positions in labour.

If using guided imagery for relaxation in prenatal sessions, the selection of music to support the imagery used should not detract from the spoken word by causing a sensory overload or cognitive shift.

Chanting

Chanting is a powerful tool for relieving stress, clearing the mind, healing and bringing us to our innermost selves. Chanting also brings the environment into sacred space or can invite celebration.

Chants are most often simple melodies with very few lyrics. The words will suggest a feeling or desire and the melodies are kept short. While singing, the whole chant is repeated several times. With repetition, the chant becomes more powerful and the desired meaning is felt at a deeper level each time it is sung. Often chants will start

---

Box 10.4

When I visit with women prenatally, I ask if there are any fears that need to be addressed. We talk about ways to cope with fear. I like to mention that music in the form of chanting can assist in turning fear into trust. I have encouraged women to write their own chant. A chant is just a repetitious little song, a few words with a short melody that is repetitious. The whole idea is about positive affirmations and for some people who are sound orientated, chanting can really help integrate that affirmation into their whole body. For instance, a woman may express that she is afraid of her perineum stretching. She may want to repeat 'I am not afraid. I will stretch and open'. She could add a melody to those words and just keep singing it over and over again. This may sound simple but repetition is powerful.

out soft, with increasing dynamics. The rising volume and repetition invoke the deeper meaning of the chant.

The beat of many chants echoes with a human heart beat. Drumming while chanting is common and really helps to sustain the energy of the chant.

'Drumming is said to be most effective for inducing trance states when the beat is synchronized at a frequency of between four and seven impulses per second. This is the same frequency as theta waves in the brain, the wavelength associated with dreams and visionary states.'

(Marks 1993, p.vii)

Perhaps we could suggest to antenatal educators that they discard the doll and pelvis and invest in a collection of drums instead.

Singing

'Singing is the first of all, the inner dance of our breath, of the soul.'

(Yehudi Menuhin)

There is little evidence to suggest why, as a species, we are able to sing. Some theorists believe that song capacity evolved as a means to establish and maintain pair and group bonding. There are other groups of mammals who share the ability to sing, such as whales and porpoises, wolves and gibbons, in whom it would appear that song was naturally selected for its capacities for reinforcing social bonds. Anthropologists find song also has this function amongst all human societies (Vaneechoutte & Skoyles 1998).

In the 1970s Michel Odent put the small French town of Pithiviers on the childbirth map when the hospital where he practised was under the microscope for its revolutionary use of water for birth. The water birth went on to gain fairly mainstream recognition and many Western hospital units now boast the offer of a pool for labour and birth. Pithiviers was pioneering for another feature which has not received the same international interest or acclaim of water birth: that is, community singing (Kitzinger 2000).

In Pithiviers one evening every week, a community of expectant parents, midwives, obstetricians, assistants, domestics, in fact anyone who had any association with the centre, would gather around a grand piano in a community singing session. The idea behind the gathering was that singing would bring those involved together in a social capacity but also that there were physiological benefits to singers, and significantly the unborn babies who attended. In an article authored in 2000, Sheila Kitzinger questioned why the water births pioneered at Pithiviers went on to gain mainstream acceptance whereas the communal singing was not notably translated into the culture of Western maternity care. She concluded that the social system in modern healthcare would not tolerate a communal activity like the singing carried out in Pithiviers, because it would blur the boundaries between staff

---

Box 10.5

It is wonderful when a mother is inclined to sing the same lullaby to her baby during pregnancy and after birth. If you pay close attention, you can see how the baby responds. It is as if the baby melts into a deeper consciousness. I often see a curious look on babies' faces when they hear their mother sing to them, especially a song they already know. It is comforting to hear a lullaby not only for the baby but for the mother as well.

and patients and disturb those who relied on a rigid social system to define their position and role and to maintain order in a hierarchically based institution.

Providing singing for parents is another way of encouraging them to engage in an activity that Odent (1999) claims enhances placental perfusion and maximises oxygen saturation levels in participants, leading to optimal growth and development conditions for the growing baby.

A starting point could be the teaching of lullabies and nursery rhymes to couples in the antenatal period. The lullaby is a fascinating, almost universal phenomenon which has a beat that mirrors that of the normal human heart rate. However, anecdotally at least, it would seem that in Western industrialised society, we are in danger of losing the tradition of singing to babies. Young parents do not appear to know the words and tunes that are traditionally associated with infanthood and although lullabies and nursery rhymes can be purchased on CDs or acquired as the musical component of a toy, the act of holding, rocking and singing to a baby is so much more than an auditory experience.

'When a mother sings to her baby a lullaby, she is not only sheltering him and providing for his safety and transmitting her love, she is also conveying to him what we human beings cherish as most essential: Our folklore, race, warmth, word, gesture, purity, silences, essences, sense of time and space, song, rhythm, gesture and our body's touch. As well as the beginning of education, the basis of our moral and ethical principles, the very essence of our life. We are strengthening an eternal link. We are transmitting feelings that have passed from one generation to another. We are transmitting the history of our humanity and we are not even aware of it.'

(Federico & Whitwell 2001, p.310)

Music in high-risk pregnancies

There are studies that suggest that music has a specific role where pregnancy may be complicated with obstetric or medical conditions. Sidorenko (2000) claims that a method known as Medical Resonance Therapy-Music was effective in reducing the number of preterm births in the cohort observed, and additionally that it had a value in preparing women for caesarean section. It was seen to provide a powerful antistress effect which led to a reduced need for analgesia. From anecdotal evidence, using music for relaxation prior to an elective section and during the administration of epidural and spinal anaesthesia would seem to be beneficial. Another study carried out by Goroszeniuk & Morgan in 1984 identified 126 women who were offered the chance to listen to music during a caesarean section and the researchers drew similar conclusions to Sidoronko (2000). Perhaps we should be encouraging women to choose the music that they would like to have played during caesarean section rather than it being left to the choice of the obstetricians and anaesthetists!

It may well be that women with complicated pregnancies, labours and postnatal experiences may benefit greatly from the use of music as a healing modality and this would certainly appear to be an area where further research would be useful.

Music in labour

Women are often encouraged by midwives and others to produce a tape of recorded music of their preference to use whilst in labour. It is generally suggested that they

> **Box 10.6**
>
> When I drive to a birth, I am so adrenaline rushed that music is the only thing that can help me adjust and calm down. And so I sing a lot ... I usually sing all the way to a birth. I have my own favourite little chants and songs that help me stay really focused. Singing helps my body stay calm because I often feel that my intuitive self and my body are really separate. My body goes berserk with so much adrenaline pumping through me so I use music as a sedative. And on the way home from a birth, I use music to keep myself awake. Sometimes when I am at a birth and things don't seem clear to me and I do not know what to think, I sit and sing or chant. Singing aloud or in my mind really helps keep me focused so that I can stay in my intuitive self. It is important for me as a midwife to stay in the deeper intuitive part of myself. When I am fearful or need focus, music, chanting and singing will help me stay in that much-needed space.

choose music that makes them feel relaxed and which may help to create a sense of familiarity if they have chosen to birth in a hospital setting. It is also believed that music may facilitate the gate control theory of pain control to help them to cope with the demands of pain which may be experienced during labour.

Music and pain

Melzack (1993), who has carried out extensive work on establishing levels and perceptions of pain, states that 60% of primiparous women and 40% of multiparous women experience severe pain in labour. We know that pain is a subjective phenomenon and that many variables may feed into an individual's perception of pain. However, there is evidence to suggest that fear of pain is now the major consideration of women in Western industrialised society who are approaching labour and birth, and we equally know that this fear can affect both the experience and outcome. Over half a century ago, Grantly Dick-Read authored the seminal text *Childbirth Without Fear* (Dick-Read 1960), in which he espoused the theory that fear increases tension, leading to a further increase in pain and the establishment of the fear–tension–pain cycle. All analgesics carry some degree of risk and affect the physiology of birth to a lesser or greater extent. Therefore, if a non-pharmacological modality can be used to negate the effects of perceived pain to some extent during labour, then it has to be given serious consideration.

The physiology of the auditory pathway and its interconnections with nuclei known to be involved in pain inhibition suggest that auditory stimuli may contribute to pain relief (Barabin 2002). Additionally, we have already discussed that the use of music may result in a sedative effect when utilised as a component of relaxation.

> **Box 10.7**
>
> A lot of the recorded music that I have heard women listen to in labour is New Age music. This music often does not have a rhythmic pattern. Instead of a beat, the music has an ethereal, sort of floaty feeling. I can see how having music with a really strong beat, especially a quick rhythm, could really take a woman out of that internal space where she needs to be in labour.

Box 10.8

The elements of music are rhythm, melody and harmony. One reason why I enjoy birth is because it is a lot like music. I like the rhythms of labour and the sounds of birth. I always find it interesting to see the pattern of how women labour and how sometimes a labour is like a waltz of 3/4 with one strong contraction and two shorter ones … The process, of course, is very individual and not like what you read in books. Or the rhythm of labour can be boom, boom, fast and furious, 1–2 1–2. Or it can seem to be without a pattern but there is one. Like Lloyd Webber's occasional 5/4 and 7/8 bars. So there is the rhythm aspect. I wouldn't say that every labour has an accent, like the first beat of each measure has an accent. Sometimes it does but sometimes it is more like the feel of it, you know, the feel of 123 123 123 or 12 12 or 1234 1234 or 123456 123456. Then there is the syncopated: **boom** boom boom **boom** boom: **one** and two **and** one and two and …Then there is the rhythm of the breath too and that really ebbs and flows and hopefully the midwife realises that the rhythm is moving forward but if it seems to get stuck, then the midwife can give the woman ideas to keep it going.

In 2003, Phumdoung & Good published a paper in the journal *Pain Management Nursing*, which reported the findings of a randomised controlled study which set out to ascertain whether music did actually act in a therapeutic manner in labour to help to reduce levels of pain. They found Western music without lyrics, with a slow beat of 60–80 beats per minute (normal heart rate), with no strong rhythms or percussion and sustained tones, to be the type of music that women most frequently demonstrated a preference for. The authors believed that the sedative effect of such music helped the women to relax and distract them from increasing levels of pain. They concluded that music acted as a mild to moderate strength intervention that consistently provided significant relief of severe pain across 3 hours of labour and delayed the increase of affective pain for 1 hour. This study was carried out in Thailand where serious attempts to find alternative methods of pain relief are being sought because of the expense of pharmacological drugs and the costs resulting from less than positive outcomes associated with the use of epidural anaesthesia, opiates, etc. It is possible that the cultural complexities relating to issues like pain perception could invalidate this study in terms of transferability. However, several other studies concur with the findings of Phumdoung & Good, including Clarke et al (1981) and Hanser et al (1983). It would appear that there is still considerable scope for further research relating to this interesting concept.

Both rhythmical sound and movement can be very soothing and therapeutic. When a small child falls over, the mother will often 'rub it better' with a massaging rhythmical action which will frequently be accompanied by a chant such as 'there, there, there'. Moaning when in physical or emotional pain may help to bring us relief in adulthood. So it is really not surprising that woman make rhythmical sounds during labour and birth. According to W Ernest Freud (cited in Whitwell 2005), 'rhythm itself provides a most reassuring "cradle" because of its promise of repetition and continuity'.

Toning

Toning, a method that has its basis in ancient religions, has recently enjoyed a renaissance in some European countries, where women and their partners are taught the principles in the antenatal period. The technique encourages the woman to focus and relax in labour by using extended breath and sound on one tone while chanting. It includes simple melodies contained within a small range of pitches, with no meter (Federico & Whitwell 2001). If we can imagine pain as a vibration that is not able to move, then a 'toning' note may converge with the stagnant vibration of pain and resonate with it, forming an entrainment, which is a process in physics whereby two objects vibrating at similar frequencies will tend to cause mutual sympathetic resonance. By continuing to use the same note, the congestion is broken down, enabling the flow of energy to continue throughout the body, thereby releasing the pressure of pain.

The Austrian birth video *Die Kraft in Mir* (Inner Strength) demonstrates the use of the method for some of the women who gave birth at a birth centre in Vienna. The women using the method, and sometimes their partners, start by making a really low sound. They do not use scales but the sound does escalate. The partners make a sound that is about a third above or below or an octave below, which seems to complement the sound that the woman is making and appears to help her to remain focused and able to cope throughout the contractions. We know that making a noise in labour stimulates endorphin production, which helps with pain relief. We do not advocate out-of-control screaming but a purposeful rhythmical chanting, such as that used in toning, may be an effective form of pain relief for some women.

The technique could be very useful because it gives women permission to make a noise whereas without such permission, they may feel inhibited, especially in cultures where the making of noise is looked upon as unacceptable or as a waste of energy. As midwives, how often have we heard women advised to contain their noise because it will strain their vocal cords, make them tired or frighten other women? It may be useful for midwives to be aware of the value of toning and other vocal coping mechanisms that women may adopt during labour, and to perhaps explore and even practise vocalisation in antenatal education. In *Birthing from Within* (England & Horowitz 1998), an exercise called Coyote Circle demonstrates how it is possible to introduce the art

---

Box 10.9

Several years ago I was the midwife for a woman who was having her second baby. She was from Africa. Her tribe had shunned her because she made a lot of noise during labour. She was forced to leave. She was so sad when she told me her story, that her own mother would reject her. But her mother didn't want to, it was just that that was what the rules were. With this baby, she was so worried that we were going to feel that way about her, so every prenatal we kept saying 'It's OK. We don't care if you are loud or what you say. You just do whatever you need to do to birth your baby'. Well, when she was in labour it would have been great to tape-record it; her vocalisations were beautiful and powerful to me. I don't know what she was saying because it was in her own language but she was chanting in this really low, deep voice while stomping her foot rhythmically. There was an amazing beat in her body and she was stomping her foot and swaying to it. She was swaying to the chant that was coming out of her mouth and to the rhythm that was consumed in her whole body. It was so amazing. She had this little apartment and she was stomping so hard that all of her little objects were falling off the walls. We took everything down and kept them in order, but she didn't care because she had her baby just fine. She was so grateful that she was able to do whatever she needed to do and make whatever noise she wanted to.

and value of making noise in labour in a structured way that is informative, fun and surprisingly liberating!

Postnatal music

'It is intuitive that there is a profound interplay of information and emotions involved in this sacred and precious dialogue [of mother singing to baby].'

[Schwartz 1997, p.3]

Within the first few days of life, without spoken language, the neonate begins to communicate with those around her or him, using sound and movement to experience and negotiate relationships.

As we have already established, the mother's voice has an impact on the developing brain of the fetus. At birth, babies react to the musical rhythms of speech which helps them to orientate to the new and hyperstimulated world that they encounter (Fifer & Moon 1994). Fascinatingly, it has been discovered that newborn babies, and even preterm babies (from 28 weeks), have similar rhythmic voice performance features as their mothers (Barabin 2002). The communication of the new baby mirrors its mother's voice pattern and features!

The language that mothers use when speaking to their infant is sometimes termed 'motherese'. This is the high-pitched musical language which mothers reserve intuitively for their babies (DeCaspar et al 1994). It is recognised that mothers expand the intonation contours of their speech to their child as soon as it is born. Compared to adult-directed speech, 'Motherese' has a higher overall pitch, wider pitch excursions, broader pitch range, increased rhythmicity, slower tempo, longer word durations and increased amplitude (DeCaspar et al 1994). It is also acknowledged that newborn babies can distinguish their own language from a foreign one (Moon et al 1993). Again, this suggests that they are increasingly able to focus upon the unique intonation aspects of their 'mother' tongue.

The importance of providing musical stimulation and singing to babies before birth takes on further significance in the postnatal period. On the basis of observations and experiments with newborns, neuroscientists now know that infants are born with neural mechanisms devoted exclusively to music. Studies show that early and ongoing musical training helps organise and develop children's brains (Gardiner et al 1996).

Babies who have been sung to, in utero and beyond, often start to sing around the eighth month, using about four notes up or down a scale. They imitate gestures and facial expressions and this encourages the development of speech as well as musical awareness. Postnatal groups could use this knowledge to inform parents of the benefits of using music with their baby from a very early stage in their lives. The boom in music sessions for toddlers in recent years demonstrates that parents value the effect of introducing song and musical instruments to their preschoolers, but are they as aware of how early the principles can be applied to enhance the learning and aesthetic appreciation of their offspring?

It has been suggested that breastfeeding may be enhanced with the use of music. Woodward & Guidozzi (1992) demonstrated that neonates would change their suckling patterns whilst breastfeeding by increasing the duration between suckling bursts to enable them to hear a lullaby that they had been exposed to during the last weeks of pregnancy. They incidentally responded even more favourably to the sound of their own mother's voice.

Music in neonatal care units

'I am hopeful that the scientific contributions of neuroscience, genetics and psychology will help to illuminate the nature of the very early musical responsiveness which appears to be an innate function of all human beings.'

(Fridman 2000)

An increasing awareness of the optimal environment required to nurture preterm babies in neonatal intensive care units has led to major reconsideration of the place of music as therapy for these tiny patients. The playing of music in neonatal units has been shown to promote weight gain and reduce movement, reduce irritability, crying and stress behaviours, stimulate development, increase blood oxygen levels and decrease length of hospitalisation (Schwartz 1997).

Music tapes timed to an adult heart beat have been used in neonatal units to assess the modulating effect of music on the pain experience of the preterm and sick neonate. It would seem that the babies who were exposed to music during procedures to obtain blood samples had lower pain ratings, detected from videotapes, and higher oxygen saturation levels (Kect et al 2000, cited in Barabin 2002).

In another study where tiny 'Walkman' type personal stereos were introduced to the babies in a neonatal unit, Schwartz (1997) concluded that the relative expenditure for music in their NICU could save $2000–$9000, simply by reducing the babies' stay by 3 days. More importantly, these infants demonstrated a trend for faster growth in head circumference, an indicator of increased brain growth. Fridman (2000) suggests putting a tape recording of the parents' own songs into the incubator.

A wonderful Israeli website (The Voices of Eden: www.voicesofeden.com/Babies. html) has photographs of a group of musicians visiting a special care baby unit and describes the effect that their ensemble has when they begin to play. The photographs and the comments of the parents and staff about the benefits of playing music (and, perhaps significantly, live music) for the challenged newborn speak volumes.

Useful trends, such as kangaroo care, that develop from experimentation in neonatal care units often prove to have a much wider benefit for all neonates. Healthcare financial managers would be wise to consider the benefits of providing maternity units with weekly visits by a string quartet!

Music and midwives

For the last 5 years or so, a small group of British midwives and students have visited The Farm Midwifery Center in rural Tennessee, the home of the group of midwives immortalised in Ina May Gaskin's *Spiritual Midwifery* (1977). Music plays an important part in the culture of The Farm and several of The Farm midwives are also members of one or two of the women's singing groups that meet to sing, laugh and cry together. When the British midwives and students arrive, they are invited to sing along with the Shamamas or The Babes in the Wood. Initially they have to work quite hard to find their voices. However, by the end of the week, they cannot be silenced and lead singing sessions enthusiastically and with little inhibition. The singing creates bonds between these women and offers invigoration, catharsis and healing.

An attempt to introduce a choral element to an undergraduate midwifery programme on return to the UK following such a visit was less well received. Although some of the group were keen to sing, and others were willing to give it a go, a large percentage of the group declined the invitation and some made it known that they felt the whole exercise to be 'unprofessional'. This leads us back to the article by Kitzinger (2000) and the supposition that the current maternity care system is so imbued with notions of hierarchy that the mere suggestion of participating in a great levelling and creative activity such as singing fills many with dread and fear. Is the problem 'professionalism'? Does being professional mean that we have to distance ourselves from each other by avoiding group activities that may lead to us connecting in a way that may be unattainable in other areas of our working lives, a connection that may touch us on a spiritual or intuitive level? Is the reticence a reflection of the risk-managed culture of fear in which we practise?

Where does that leave us in relation to our role 'with woman'? Where does it leave us with regard to our relationship with ourselves?

Perhaps we could begin by introducing music and song with confidence and with conviction. Think of the public health opportunities to teach client groups about the physiological benefits and pleasures of music as therapy.

If singing is seen to be part of the culture of birth, then we may find it easier as practitioners to introduce nursery rhymes and lullabies to parents in the antenatal period, and perhaps even encourage them to create their own. If we inform parents of the benefits of playing Baroque music during pregnancy, then we offer them the opportunity to do something that may help their child to grow into an individual who is well integrated in their physical, emotional, cognitive and spiritual self.

We can acknowledge that 'toning' may be useful as a prophylaxis or form of pain relief in labour, and that it is not just something that 'alternative' clients may like to do.

We could be more mindful of the music that we choose to play during childbirth preparation or lead a Coyote Circle to get women to vocalise and moan their way through labour. We could play calming music in antenatal clinics and GP surgeries to relax women awaiting antenatal appointments. Who knows, this action alone could save a strapped-for-cash health service the expense of antihypertensive medication for some women.

Lynch & Bemrose (2005) have developed a way of encouraging pre- and postbirth interaction by using information cards which include an action song for pregnant mothers, and have concluded that by learning to communicate with their babies during pregnancy, the parents-to-be are more likely to set up patterns which help to form positive attachments once the baby is born.

We could follow the lead of our Tyrolean sisters who formed the Austrian Midwives Choir and discovered that they could make wonderful music together and, in doing so, form collegial bonds. We could welcome student midwives to the profession by singing them a greeting. The opportunities to use music in practice are manifold.

Above all, however, we need to embrace the sometimes inexplicable enchantment of music as a powerful and therapeutic modality in the world of birth, and as Andsell rightly states:

'We need to begin to think of ourselves as symphonic beings, rather than the mechanical ones that reductionist scientific medicine would often have us.'

(Andsell 1995, p.8)

A more harmonious approach to practice and to life generally may lead to stronger and more meaningful relationships with women and their families and give us a greater sense of worth in our own role.

References

Aitchison J 1997 The seeds of speech: language origin and evolution. Cambridge University Press, Cambridge

Andsell G 1995 Music for life: aspects of creative music therapy with adult clients. Jessica Kingsley, London

Barabin B 2002 Music during pregnancy. Ultrasound in Obstetrics and Gynaecology 20: 425–430

Browning C A 2000 Using music during childbirth. Birth 27(4): 272–276

Clarke M E, McCorckle R R, Williams S B 1981 Music therapy assisted labor and delivery. Journal of Music Therapy 18: 88–100

Davis C A 1992 The effects of music and basic relaxation instruction on pain and anxiety of women undergoing in-office gynecological procedures. Journal of Music Therapy 29(4): 202–218

DeCaspar A J, LeCanuet J-P, Busnel M-C, Granier-Deferre C, Maugeais R 1994 Foetal reactions to recurrent maternal speech. Infant Behaviour and Development 17: 159–164

Dick-Read G 1960 Childbirth without fear, 4th edn. Heinemann, London

Emoto M 2004 The hidden messages in water. Beyond Words Books Hillsboro, OR

England P, Horowitz R 1998 Birthing from within: an extra-ordinary guide to childbirth preparation. Partera Press. Albuquerque, NM

Federico G F, Whitwell G E 2001 Music therapy and pregnancy. Journal of Prenatal and Perinatal Psychology and Health 15(4): 299–310

Fifer W P, Moon C M 1994 The role of the mother's voice in the organisation of brain function in the newborn. Acta Paediatric 397(suppl): 86–93

Fridman R 2000 Life before birth: prenatal sound and music. Available online at: www.birthpsychology.com/lifebefore/sound2.html

Fried R 1990 Integrating music in breathing training and relaxation: I. Background, rationale, and relevant elements. Biofeedback and Self Regulation 15(2):161–169

Friedman R 1993 Proto-rhythms: music in prenatal and postnatal life. In: Blum T (ed) Prenatal perception, learning and bonding. Leonardo Publishers, Berlin

Gardiner M F, Fox A, Knowles F, Jeffrey D 1996 Learning improved by arts training. Nature 381: 254

Gaskin I M 1977 Spiritual midwifery. Book Publishing Company, Summertown, TN

Gaynor M 1999 Sounds of healing: a physician reveals the therapeutic power of sound, voice, and music. Broadway Books, New York

Hanser S B, Thompson L W 1994 Effects of a music therapy strategy on depressed older adults. Journal of Gerontology 49(6): 265–269

Hanser S B, Larson S C, O'Connell A S 1983 The effect of music on relaxation of expectant mothers during labor. Journal of Music Therapy 20: 50–58

Hepper P G 1991 An examination of fetal learning before and after birth. Irish Journal of Psychology 12(2): 95–107

Kitzinger S 2000 Waterbirth and song. Practising Midwife 3(9): 14–17

Lane D, Wilkins R 1994 Music as medicine: Deforia Lane's life of music, healing, and faith. Zondervan Publishing House, Grand Rapids, MI

Langer S 1942 Philosophy in a new key. Harvard University Press, Cambridge, MA

Lynch L, Bemrose S 2005 It's good to talk: pre and post-term interaction. Practising Midwife 8(3): 17–20

Marks K 1993 Circle of song: songs, chants, and dances for ritual and celebration. Full Circle Press. Amherst, MA

Mellor D 2005 Onset of sentience: the potential for suffering in fetal and newborn farm animals. Conference proceedings, Compassion in World Farming Trust, London

Melzack R 1993 Labour pain as a model of acute pain. Pain 53(2): 117–120

Meyerowitz S 2001 Water: the ultimate cure. Book Publishing Company, Summertown, TN

Moon C, Cooper R, Fifer W 1993 Two-day-olds prefer their native language. Infant Development and Behaviour16: 495–500

Odent M 1999 The scientification of love. Free Association Books, London

Phumdoung S, Good M 2003 Music reduces sensation and distress of labor pain. Pain Management Nursing 4(2): 54–61

Rider M S 1985 Entrainment mechanisms are involved in pain reduction, muscle relaxation and music mediated imagery. Journal of Music Therapy 22(3): 183–192

Sansavini A, Bertoncini J, Giovanelli G 1997 Newborns discriminate the rhythm of multisyllabic stressed words. Developmental Psychology 33: 3–11

Schwartz F 1997 Perinatal stress reduction, music and medical cost savings. Journal of Prenatal and Perinatal Psychology and Health 12(1): 19–29

Shahidullah S, Hepper P 1992 Hearing in the fetus: prenatal detection of deafness. International Journal of Prenatal and Perinatal Studies 4 (3 and 4): 235–240

Sidorenko V N 2000 Clinical application of Medical Resonance Therapy (MRT-Music) in risk pregnancies. Integrated Physiological Behavioral Science 35(3): 199–207

Spintage R, Droh R 1987 Effects of anxiolytic music on plasma levels of stress hormones in different medical specialties. Fourth International Symposium on Music, Rehabilitation and Human Well-Being (pp. 88–101). University Press of America, Lanham, MD

Vaneechoutte M, Skoyles J R 1998 The memetic origin of language: modern humans as musical primates. Journal of Memetics – Evolutionary Models of Information Transmission 2. Available online at: http://jomemit.cfpm.org/1998/vol2/vaneechoutte_m&skoyles_jr.html

Whitwell G E 2005 The importance of prenatal sound and music. Life before Birth. Available online at: www.birthpsychology.com/lifebefore/sound

Woodward S C, Guidozzi F 1992 Intrauterine rhythm and blues? British Journal of Obstetrics and Gynaecology 99: 787–790

Zentner M R, Kagan J 1998 Infant's perception of consonance and dissonance in music. Infant Behaviour and Development 21(3): 483–492

CHAPTER ELEVEN

Dancing Birth:
Choreography and Improvisation

CAROL BARTLE

Rise, baby, rise!
Let's dance
Arm-in-arm, hand-in-hand with everyone!
Be forbidden from now on
Kiss of lips and kiss of cheeks,
Let the names of lovers
Kiss each other,
Let the wings of garments,
The tunes of feet flying high,
And the breath of fingers
Swinging light,
Kiss one another.
All dancing
Face-to-face, eye-to-eye,
Let's cross beyond countries
And over the seas, all dancing,
Let's go beyond this world

(Vagif Bayatly Oner*)

Floating, wriggling, stretching, bouncing, pushing, rebounding, flexing, turning, bending, swaying, touching, contracting, descending, rotating, opening, crawling, gazing, embracing, connecting. Movement words associated with dance and birth. As a midwife who dances, these words have multiple meanings for me, connected to both birth movements and dance movements. They are words which describe the baby moving and floating languidly inside the womb and then more forcefully descending in synchronisation with the mother's uterine contractions. Words which also describe the baby entering the world

*From a poem entitled 'Let's Dance from Birth to Death' by Vagif Bayatly Oner who was born in 1948 in Jabrayil, a district in Karabakh now militarily occupied by Armenia. Vagif studied construction engineering and architecture at Azerbaijan Construction Engineering University. This section of poetry is gratefully used with permission from Vagif Bayatly Oner whose works are published in the Azerbaijan International Magazine. Grateful thanks for permission to the publishers also. Search Oner at AZER.com.

outside the womb and words which have meaning for the woman labouring, giving birth and meeting and embracing her baby physically for the first time. I have also used these same words when guiding students and lovers of dance and movement of all ages, ethnicities, abilities, shapes and sizes through classes in movement improvisation and semi-structured choreography. As a midwife with a long history as a dancer and choreographer, this is a glorious opportunity for me to explore birth and dance and blend together a discussion about the interconnectedness of these choreographed and improvised movement celebrations of life itself.

Dance is an expression of life and birth is a beginning of life. Performing dance acknowledges the wonder that is life and body. Dance is concerned with the relationships of bodies, always between a performer and her body or her body involved in making connections with other bodies. The Birth of Dance, the Dance of Birth. Inseparable. Rituals which have existed since the inception of human life; rich with expression and choreographic content, improvised, structured, semi-structured and instinctive performances. Birth choreography can never be a solo performance for even without birth attendants, there will always be a baby or babies and a mother, mother and baby intrinsically connected. The baby practising flexion, gradually reducing movements and descending lower as the time of birth draws ever closer. The baby who emerges using a beautifully choreographed sequence of movements and who in turn contributes to the choreographed movements of the mother during the strong passage of movement created by labour contractions. Walking, leaning, swaying, crouching, bending, rhythmically pushing, supporting, holding, clutching, touching and being touched. The dance of labour. Fathers, midwives, doulas, support people, family and friends join in the dance and make up a chorus of caring performers, taking their cues from the leading couple, the starring duet, the mother and her baby.

The baby in the warm liquid womb, dancing like a fish, floating in a warm bath of fluid, touching the womb, a touching of two bodies, one does not end and one does not begin, impossible to separate and say where baby ends and mother begins. A physiologically, physically, psychologically and emotionally interconnected duo. An intimate duet which dances from the inside world to the outside world, with an eventual loss of the physical umbilical cord connection between mother and baby, but with the emergence of a psychological umbilical cord, to maintain the mother–baby dance connection.

The psychological umbilical cord was conceptualised by Professor Adik Levin, a neonatologist from the Tallin Children's Hospital in Estonia. He pioneered a form of neonatal intensive care which he called the Humane Neonatal Care Initiative (Levin 1999). The principles underpinning this care include providing facilities for mothers to stay with their sick babies twenty-four hours a day, reducing psychological stress for mothers and caring for mothers as well as babies. Professor Levin was concerned with the importance of protecting a link between mothers and their babies in situations where babies are admitted to neonatal intensive care units (NICUs). The significance of the mother–baby connection is respected, valued, supported and maintained by making it possible for the mother to stay in close contact with the baby despite an intensive care admission. The postbirth mother–baby dance is supported by maintaining the link between these two connected beings and the optimal means of ensuring that this connection is valued, nurtured and protected is to provide caring facilities for mothers and to enable them to stay near their sick newborn babies. Separating mother and baby because of a NICU admission has not been one of the most astute practices our Western health systems have pioneered. In the United States there is now a move to provide individual NICU rooms to enable families to stay close to their babies for the benefit of babies, mothers and families. The loving duet, although derailed by illness and, by necessity, having unexpected others joining in the postbirth dance, can still have the crucial connection preserved. Rather than mother becoming an understudy and facility staff becoming the 'stars', this system retains mother securely as lead and most essential/ significant and others as supporting chorus and guests in the mother–baby space.

Enabling mothers and babies to stay close supports the postbirth mother–baby dance. It positively affects emerging postnatal issues such as the urgent provision of breastmilk for the sick baby and alleviation of the high degree of emotional distress experienced by the mother and the baby. Creative ways of ensuring that the mother–baby bond is not broken have to be found in these situations.

At the time of writing, there are in existence, to my knowledge, two other humane neonatal care units in the world: one at High Wycombe in England and one in Buenos Aires, Argentina. In the North Island of New Zealand's Waikato region, a new consumer lobby group has been formed. Its prime motivation is to agitate for neonatal intensive care units (NICUs) to make provision for mothers to stay with their babies if they wish and/or are able to do so. This group has a website and collects mothers' and health professionals' stories, displays relevant research and provides a supportive forum for families with NICU babies (www.numb.net.nz).

Kangaroo Mother Care (KMC) restores the contact between the mother and her baby. Dr Nils Bergman defines Kangaroo Mother Care as 'a universally available and biologically sound method of care for all newborns, but in particular for premature babies, with three components: skin to skin contact, exclusive breastfeeding and support to the mother–infant dyad'. Dr Bergman maintains an active website with research, references, photos and stories about Kangaroo Mother Care (Bergman 2005). He considers that separation of the mother and baby, although common, is abnormal and harmful. Skin-to-skin care is, and has been, practised by mothers in many countries and in many situations but KMC, as a positive intervention in neonatal intensive care environments, is reported to have been started in Bogotá, Colombia, by Drs Rey and Martinez, as a response to a shortage of incubators and an incidence of severe hospital infections. KMC restores the contact between mother and baby and places the baby back into a somatosensory maternal environment where beneficial tactile, auditory, visual, rhythmic and vestibular components are reestablished. A homecoming for the baby nestled naked against the mother's skin, a haven in a warm place of safety, which acts as a buffer to overstimulation and restores connection and responsiveness. Perhaps protecting this mother–baby connected dance in all its show-stopping, breath-taking beauty and special intimacy may provide more benefits than we can imagine.

In a neonatal intensive care area, where technology reigns supreme, it is sometimes difficult to comprehend how simple minimalist actions requiring no technology or invasive procedures can result in extraordinary moments of far-reaching significance. Neonatal intensive care staff anticipate that NICU babies, and preterm babies in particular, will be sleepy and unresponsive and have difficulties with feeding. Animal studies indicate the deleterious effects of separation of mothers and babies. Piglets exposed to intermittent contact with their mothers show significant decreases in locomotion and activity (Kanitz et al 2004) and isolated rodents and monkey babies become steadily more lethargic and passive (Hennessy et al 2001). Interrupting the mother–baby dance by separation may have far-reaching consequences and negative developmental implications. A simple practice such as skin-to-skin contact between mother and baby can reduce mother and baby distress, stabilise the baby physiologically, have positive effects on lactation and later breastfeeding and protect the continuum of the mother–baby dance. Kangaroo Mother Care, as described by Charpak et al (2001), 'would humanise the practice of neonatology, promote breastfeeding and shorten hospital stay without compromising survival, growth or development' (p.1072). The psychological umbilical cord is not only maintained but actively supported and the mother–baby dance continues to give pleasure, support mother–baby responsiveness, make lactation more robust and promote a loving relationship.

The Early Childhood Education curriculum in New Zealand, or Te Whāriki (Ministry of Education 1996), presents a framework providing for children's early learning and development within a sociocultural context. The emphasis is on learning partnerships between parents, teachers and children. Te Whāriki, which symbolises a woven mat for all to stand on (Carr & May 1992), weaves together five strands considered crucial for education. These strands are well-being, belonging, contribution, communication and exploration, and signify a weaving together of a holistic curriculum respectful of the diverse needs of parents and respecting differences in sociocultural context. Te Whāriki is a useful model to consider when confronting crucial issues in other spheres, such as maternity and postbirth periods, when normal events become derailed and plunge mothers and babies into unfamiliar and scary landscapes. To maintain well-being in baby and mother, to foster a sense of belonging, to ensure the mother feels that she is contributing, to ensure that the communication and exploration between mother and baby are not interrupted means that separation is not an option. The dance must continue and this means supporting the togetherness of the mother and baby even through adversity.

Dance affects all the senses and, indeed, so does birth. Louise Steinman (1986), writing about dancing bodies, discusses the concept of proprioception, which is an explanation for how we 'sense' ourselves. The proprioception system has three main sources of input which are kinaesthetic, visceral and labyrinthine/vestibular. Kinaesthetic refers to the feelings of movement derived from skeletal and muscular structures, which include feelings of pain, orientation in space and time, and rhythm. Visceral feedback comes from the internal organs and how we sense the feelings that derive from these organs. Labyrinthine/vestibular is the feeling of our position in space. Steinman studies the relationships between performers, their bodies and their audiences and she considers that during the energy exchange between the performer and audience, there is a 'potential for a tremendous amount of learning, potential to stir up powers beyond evident human capacity' (Steinman 1986). Steinman also discusses experimental or 'avant-garde' work where she considers 'one is likely still to find the values that are at the root of traditional art forms'. Steinman notes that the playwright Ionesco commented that to be 'avant-garde is not to be far out, but to return to our sources, to reject traditionalism in order to find again a living tradition' (ibid). Steinman then comments that this living tradition is 'rooted in our first breath, in the transformation of childhood and dream, in the acknowledgement of our ancestors and our animal selves'. There too exists birth. Birthing without interventions, supporting the release of all the powerful potential from within the mother. The living tradition of birth. A celebration of movement and woman's powerful and magical capacity. Rather than being considered 'far out' when insisting that birth should take place out of hospital birthing environments, one is, of course, going back to the living tradition of physiological birth and rejecting the traditional, much more 'acceptable' version of medicalised techno-choreographed birth and the scripted, controlled dance of technology.

Susan Leigh Foster (1996) is the editor of a book about dance choreography which theorises the relationships between body and self. This book is a collection of essays on the study of bodies, 'through a consideration of bodily reality, not as natural or absolute given but as a tangible and substantial category of cultural experience' (p.xi). Foster, and other contributors, state in the introduction that, 'the essays [in this volume] refuse to let bodies be used merely as vehicles or instruments for the expression of something else'.

> 'Bodies develop choreographies of signs through which they discourse: they run (or lurch, or bound, or feint, or meander) from premise to conclusion; they turn (or pivot or twist) through the process of reasoning; they confer with (or rub up against, or bump into) one another in narrating their own physical fate.' (p.xi)

This book considers dance as a cultural practice which provides rich resources for any study of embodiment. If we examine the role bodies play in producing rich narrative, then consider birth through a study of movements or as a performance of movements, it can provide us with an abundant source of accessible metaphors to describe the dance of birth which launches a platform for greater understandings of birth spirituality and birth as 'not-illness'.

The dance of birth and its choreography involves two bodies and their relationship to each other and to the dance/birth process. The body as an instrument is capable of creating its own language and during pregnancy and birth, two languages and movements are combined, so that the growing baby affects kinaesthetic, visceral and labyrinthine sensations in the mother and changes movements and everyday choreography. 'Inside' the mother becomes a 'different' space, incorporating 'inside' the baby, 'outside' the baby, 'outside' the womb and a curious mix of twice as many organs as the usual 'single' state, all performing together in the pregnant body, with the associated sensations of weight, rhythm and spatial changes. The baby inside experiences the mother's movements and choreography and goes along as a small and connected passenger, taking part in the dance and inspiring changes to the mother's day-to-day movement choreography by virtue of just growing and by performing baby-choreography within mother-choreography. Visible internal baby-choreography is noted on the outside and a source of wonder and pleasure to the mother and father and other close privileged people. The baby also quietly performs choreography with only one exclusive audience member, the mother, who feels the baby moving, kicking, stretching, swimming and growing.

Bartal & Ne'eman (1975) provided inspirational insights into movement, awareness and creativity when they published their book a few years prior to my joining a team of dance and movement improvisation teachers and commencing teaching or facilitating movement classes on a regular weekly basis for 10 or so years. Bartal & Ne'eman consider that movement is an instrument of human creativity even more important than literature, art or music because it is a form of expression used by every human being every day, regardless of gender, ethnicity, language, culture or circumstances. Their book presents a programme of techniques designed to help with developing the language of dance, human movement expression, awareness, imagination and creativity. This approach leads to the development of a unity of mind and body which releases the expressive qualities of the body. With their approach, Bartal & Ne'eman aim to assist an increase in 'human perceptiveness through the development of imagination and creativity' (p.3). Physiological birth supports a unity of mind and body and is a glowing example of how a mind/body unity enables a labouring woman to travel inwards towards a deep connection with her body and her baby, facilitating the profound expression of physical birth through a journey of movement, vocalisation and physiological choreography.

Now re-reading this book many years later, I am drawn to a paragraph which has powerful meanings for the dance of birth.

'The nearer a person is to his [sic] own instincts, the more aware of his own archetypal roots, the better will he be able to turn himself into a free flowing instrument in touch with the inner nature he has in common with all other human beings.' (p.5)

Physiological birth supports a labouring woman to come closer to her own instincts, enabling the transformation into a 'free-flowing instrument' which in turn scaffolds the birth choreography, resulting in intensely powerful feelings, maternal satisfaction and empowerment. How is it possible to become a 'free-flowing instrument' when all sensation and feeling is lost in the body below the waist? When movement sensations are derailed, one arm is busy being attached to an intravenous infusion, pregnant tummy surrounded by straps and monitors, choices of movement and position severely restricted, birth chorus expanded to include performers who have inserted themselves into the performance without being at any rehearsals? Physiological birth choreography distorted into techno-choreography with a medical director. The dance-theatre of techno-birth. Interfering with the dance sequences of baby and mother and distorting the natural pathways of mother–baby connectedness.

Maggie Banks, an inspirational New Zealand home birth midwife, researcher and writer, presented study days during 2005 entitled 'The Spirit of Birth: Nature, Nurture and the Evidence'©. These days were created in response to 'escalating levels of intervention during childbirth and a declining "normal" birth rate'. Banks presented figures from the New Zealand 2004 Report on Maternity which found that 'normal' birth now represents less than 68% of all births, with labour induction at 20.1%, epidural anaesthesia at 25.3% and episiotomy at 10.5%.

Proponents of physiological birth such as Sheila Kitzinger, Marsden Wagner and Michel Odent have been talking about the importance of restoring the 'normal' paradigm of birth for many years. Odent's *Birth Reborn* (1984) has a foreword written by Doris Haire, who was President of the American Foundation for Maternal and Child Health and Chairwoman on the Committee on Maternal and Child Health at the time of writing. Haire hailed the book as possibly being the one that might 'bring[s] about a new direction in obstetrical care. Into a world where childbirth in most hospitals has become a nightmare of chemical and technological interventions in the name of safety but without sound scientific evidence to demonstrate that such interventions are necessary' (Odent 1984, p.xi). Sadly, more than 20 years later midwives and women are still facing the same issues, nightmares and dilemmas. Sheila Kitzinger, in the introduction for the same book, describes how tempting it is for an obstetrician 'to become the stage manager of the drama of birth' (Odent 1984, p.xv). Obstetrician as the lead choreographer for the dance of birth with the mother as a passive recipient of medicalised techno-care. Michel Odent provided birth settings where women could perform birth in their own unique ways, restoring the capacity of the mother to become a 'free-flowing instrument', in touch with the baby's movements and with her own bodily messages. Dancing birth, co-constructing and co-choreographing the events of labour and birth with her baby and her own body. A creative movement and moving experience for birthing women. Kitzinger points out that 'professionals with special skills' (Odent 1984, p.xviii) take their parts at the birth but these professionals, and the environment provided for the birth, support the women to experience a physiological birth and perform their own birth dance. Something that home-birth midwives quietly provide for women in countries all around the world.

Rudolf Laban wrote about human movement in his book *The Mastery of Movement* which was first published in 1950. In a revised and enlarged fourth edition, Lisa

Ullmann (1980), who was formerly the Director of the Laban Art of Movement Centre, explains that movement may be influenced by the environment of the mover. The milieu will colour the movements of the actors moving within it. Laban/Ullmann also suggest that movement is a result of 'the striving after an object deemed valuable, or of a state of mind' (p.2). There is a richness of language in this book to apply to both dance and birth and stimulating sections of writing discussing the meeting of dancers on the stage, their approach, and later separation. Laban/Ullmann describe how members of the group move, 'in order to show their desire to get in touch with each other' (p.2). Visualising the scene of a home birth and the movements of the labour supporters around the labouring woman, the choreography presents itself as one of connection and sensitivity to the flow of the woman's labour. The environment supporting the labouring woman and providing the comforting milieu of a known space. Supportive choreography may also occur within maternity facility settings if enlightened midwives and other health professionals can facilitate the mother to take centre stage, support physiological movement and also resist the use of intervention and techno-choreography.

Laban/Ullmann distinguish between an 'unhampered or free flow' of movement and a 'hampered or bound flow' (p.18). In Laban movement philosophy, the movement flow of a human body is influenced by how and in what sequence the various body parts start to move. Therefore, by restricting natural body movements, the physiological flow of movements becomes bound, leading to interruptions or derailments of this natural flow. How many labouring and birthing women have their natural movement sequences restricted by imposed body positions and structural interventions, which then lead to a further derailment and additional difficulties? Obstructed labour, failure to progress, delay in second stage, fetal distress, episiotomy, forceps, Ventouse extraction, caesarean birth to name a few of the common terms associated with techno-birth.

Founded by dancer Steve Paxton over 30 years ago, contact improvisation is a fluid dance where two or more dancers connect with each other and listen and support each other's movements. Paxton describes the body as a tool which explores the spaces around it. Contact improvisation emerges when contact or touch occurs between dancers and this contact is viewed as 'the uniter'. Who touches, and how they touch, and what touches the labouring and birthing woman shapes what Paxton describes as the 'third entity', which is a term used in contact improvisation to conceptualise the connections formed between the people who are touching and being touched. This third entity is described in contact improvisation as 'the dance'. Paxton called the awareness of the smallest motions and workings of the body 'small dance', in which dancers have to be in tune with their bodies, 'listening' to what their bodies are quietly performing, with their minds being aware of the movement but not dictating the movement. The three main communicators in this contact dance form are touch, pressure and weight.

Contact improvisation principles may be transformed into meaningful descriptors for the dance of birth. The baby's body exploring the space around it, at first luxuriously roomy, supporting unrestricted stretching and floating and later becoming cosy and providing a supportive scaffold of soft surfaces to rebound from and to push against. A unity between the baby who physically touches the inner-mother. The outer-mother who feels the movements of her inner-baby touching her inside-spaces. 'Small dance', with the mother and her baby in tune with each other and listening with their bodies to their performances. The baby is never isolated from touch and her movements may be spontaneous or provoked by external events. The first communication through movement is in the womb. The womb as the first stimulating interactive environment complete with sound, vibration and movement experiences to support baby development. The mother who supports the baby through pregnancy and birth, feeling touch, pressure and weight. Birth supporters touching the labouring woman, connecting and supporting weight and movement. How the woman moves or responds to contractions or touch, giving cues for the next movements of her supporters. Contact improvisation supporting the choreographed sequence of the inner-baby dance. Contact improvisation performed in its most intimate form between the mother and her unborn baby.

The ancient movement art of Oriental dance, or what has come to be known as 'belly dancing' in the Western world, has origins as a religious rite to worship motherhood. Tribeswomen perform this dance in a circle around the bedside of a labouring woman who also imitates their rolling pelvic movements intermittently. A woman known as Morocco has been studying and researching Oriental dance for over 40 years. Morocco has written many articles about 'dancing the baby into the world' and describes this Oriental dance as the 'oldest form of natural childbirth instruction' (Morocco 1996). Morocco was once smuggled into the birthing room of a friend's cousin where she observed the ritual dancing of the childbirth supporters and the undulating movements of the labouring woman. She describes the hypnotising effects of the dancing circle of women and explains the technique which requires the skills of allowing the abdominal muscles to contract while other muscles not involved remain relaxed. The dance reduces pain from labour contractions and facilitates the birth of the baby. The birthing woman is supported to move with the contractions rather than fight against them. Natural body movements with body parts moving in a sequence which supports the birth process.

Taking us back to the concept of unhampered free-flowing movements and the body as a free-flowing instrument connected to and in synchrony with the baby and the birth process. Dancing birth, 'dancing the baby into the world'. Relationships, contact, connection, ritual. Words associated with movement, dance and birth. Well-being, belonging, contribution, communication and exploration. Words associated with a scaffolding of the birth process and a physiological birth and postbirth choreography which supports the continuation of a remarkable form of choreography and dance. One which begins long before labour commences, when the baby starts to awaken in the womb and the mother feels the first stirrings of her baby dancing.

References

Bartal L, Ne'eman N 1975 Movement, awareness and creativity. Souvenir Press, London

Bergman N 2005 Kangaroo Mother Care Promotions. Available online at: www.kangaroomothercare.com

Carr M, May H 1992 Te Whāriki: Early Childhood Curriculum Development Project. Final Report to the Ministry of Education. University of Waikato, Hamilton, New Zealand

Charpak N, Ruiz-Pelez G, Figueroa de Calume Z, Charpak Y 2001 A randomised controlled trial of Kangaroo Mother Care: results of a follow-up at one year corrected age. Pediatrics 108(5): 1072–1079

Hennessy M B, Deak T, Schiml-Webb P A 2001 Stress-induced sickness behaviours: an alternative hypothesis for responses during maternal separation. Developmental Psychobiology 39(2): 76–83

Kanitz E, Tuchscherer M, Puppe B, Tuchscherer A, Stabenow B 2004 Consequences of repeated early isolation in domestic piglets (*Sus scrofa*) on their behavioural, neuroendocrine and immunological responses. Brain, Behaviour and Immunity 18(1): 35–45

Laban R 1950 The mastery of movement. Macdonald and Evans, London

Foster S, Franko M, Gilpin H et al 1996 Introduction. In: Leigh Foster S (ed) Corporealities: dancing knowledge, culture and power. Routledge, New York, pp.xi-xvii

Levin A 1999 Humane Neonatal Care Initiative. Acta Paediatrica 88: 353–355

Ministry of Education New Zealand 1996 Te Whāriki: He Whāriki Mātauranga mō ngā Mokopuna o Aotearoa: Early Childhood Curriculum. Ministry of Education, Wellington, New Zealand

Morocco 1996 Giving to light: dancing the baby into the world. Habibi 15(1). Available online at: www.casbahdance.org

Odent M 1984 Birth reborn. Pantheon Books, New York

Steinman L 1986 The knowing body: elements of contemporary performance and dance. Shambhala, Boston

Ullmann L 1980 The mastery of movement, by Rudolf Laban, 4th revised edn. Macdonald and Evans, London

CHAPTER TWELVE

A Soulful Journey:
Creativity and Midwife Educators

—————————(•)—————————

JANICE BASS

'During the birth process there is a period when the mother behaves as if she were "on another planet", cutting herself off from our everyday world and going on a sort of inner trip. This change in her level of consciousness can be interpreted as a reduction in neocortical activity ... (Midwives) who understand this essential aspect of the physiology of labour and (birth) would not make the mistake of trying to "bring her back to her senses".'

(Odent 1999, p.28)

The debate about whether midwifery is an art or a science becomes rather academic after reading Odent's account of birth physiology. Clearly, the interaction of both art and science, represented as synergy between the body and mind during birth, is evidence of the importance of integration and not separation within midwifery. The argument is not about whether midwifery is art or science; both inform our understanding of birth. Science implies rationality yet can also be used to provide evidence that supports natural birth. Art engages all of our senses as we experience birth as a bio- psycho-socio-cultural- spiritual journey. Yet neither captures fully the mystery of life and death, our essence, our soul.

Odent (1999) suggests a higher level of consciousness during birth where spirit and nature complement each other perfectly. The point at which we transcend the physical or material confines of our body to surrender ourselves to spirit is where we experience the merging of soul and body consciousness. How, then, can we honour the mystery of birth, the perfect dance between nature and spirit, the role of the mother and father in weaving birth's tapestry and also support the baby's highest intentions?

Many of these philosophical questions also lie at the heart of what it is to be a midwife, to truly be 'with woman'; as guardians of natural birth and as gatekeeper, 'acting as the bridge between the heavens and earth, spirit and matter' (Karll 2003).

How do we 'midwife the midwife' (Taylor 1996) and facilitate the birth of aspiring midwives to practise this ancient art steeped in mystery? The analogy here of the role of the midwife as also 'being with student' is powerful if we consider how we role model the very qualities that we wish aspiring midwives to share with women and babies. Central to this is a respectful relationship which values the spiritual awareness of each woman, midwife and student.

This issue represents a challenge to midwifery, especially considering the dissonance students experience whilst aspiring to achieve the ideal of holistic midwifery practice, yet living the reality of the existing 'techno-medical hegemony' (Benoit et al 2001). The rise of the technocracy and the technico-rational paradigm has influenced midwifery practice such that the majority of midwives no longer practise real, authentic midwifery or actively promote the 'unique normality of birth' (Downe & McCourt 2004).

Personal experience as a midwife and midwife teacher led me to question the success of existing approaches within midwifery education. How can we prepare aspiring midwives as autonomous and independent practitioners committed to holistic, woman-centred care? As a midwife and educator, I have been concerned about the deepening 'gulf' between midwifery theory and practice and the continuing professional socialisation of aspiring midwives into the role of obstetric nurses. This occurs despite opportunities to experience a midwifery philosophy of care amidst programmes that advocate woman-centred, holistic approaches and promote the role of the midwife as guardian of normal birth. However, this suggests that aspiring midwives lack spiritual awareness and need to be educated. From a humanistic perspective, it must be acknowledged that students may in fact achieve higher realisations about their practice than those midwives/midwife educators around them. Similarly, some aspiring midwives may not be able to acknowledge that birth is more than physical and this must be accepted in a respectful way that upholds spiritual development.

Central to this is the debate about how we best facilitate the development of aspiring midwives who are 'able to think not only about what is but also about what could be ...' (Bass 2001).

Midwives make a difference to the lives of women, their partners, their families and the wider community. Recent evidence supports the long-held belief that 'the most important determinants of a woman's birth are the attitudes and ideology of her primary caregiver' (Hodnett 2002). These attitudes are experienced first hand by aspiring midwives during the programmes that prepare them for practice. Midwifery education provides the foundations for best practice, fostering the personal and professional growth and development of each midwife. This is imperative to creating and sustaining any cultural or paradigm shifts which could make a difference to the experiences of women. Can midwifery educators help facilitate these shifts?

A different kind of educator?

'We have to recognize that the "ways of knowing" offered by the dominant rational/experimental model are severely limited in situations of social change.'

(Schon 1987)

Whilst observing midwife educators over a period of years, it became clear to me that some utilised creative approaches in addition to traditional learning and teaching strategies to support facilitation of aspiring midwives. These educators appeared able to facilitate the notion of holistic midwifery practice, bridging the theory–practice gap through creative approaches to learning and teaching. They often referred to activities that employ cognitive, emotional and spiritual intelligence and openly encouraged students to think in imaginative ways about themselves as individuals as well as midwives.

They seemed to manage to incorporate creative approaches to learning and teaching that develop the power of individuals and groups to learn more effectively. This was further evidenced by students evaluating preregistration programmes, who would comment that certain educators influenced their thinking more than others. These teachers are variously described by students and colleagues as 'creative', 'artistic', 'radical', 'challenging', 'out of the box' and 'innovative'.

'What transforms education, is a transformed being in the World.'

(Parker 1998)

It is widely acknowledged that the skill of the educator and the practice of teaching are central to effective facilitation of learning (e.g. Kelly 1995). I began to wonder if there was something about how these educators think about what they do and how they approach their role as teachers that might make a difference to the development of holistic midwifery practice. Are they doing more than teaching and facilitating learning? To consider this further, it is necessary to explore the values and beliefs of educators who use creative approaches to learning and teaching.

One summer's journey...

The remainder of this chapter offers a discussion of some of the findings drawn from a study of midwife teachers who debated such issues with me in a series of focus groups and interviews during the summer of 2003 (Bass 2003). While this chapter is not intended to constitute a conventional research report, and does not include all of the themes that emerged, due to space constraints, the following points may be of interest.

- The focus of the study was to explore the creative teaching and learning approaches used to facilitate aspiring midwives and consider how this was affected by personal philosophy.
- The participants in this study were all midwife teachers working for one university and contributing to the midwifery programme. Further to this, they were all, to a greater or lesser extent, identified by students and their peers as being 'creative'. Having said this, my selection was sufficiently broad to include those midwife teachers who may not consider themselves as being as creative as some of their colleagues, and to accommodate differing levels of teaching experience.
- In all, seven participants took part in the study. All of the participants are women and midwives and their ages ranged from 31 to 52. Their experience in midwifery education ranged from less than 1 year to over 15 years. Two of the participants had significant experience as independent midwives, and all but one are currently engaged in midwifery practice, albeit mostly on an occasional rather than a regular basis. Three of the participants worked part-time and four worked full-time. One participant was a first-year student tutor, one was in the final stages of completing the preparation for teaching programme, and one recently qualified as a tutor; the remaining participants have been qualified as tutors for 3 years or more.
- Grounded theory was used as a method of research and data analysis.

The stories shared, and reproduced here with permission, provide some insight into the values and beliefs of midwife teachers who use creative and imaginative approaches to facilitate aspiring midwives to develop holistic midwifery practice. The journey is only really just beginning; this exploratory study represents the first step along a winding road. However, at this juxtaposition between what has been and what is yet to come, it is possible to make some tentative connections around the concept of creativity in midwifery education and what, as I will explore below, might be termed Soulful Midwifery.

'That indefinable quality'

A fundamental starting point was to establish what creativity actually meant to the participants; the way in which creativity is structured and how it is expressed.

The term 'structure' is used deliberately to reflect the existing model of Western society as expressed by participants and this represented a recurring theme throughout the study. During the early stages much of what was expressed about creativity was couched in language that reflected the dominant culture.

This is the reality that represents part of the challenge that we face as midwife teachers in preparing aspiring midwives for the reality of what is, and the possibility of what could be. The significance of this in relation to the research is the extent to which midwife teachers exercise creativity as part of their role and enable aspiring midwives to realise both the reality and the ideal.

Defining creativity stimulated much debate and the diversity of views expressed explains the complexity and the multidimensional nature of creativity. Participants frequently described creativity in terms of novel ideas that are useful...

> '[It's] about making something new. Because if you create something – whatever it is – if you're creating a recipe to make something or a quilt or something that you're making in craft or whatever it's about making something new isn't it?'

...or taking something that already existed and developing a new or different angle.

> 'Creativity involves creating something that is different'
>
> 'Taking a new angle on something'
>
> 'Making something new ... take something and come out with something different at the end'

For others, this also included the concept of creation...

> 'I think about creation ... for me it's like linked to, I was going to say the act of creation but I don't quite mean it in maybe the way it sounds.'

... or generativity.

> 'I was thinking there's something about creativity that, it's like if you do anything else creative like draw or cut out pictures or I was thinking knitting or whatever or making quilts, it's something about the generativity of creating like that which almost stimulates another level of creativity. So I know that if I don't engage in those creative activities it stifles my overall creativity, so there's generativity about it.'

Interestingly, these notions of creativity each shared a common theme, that of doing or producing. In the creative process there are always two different, yet interrelated dimensions (Herrmann 1996).

Expressions of creativity

In the domain of creativity there seem to be those who are idea generators and those who are problem finders.

'I don't know if for me that's an essential element of creativity, that you perhaps take stuff that's already been there and you mix it together in a new way and come out with something new and different at the end.'

In this statement, the participant is differentiating between original and applied creative thinking. 'The original thinker comes up with a stream of ideas on a given topic and the connector sees their ideas as pieces of the jigsaw puzzle that suddenly fit and bridge together, two thoughts that have been adrift but are now interconnected and whole' (Herrmann 1996).

There is a myth that creativity is the exclusive domain of artists, scientists and inventors – giftedness not available to ordinary people going about the business of daily life – and this was evident in some responses.

'I think it's interesting if you use that term creative and try and apply it to famous people or types of people, in my mind anyway I would think about artists and poets, what I wouldn't think about would be famous scientists for example, people bound by rules. But I'd think about people who've thrown away the rules and gone beyond the boundaries and looked for new forms of expression.'

Because of the strong association of creativity with the arts, participants did not always recognise when they were being creative. I also found that people tended to refer to others as creative but were not always able to recognise this within themselves until they reframed the meaning.

'I don't think I'm creative, because I think of creativity as something to do with arty stuff, I'm not particularly confident with arty kind of stuff … and then I thought no, creativity for me is about making something new. And then I started to think … I do create new things, and I look back at just over the past year and thought, yes, I've created lots of new things and they're things that are new in terms of the way that they're taught … Then I thought, OK, maybe I can be creative.'

'So in terms of work, being creative I don't think I have the time, and when I'm at home I think I have to make time to do things, to relax and de-stress and chill out, so when I think about being creative at home and I do things in the garden. So whereas some of the others might have philosophical thoughts, I just think creation as in planting and growing things, and in terms of drama and doing the acting and being different roles.'

Perceptions of creativity

There is a widely held belief that creativity is associated with right-brain thinking and this was endorsed on several occasions by many of the participants in the study.

'To me creativity is about right-brain thinking, it's about getting away from a standard reductionist approach really is what we're talking about in terms of the written word …'

Another shared perception is that creativity is associated with being 'mad or wacky'. Again, this may overlook the potential creativity that is expressed in different ways.

'That's how I know I am creative, I come up with these entirely mad ideas, crazy ideas about how I can do it. The next stage of course is how you capture that and make them reality and get a product at the end and that's the other side ... the logical working through step by step part of the brain, but the creative side is trying to stand outside anything you have ever done or seen or imagined before and come up with something entirely new or different.'

Factors affecting creativity

What was striking was the fact that all participants considered that creativity is more likely to be expressed in certain situations (see Fig. 12.1). The environmental atmosphere and supportive culture in the workplace can influence the conditions that support the creative process.

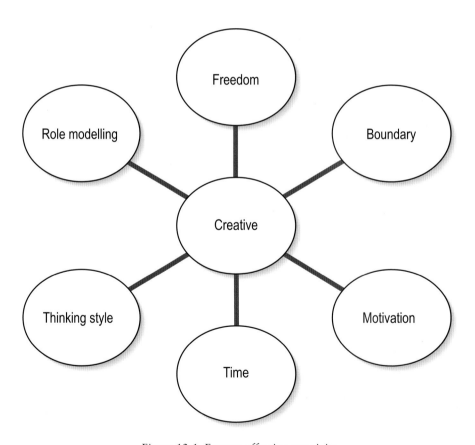

Figure 12.1 Factors affecting creativity

Freedom

A key factor in the ability to express creativity was the extent to which the midwife teachers experienced a sense of freedom within the organisation. Participants stated that this almost felt like permission to be creative. This was expressed as freedom to be creative and boundaries that may hinder facilitate creativity, both of which are experienced at a cultural and personal level.

'But you need a kind of freedom don't you?'

'You can't be constrained by too many rules and regulations and protocols, you actually need a space and freedom to be able to think creatively before you can actually do something creatively.'

However, this may not mean removing all structures; rather, it is about establishing safe, supportive environments in which people are encouraged to be creative, with minimal interference. In fact, the importance of balance between boundaries and freedom was surprising.

Boundaries

Boundaries may also be expressed as having clarity about expectations, imposed by either self or others.

'Yes, the things I thought about were space, that was a big thing for me was having space ... I also feel boundaries are important because somehow you respond to boundaries, they're a stimulus, you might not like them, you might need them, but somehow they get you going.'

'But there's also something about acceptance ... if I'm feeling criticised or judged or the expectations feel too high for me to attain or I'm just too aware of them then I tend to get a bit tied up. Or even if I'm just putting high, unrealistic expectations on myself.'

'I think sometimes it's about knowing about where the edges are because if the space is too big and doesn't feel safe ... It's about having a container within which to be creative, and if they're too constraining that can be positive in the sense that you kind of want to make them bigger but it can also be completely stifling and just take the breath out of it.'

Boundaries for some may appear safe and for others something to be pushed back – almost like a level to go beyond, take risks and challenge current thinking.

'It's risk taking isn't it, creative people are risk takers.'

'In a way that's what some scientists do, they push back those boundaries and produce new thinking which is outside of the realms of normal possibility isn't it, so in a way it is creative I mean art and science are intrinsically linked.'

Motivation

A key theme consistently raised was the issue of motivation to be creative. Initially I explored this in respect of why the participants were in education, leading into reasons why they chose creative teaching and learning approaches.

'...because you want to enthuse the (students) you want them to have a feel for the subject and to have an enthusiasm for it, to grab them. Even if it's something that's a bit dull there are ways of making them enjoy it and to remember it.'

'It's very constrained and, you know, there's no space for fun and the only way you learn is if it's fun. The things that I remember from school or from university are things that you did that were fun, that got you thinking and that got you active. I suppose that's where my philosophy probably comes from – you do what you think you enjoyed in a way.'

Another reason why midwife teachers may be motivated to explore different ways of doing things and coming up with new ideas may be linked to intrinsic motivation. Certainly boredom appears to be an issue expressed by some participants.

'It's keeping it exciting, keeping it alive and that comes down to me being a butterfly again, I need a lot of stimulation and I know that and I know it's a shortcoming in many ways as well. But I deal with it.'

This can also be about ensuring that learning is not boring for learners.

'I think they remember people who are like that and who bring it alive for them, as opposed to the death by overhead. I think that's the difference, you can have the overheads and they do need some of the material in that way, but you've got to have the energy and enthusiasm to do that.'

Many participants expressed a desire to make a difference and saw creative approaches as attempts to think differently about some of the challenges in midwifery.

'I think the difference I would want to make, would be to get them to think for themselves, to be creative thinkers.'

Other constraints appeared to relate to the nature of the work involved, including rather pragmatic factors such as group size, stage of programme, learner's expectations and subject. Although again, this may be more a reflection of the perception of the relevance of the work rather than the work itself.

'What makes that very difficult though is group size, and that's a huge constraint because I believe that to work creatively it needs to be an acceptable size. Working with groups with 40 plus is really difficult.'

'It's interesting because I kind of feel with the subjects that I teach that they are, not superficial level, but I do tend to teach them almost like a set of rules, because I feel like that's what they (students) can manage at that point.'

Time

Time featured prominently, particularly in relation to the way in which creativity is expressed and experienced. Lack of time to be creative appeared to be a factor for some. However, when I explored this further I began to consider that this may be less about time and more about experience or confidence and perception of role as midwife teacher.

'I don't feel I have the time to put into doing things creatively at work. I think that's because I do so many different things and it concerns me that a year goes by and I'm back to doing the same teaching sessions and I haven't really had the time to make them that much different or to revamp them or to make them more interesting.'

Some of the participants considered creative teaching to be a natural element of all their work and in effect no extra effort was invested, whereas for others this did require additional work, hence time factors may become important. In this way we begin to glimpse personal values and beliefs that may influence perceptions about their role as educators.

'I do think that this is a lifestyle … It's not a job it's a lifestyle and it's integral. And you can't pin it down to hours. I'm constantly looking and reading and assimilating and talking to people and it's there…'

Some participants spoke of actually experiencing creativity in real time, i.e. spur of the moment or output in a short space of time. Some situations require spontaneity and the skill of the educator is to be able to respond quickly as well as creatively.

'I remember doing one thing … and I ended up, because I had something on a theoretical level which I planned to do with them which they should have been able to cope with about blood clotting and they couldn't. And I ended up at the end of the day doing a thing about cowboys and Indians and I had them all running round the room being different things.'

Others experienced creativity as a multi-stage process where sufficient time is allowed for the generation and selection of ideas. Clearly, if there is a mismatch between the nature of the creative process and the time available, this may in fact stifle creative energy or manifest as disruption.

'Because you need to have the space and the time … I think some organisations obviously do create an environment that enables staff to be creative, whether that's through research or through new developments. And I think that it does feel like you're battling to make that space to enable you to do it.'

Thinking styles

The combination of freedom, boundaries, space and time seems to allow people to mull things over, revisit thinking over and over, and allow ideas to evolve. Whilst this may relate to the nature of the activity involved, it also reflects the non-linear thinking that accompanies creativity, what Herrmann (1996) refers to as 'zig zag thinking'.

'There is no manual, creativity is not linear or logical steps; you make leaps in your understanding.'

Many participants stated that the form of creative thinking that involves 'originality' evolved more slowly, then suddenly there was a 'leap' forward accompanied by the 'a-ha' phenomenon. This slow unfolding of ideas is an essential quality of creative thinking and typifies unpredictable situations, allowing for spontaneity.

'An idea occurs and acts as a catalyst that builds and builds.'

'Mull over then suddenly from nowhere, a-ha occurs.'

Interestingly, many of the participants described the creative process as slow and reflective, followed by a 'leap forward 'in their understanding of the situation. This has significant implications for the way in which midwife teachers work; without the time and space for the more reflexive and contemplative aspects of our work, the creative potential of a person or organisation may remain untapped.

Role modelling

The majority of participants were able to identify significant people along the way who had influenced their attitude to education and, quite literally, their teaching style.

' …and you know, you do look back to your own experiences of teaching and learning. And my very first teacher, I remember her now … and she was an amazing teacher and she was doing almost inquiry-based learning when I was nine … And for that to be a lasting memory of my school days speaks volumes about that woman's ability to engage and she was fantastic and she's one of those people … Probably the most vivid memory in terms of learning and teaching as a role model.'

However, a number of participants could not recall such good role modelling when it came to the experience of preparing for their role as professional educators.

'I never learnt anything on that; to be honest, I actually learnt how not to do things.'

'I do think that the education about teaching that we get, is very restrictive in some way and it would be really useful to explore things like … what that means and how we can put that into practice. But there isn't anywhere to exchange that stuff and talk about how it might work for this subject or that subject, and in some ways it's a bit sad …'

This is an important consideration if midwife teachers are to develop their potential creativity as well as gain confidence in trying new teaching approaches.

Creativity: from dichotomy to metaphor

'Creative thinking deals with shades of grey, not with blacks and whites.'

(Anon)

The first theme revealed that participants attempted to explain creativity from many different perspectives, without offering formalised or concrete definitions. I was very conscious of this and the resulting need to avoid 'in the box thinking' about what creativity is, who is creative and how it is expressed. It seems from the data that creativity means different things to different people and attempting to define creativity may limit our understanding. The very essence of creativity is the universality and individuality that are characteristic of the dichotomies manifest within creativity. It seems to be multidimensional and multifactorial.

This was perhaps best captured when the participants talked about their experience of 'being creative' during the second focus group. A range of dialectics was revealed, almost as a creative continuum that is perhaps inevitably difficult to convey in written form. As an observer, I began to sense a shift in thinking, as well as in group relationships, between the first and second focus group. It was apparent to me that we were beginning to engage in something much more fundamental, exploring personal philosophies in an open and meaningful way. This was characterised by an expression about what creativity actually meant on a personal level. The language had softened and assumed a much more free and feminine feel. There was evidence of a distinct transition from fixed meanings to fluidity.

The dichotomies expressed included the comparison of left- versus right-brain thinking, midwifery as art versus midwifery as science and rationality versus imagination. However, while describing these dichotomies, the midwife teachers used highly imaginative and creative forms of expression. The metaphors were accompanied by animation and the educators almost became like actors on a stage. It is impossible to convey the meaning behind the words and capture the collective energy that was unleashed. It was as if a touch paper had been lit and then 'Whoosh' ...

'To have those ideas milling round, bubbling up and having coloured visions of how it could be.'

Metaphors allow a person to express feelings, thoughts, experiences for which there are no easy words; in this way, we know more than we can tell. The use of metaphors by the participants during the study could be interpreted as part of the process of praxis (Mezirow 1990).

During the focus groups creativity was frequently expressed as being fluid-like and evolutionary. This generated a sense of movement that was confirmed by the metaphors and dichotomous statements. One of the most powerful metaphors that stimulated the most debate and unleashed the creative energy in the group was 'creativity as fireworks' (Fig. 12.2).

'I think that's for me that's what it is, it's about this release of energy, they talk about creative energy don't they, it's about, and you feel stimulated and excited and energised.'

It is possible to situate creativity within the context of the soul, particularly when we consider the energy that is so characteristic of the way in which midwife teachers expressed creativity during the study. The creative energy was flowing and art was used to capture this moment to say more than we can tell (Fig. 12.3).

Some of the metaphors used are expanded upon in Box 12.1 and included:

* teaching is like making a cake
* becoming a midwife is like being in a war zone
* being a teacher is like being an artist
* preparing students is like preparing a woman for birth.

It is interesting to note that at this stage of the research, the polarisation associated with the right/left-brain thinking model was apparent only in the ways in which the participants defined creativity. Initially, I was aware of a level of divergent thinking that may be indicative of the rather subjective assumptions about what constitutes creativity in midwifery education. This is understandable given the diversity of creative thinking and range of experience within the group. When the wider issue of values and beliefs

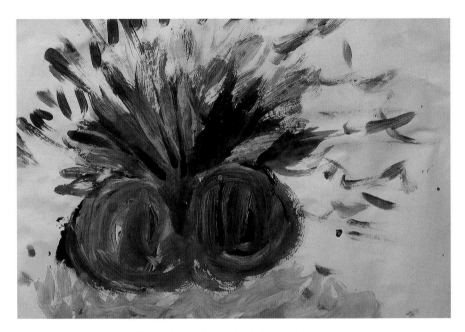

Figure 12.2 Creativity is like a firework

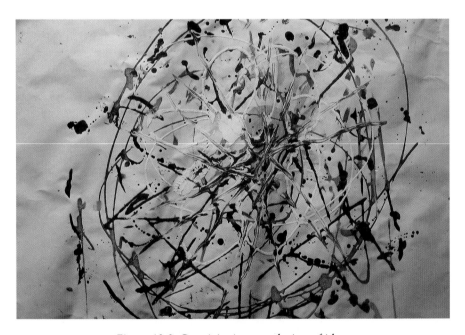

Figure 12.3 Creativity is an explosion of ideas

Box 12.1

Creativity as metaphor

Teaching is like making a cake
- It is a mix like a cake
- Has to be a good mixture
- If you don't have all the right ingredients, it falls flat
- Like a cake when it's divided up, we lose something
- We get caught up in all the structures
- It starts to feed itself and gets bigger and bigger
- Fit student into a mould
- Units of production in a factory
- Creating a recipe to make something new

Becoming a midwife is like being in a war zone
- They have to conform to survive
- The health service is like a war zone so you need to be good at survival
- Even if they could be creative, you see it driven out of them
- Until they give up
- It's beaten out of them or suppressed
- Midwifery is quite violent for students
- We crush their spirit early on
- Because they have to do that surviving thing, they're not just learning how to be a midwife, they're learning about other stuff

Being a teacher is like being an artist
- Teacher as artist
- If you're in a theatrical performance and go on stage, you get butterflies, don't you? Well it's the same in teaching
- Creative tension/energy
- Alternative way of being creative
- How do I do the dance of being compassionate with the students and recognise they are on an incredibly tough journey?
- Sew the seeds and watch them cracking out of their seed shell things
- To do your birth art
- When I think of creativity, the first thing that came into my head was about drama and theatre

Preparing students is like preparing a woman for birth
- Feels like you are getting them through
- Like giving birth then – you work past the pain
- Don't raise their expectations
- We'd forgotten the enormity of what it was that we were facilitating. It was about letting spirit out
- Motherhood and midwifery the whole transformational nature
- It's like is labour: particularly pleasant, no, but it's how you get your baby out

that underpin individual approaches to midwifery education were explored, similarities emerged.

The reality of those similarities was marked by the sense of dislocation and separation within midwifery as a whole. The midwife teachers may experience this far more acutely as a result of the geographical dislocation from the practice of midwifery. Although these were expressed as dichotomies and metaphors, this appeared to be an indication of dissonance within the role rather than between midwife teachers.

It is perhaps interesting to note that creative thinking appears to only partly explain any difference in the approaches to teaching and learning that the participants used. There was something else happening on a much more fundamental level that may elucidate this issue further. From the data analysis, it was possible to identify where each of the participants is currently in relation to a continuum of creative teaching and learning. This represents the juxtaposition between where they are now, where they may be going and why.

This forms the basis of the third theme, 'Integration', and charts the next leg of the journey, as we travelled away from discontinuities and separation towards continuation and integration.

Integration: from separation to holism

The dichotomies referred to earlier suggest that midwife teachers may be experiencing a sense of separation on a number of levels. The creative approaches used appear to be in response to the need for integration and reflect a sense of movement. Achieving an integrative approach is challenged by separation of the curriculum into parts (i.e. modules), although this may be balanced by a shared philosophy that seeks to overcome the separateness.

'[It's] important to achieve a seamless approach … a community of spirit.'

Achieving a shared philosophy within a curriculum is challenging, particularly where a curriculum is based upon a model that is primarily grounded in a humanistic philosophy but that fails to provide a specification about the practice of teaching (Stenhouse 1975). The quality of the curriculum is dependent upon the skill of the midwife educator to translate and act as mediator between the vision of what may be achieved and the aspiring midwife, by creating the right opportunities.

'And the thing is when you were saying about your pictures, I can remember
that actually created a very good response from students because it was
something very simple, they were allowed to be creative and think differently
and to verbalise, it just had much more impact than the written word, and … the
joy of doing that is that every time I do it it's different, it's always a surprise.'

There is a sense here of the midwife educator engaging in the role of knowledge making rather than knowledge telling. Acting as navigator whilst the aspiring midwife finds her own path through, making sense of the reality of practice and making choices about how she will practise as a midwife, based upon her own preferences and not those prescribed by others.

'I think the fact that I make it very, very explicitly clear to them, given any
opportunity to do so that it's OK, whatever they think is OK. I think that's quite
important because they need to feel safe to be able to explore stuff … I give them

lots of opportunities to practise and look at scenarios that are pretty open and blank actually and give them as few details as possible.'

This is the difference between espoused theory and making it happen – the difference between the theories in use, i.e. what we actually do, and those that are espoused theory, i.e. what we say we do. The distinction is, according to Schon (1987), a matter of the difference between professional and organisational practice. This may also influence the theory–practice gap and the dissonance between the formal and actual curriculum, between what is and what could be.

From the data, there is a sense in which the creative midwife teacher is actively working with the theory–practice rub, using the energy to spark ideas and challenge practice through facilitating aspiring midwives to think holistically about contemporary midwifery. This is important to aspiring midwives who encounter conflicts on a routine basis between what is taught and what is seen in practice.

For aspiring midwives, integration is important to making sense of the world of practice and one approach that the midwife educators appear to use is promotion of deep personal learning. It is important to prepare students for professional practice in a way that enables them to distinguish between different theories of action.

'...and you know that whatever comes up, even if you've never met it before, because the whole thing about being an expert is that you can operate in complex situations that you've never come across and you can actually manage it and deal with it creatively and effectively and competently.'

'And that's the difference between allowing students just to learn the skills and drills, you know you go through it, they learn that and that's fine and you can assess them and yes they can take a temperature properly, that's fine, but what if they haven't got a thermometer? It's when you take away and put them into situations where they can't use those skills that it becomes dangerous.'

'I try and engage them on a level that makes them relate everything we're doing to practice and to the woman. Although we might be looking at theoretical stuff and it might be related to physiology but trying to bring that down so that they can see how it locks in to their clinical practice and to working with women and families, trying to make it real for them, I suppose.'

It appears that some midwife teachers manage to incorporate creative approaches to learning and teaching that not only develop the power of individuals and groups to engage in learning on a more personal and much deeper level, but also introduce freedom to push back the boundaries.

'A good way to teach is to be constantly engaging with the learner ... the teacher gives an idea, the student comes back and says is that what you mean and back again, backwards and forwards, and that feels right to me that that should be constantly going on, whether it's on a verbal level or a non-verbal level. Are you understanding that, is it like this, is it like that, all the time constant dialogue going on.'

Learning is fundamentally a social phenomenon; people organise their learning around the social communities to which they belong.

'I genuinely don't think that we learn alone, I think what you can do is bounce off, one idea links to another, and it starts creating different ways of thinking and you need to do it in communities ... of practice and of learning that actually can foster, you can delve much deeper in that process than sitting at home, looking in the mirror and saying I'm reflecting now.'

This approach is based on the principle that midwife teachers not only understand but also belong to the community of practice and acknowledge the learning that takes place within this community. Midwife teachers can then structure learning opportunities that embed knowledge in both work practices and social relations, as occurs with the apprenticeship model (Davis-Floyd 1998).

'Yeah and maybe that's what they [other educators] are doing, they maintain the barriers and these are the students and we are the teachers instead of trying to, we're all women at the end of the day.'

Perhaps part of the dichotomy that faces all midwives is the extent to which we feel disconnected from the wider community of women. In education, this 'separateness' may be experienced even more acutely due to the physical distance as well as the professional dislocation that the midwife teachers expressed. As we change, so does our learning, our identity, and our relationship to the community or group changes.

'That's one issue that we're not providing the practice areas with the kind of midwives they want, but then as educators that's not necessarily our job ... a lot of people moved into education to get away from the system and concurrently to try and do something to enable midwives to be different from that system.'

During the focus groups the participants frequently referred to the importance of enabling aspiring midwives to make connections and provide a holistic model of care to women during childbirth.

'I don't think of it as being deep though, to me it's integrated, it's holism Because you're not just looking at reduced parts, you're looking at a situation with a woman and a baby and a midwife and you're putting that reductionist information into a human situation and it's about integration.'

In part, this seems to arise from a genuine desire expressed by each of the midwife teachers to make a difference in midwifery. This was expressed on different levels, ranging from the individual woman or the aspiring midwife, to the community and wider society.

'It is interesting actually that when I think about it as a midwife ... one of my aims was to help women to get to a point where actually they didn't really need me. I always used to think that's what you should be trying to do as a midwife. To empower somebody and give them the confidence to do it, not unsupported but to feel like they could do it. And I suppose teaching is the same thing.'

From this perspective, the process becomes as much about our role as educators making judgements about the direction that our work is taking, as it is about the aspiring midwives preparing themselves for practice and women preparing themselves for birth and their role as mothers.

'So if we're not training them to fit into the system, are we training them to cope with the system? I'm not entirely convinced that we are because I think what we're trying to do is to train them to rise above the system and I think our expectations of them are enormous and I think that a lot of the time we're expecting things of them that we're not always doing ourselves.'

In effect, the actual curriculum may be vastly different to what is formally written, influenced by the powerful factors normally referred to as the 'hidden' curriculum, including the values and beliefs held by educators.

'I think the problem is to survive they must conform to the work culture. So even those that would have that creative flair that you can perhaps see at the beginning, as time goes on it's almost driven out of them.'

The tension that we appear to experience as midwife teachers is located somewhere between the expectations of what health service employers require from curricula that prepare aspiring midwives for practice, and the educator's personal philosophy about the purpose of education and how these influence teaching styles that foster conformity or empowerment (Grundy 1987).

'You engage with the woman and we know that a lot of problems in midwifery stem from not being able to throw away the mantle of Nurse and, you know, caring for this person in a nursing sense as opposed to caring for her in a reciprocal mutual way.'

During the study, the sense that midwife teachers are also engaged in some form of survival emerged as they swayed between wishing to make a difference by preparing aspiring midwives for what is, as well as what could be

'I think one of the big drawbacks is we sometimes can set people up to fail by introducing a more holistic approach in contrast with what they see in practice where it's very reductionist, constant push me pull you, isn't it?'

Clearly, the skill of teaching is central to this, informed by the personal values and beliefs that influence approaches to midwifery practice and education. It would appear that midwife teachers use a number of strategies to manage the inherent tensions in contemporary midwifery. These include providing an integrative approach to accommodate the inherent diversity of midwifery practice and education, including creative thinking and creative teaching. To achieve this, some midwife teachers are prepared to take risks and introduce dimensions that are rarely considered in midwifery education, such as the spiritual or psychic domain.

'...there could be a more creative way or a more satisfying way for me or the learners, whoever ... doing something challenging and different that is going to stretch them or excite them or delight them would be much more satisfying and I get these from these imaginative and creative leaps ... like reading a story – because I was trying to capture different parts of ... linking into the emotional life as well as their imaginative and physical lives...'

The soulful dimension

'From the time we are born, there is a wildish urge within us that desires our souls to lead our lives, for the ego can only understand just so much.'

(Pinkola Estés 1992)

The terms 'spirit' and 'soul' are often used as if they had one meaning.

> 'Some people use the words spirit and soul interchangeably. But in fairy tales the
> soul is always the pro-gynitor and the progenitor of spirit. In arcane hermeneutics,
> the spirit is a being born of the soul. The spirit inherits or incarnates into matter
> in order to gather news of the ways of the world and carries these back to the
> soul. When not interfered with, the relationship between soul and spirit is one
> of perfect symmetry; each enriches the other in turn. Together the soul and spirit
> form an ecology as in a pond where the creatures at the bottom nourish those at
> the top and those at the top nourish those at the bottom.'
>
> (Pinkola Estés 1992, p.272)

In the New Testament, the word for spirit is 'pneuma' while the word for soul is 'psyche'.
The Bible tells us that we are made up of three distinct parts: soul, spirit and body.
However, this view contrasts sharply with Bohm's (1957, cited in Zukav 1979) theory
of unbroken wholeness, 'which instead of starting with parts as in the Cartesian order,
begins with the whole which includes space, time, matter are all included as forms of
an implicate order in the Universe, "that which is"' (Zukav 1979). Such an approach
demands a different worldview as our current thinking is based on a reality which
essentially means all that you can think about.

During one of the focus groups, the group chose to express what creativity meant
to them through art rather than verbally. The paintings revealed a glimpse of something beyond words or even thoughts. Through art, as with the use of metaphors and
symbols, the midwife teachers were able to express more than they know.

> 'It is possible that this experience revealed a glimpse of the soul, the true essence
> of who we are, the part that remains unaffected by physical life events and learns
> our life lessons. Our spirit is part of the soul that reacts to our life experience, so
> that is why we become dis-spirited or spiritual.'
>
> (Skinner 2005, personal communication)

> 'I think using these settings and the arts is touching the circle in a way that
> is quite difficult to achieve, aiming for not transcendence, but a spiritual
> dimension.'

At the heart of holistic learning are midwife teachers taking charge of their personal and
professional growth by developing reflective, insightful practices rooted in transformative principles. In studying their work, we are able to discover the value of spiritual
learning activities that restore wholeness and wonder to learning.

> 'We'd forgotten the enormity of what it was that you're facilitating but it was
> about that, letting the spirit out.'

> 'Personal inquiry for me is my alternative way of being creative – in a way it's
> a deeper kind of inquiry than what I did in midwifery – spirituality inquiry – I
> don't know whether that's deeper, it feels more challenging. So midwifery is built
> on the spiritual.'

It is important to note here that as each of the participants expressed a strong identification with a holistic approach, this may influence perception of the irrational or spiritual
dimension of their role, whereas those who are more closely aligned with a humanistic
model may describe their role in more rational terms.

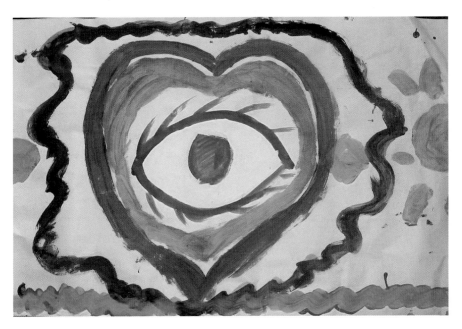

Figure 12.4 Unity

Recently, the terms 'holistic' and 'soul' have entered the language of education and educational research. Holistic education is a new paradigm, with a strong body of research and praxis that supports the development of more integrated modes of consciousness. This is possibly best demonstrated when midwife teachers talk about the purpose of what they are doing and relate this to that of the aspiring midwife.

> 'I was just thinking about that question, what are we preparing them for? And it comes back to this whole thing that we're preparing them, and why aren't we facilitating their preparing themselves? And saying to them at the outset, meet somebody individually and sit down and look at what their needs are and say to them, what kind of midwife would you like to be?'

In this way it becomes their journey not ours and the skill of the midwife teacher is in enabling the aspiring midwife to navigate her own journey.

> 'I remember sitting at graduation and there were particular students that went up there to get their degrees and you think you know, you think back to what that student was like and there are one or two of them that you feel really sort of proud that they've achieved that and managed to navigate their own way through.'

> 'So there's something about it being the sort of lifeblood of our souls to be creative. And I think it's really inspiring, I think creativity's inspiring and it's quite uplifting, good for the soul.'

When I reflected upon the soulful ways in which the midwife teachers had expressed creativity, I was struck by the following elements.

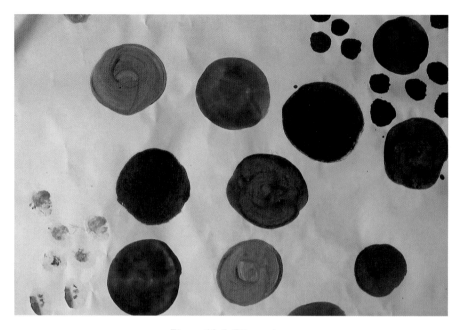

Figure 12.5 Dimensions

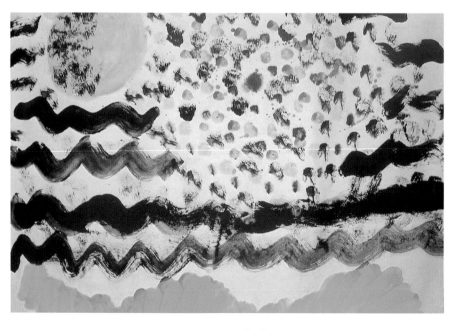

Figure 12.6 Fluidity

- *Spiral shape*, reflecting the cyclical nature of life; denotes the human spirals that wind through individual minds, also non-hierarchical levels represented by colours (Beck & Cowan 1996).
- *Fluidity* as expressed by the midwife educators when responding creatively to the dichotomies within their role.
- *Unity* expressed as mind, body, spirit and soul and represented by Wilbur (2000) as 'I/It/ We/Its' dimensions of 'being' in the world.
- *Dimensions* that connect mind, body, spirit and soul within a continuum.
- *Integration* of the technocratic, humanistic and holistic paradigms (Davis-Floyd 2001).

Continuing the journey ...

When I first decided to plan this journey, I was motivated to do so by a desire to understand what it is that some midwife educators do that makes a difference to aspiring midwives. Having decided upon a possible destination, I mapped the journey, including who else would accompany me. I endeavoured to maintain an open mind, possibly a one-way ticket, about the final destination. It was important from the outset not to define what creativity was so as not to limit the potential interpretation by participants. However, it soon became clear that the general assumption that 'right-brain thinking equates with creativity' was not broad enough to accommodate the diverse ways in which creativity is both expressed and experienced.

In response, the concept of whole-brain thinking and connections to holistic midwifery emerged as possible destinations. Each of the participants demonstrated creativity in their teaching within a continuum that represented whole-brain thinking. The comparisons between these and the technocratic, humanistic and holistic paradigms of childbirth, described by Davis-Floyd (2001), were striking but the data analysis appeared to offer up more than a holistic model of education could accommodate. As Polyani (1967) would suggest, 'we know more than we can tell'.

The sense of movement that the midwife teachers were experiencing was not explicit and in fact, did not actually unfold until the final stages of data analysis. Indeed, work on this is still ongoing. The sense of fluidity was clearly apparent as expressed through the way in which midwife educators responded to the dichotomies in their role and were creative in multidimensional ways. I was able to gain insight into the spiritual dimension of the work that some midwife teachers are also involved in. The way in which this was expressed was different within the group and emerged as a possible factor in explaining why some midwife teachers may be perceived as more creative than others.

The connection with the soul was quite dramatic when considered on the mind–body–spirit–soul continuum. When I completed a literature review, it was interesting to note the alliance of this with spiral dynamics. Beck & Cowan (1996) propose a spiral developmental model of worldviews characterised by patterns of thinking; the authors suggest that currently eight levels of thinking exist. Significantly, they are not presented as a hierarchy, as one better than the other; rather, they are fluid and capable of transformation. The essential quality is fluidity, as represented by a spiral.

Another analogy that springs to mind here is that of dancing.

'Wu Li Masters perceive in both ways, the rational and the irrational, the assertive and the receptive, the masculine and the feminine. They reject neither one nor the other. They only dance.'

(Zukav 1979)

'Midwifery education is like a dance. I feel like they are always doing a dance, so the two are almost like not separate again.'

The tentative destination

- Creative teaching involves whole-brain thinking and is embedded within a continuum of creative dimensions.
- Midwife educators who use creative teaching approaches appear to have values and beliefs that fit with a holistic midwifery model.
- The relationship between each of the dimensions of creativity appears to be connected in some way to the mind–body–spirit–soul continuum. This may explain the way in which midwife teachers make a difference to aspiring midwives.

A breakdown of the key issues which arose from this study has been summarised in Box 12.2, for the purpose here of charting the journey as it unfolds. These issues are not intended to provide a definitive list; indeed, the points made here simply provide the basis for further study.

I am aware that I have not arrived; rather, I am only just beginning the journey. What the midwife teachers who participated in this journey have offered up, and grounded theory made sense of, represents the first step along a winding road. However, at this juxtaposition between what has been and what is yet to come, it is possible to make some tentative links between creativity and factors that influence midwife educators' ability to be creative in their teaching.

Soulful Midwives

'Be soft in your practice – think of the method as a fine silvery stream, not a raging waterfall. Follow the stream, have faith in its course. It will go its own way, meandering here, trickling there. It will find the grooves, the cracks, the crevices. Just follow it. Never let it out of your sight. It will take you.'

(Sheng-yen 2004)

Box 12.2

Factors identified by midwife educators as key influences upon creativity

- Creativity and innovation are different approaches in curriculum design
- Creative thinking involves whole-brain thinking approaches, not just right-brained
- Educators who use creative teaching approaches appear to have values and beliefs that fit with a humanistic education model and holistic midwifery model

---

Continued

Box 12.2—cont'd

Factors identified by midwife educators as key influences upon creativity

- Teachers who use creative teaching appear to be both right- and left-brained in thinking orientation
- Teachers who use creative approaches can all identify the arts as influential in their formative or later years
- The motivation to make a difference to the lives of people appears quite strong, i.e. it is not just a job, etc.
- Those teachers who used different forms of expression during their teaching could identify a role model/mentor who influenced them
- The organisational culture is considered to be of great significance in the ability of teachers to feel free or safe to take risks and step out of the box
- Having time to plan and reflect upon different approaches is important
- Creative problem solving requires time to mull things over
- Preparation for midwives to become professional educators should include opportunities to explore the purpose of education, including creative approaches
- Collective creativity works for development of ideas and is best undertaken in a supportive team
- All the midwife teachers strongly identified with the holistic model in their midwifery practice
- There appears to be a relationship between creativity and spiritual dimensions that is not fully explained by holism

References

Bass J 2001 A partnership curriculum. Anglia Polytechnic University, Chelmsford, UK

Bass J (2003) An exploration of creative approaches to learning and teaching used by midwife educators in facilitating the preparation of student midwives for midwifery practice. Master's dissertation thesis. Anglia Polytechnic University, Chelmsford, UK

Beck D E, Cowan C 1996 Spiral dynamics: mastering values, leadership and change. Blackwell, London

Benoit C, Davis-Floyd R, van Teijlingen E, Sandall J, Miller J 2001 Designing midwives: a comparison of educational models in birth by design. In: DeVries R, Benoit C, van Teijlingen E, Wrede S (eds) Pregnancy, maternity care and midwifery in North America and Europe. Routledge, New York

Davis-Floyd R 1998 Different types of midwifery training: an anthropological overview. In: Southern J, Rosenberg J, Tritten J (eds) Pathways to becoming a midwife: getting an education. Midwifery Today, Eugene, OR

Davis-Floyd R 2001 The technocratic, humanistic and holistic paradigms of childbirth. International Journal of Gynaecology and Obstetrics 75(1): 5–23

Downe S, McCourt C 2004 From being to becoming: reconstructing childbirth knowledges. In: Downe S (ed) Normal childbirth: evidence and debate. Churchill Livingstone, London

Grundy S 1987 Curriculum: product or praxis? Falmer, Lewes

Herrmann N 1996 The whole brain business book. McGraw-Hill, New York

Hodnett E D 2002 Pain and women's satisfaction with the experience of childbirth: a systematic review. In: The nature and management of labour pain: peer reviewed paper from an evidence-based symposium. American Journal of Obstetrics and Gynecology 186: 171

Kelly A V 1995 Education and democracy. Paul Chapman Publishing, London

Karll S 2003 Sacred birthing: birthing a new humanity. Trafford, Canada

Mezirow J 1990 Fostering critical reflection in adulthood. Jossey Bass, San Francisco

Odent M 1999 The scientification of love. Free Association Books, London

Parker P 1998 The courage to teach. Jossey Bass, San Francisco

Pinkola Estés C 1992 Women who run with the wolves. Rider, London

Polyani M 1967 The tacit dimension. Routledge and Kegan Paul, London

Schon D 1987 Educating the reflective practitioner: toward a new design for teaching and learning in the professions. Jossey Bass, San Francisco

Sheng-yen 2004 Creating sacred space. In: London E, Recio B (eds) Sacred rituals. Fair Winds Press, London

Stenhouse L 1975 An introduction to curriculum research and development. Heinemann, London

Taylor M 1996 An ex- midwife's reflections on supervision from a psychotherapeutic viewpoint. In: Kirkham M J (ed) Supervision of midwives. Books for Midwives Press, Hale

Wilbur K 2000 The theory of everything: an integral vision for business, political sciences and spirituality. Shambhala, Boston

Zukav G 1979 The dancing Wu Li masters: an overview of the new physics. Rider, London

Feeling the Fear and Doing it Regardless! Creative Ideas for Midwifery Education

$\longmapsto$ —————————— (•) ———————————— $\longmapsto$

LORNA DAVIES AND SARA WICKHAM

'The most important developments in civilisation have come through the creative process, but ironically most people have not been taught to create.'

(Fritz 1994)

Introduction

This is intended to be a chapter about doing rather than saying. There are numerous texts espousing educational theory but fewer that give practical, creative ideas for use in midwifery education. This chapter offers some of the ideas that we have developed, begged, borrowed or adapted during our time working as midwife teachers. We hope that it will pull together some of the theory explored within the other chapters and offer further perspectives. By outlining a selection of activities that we have utilised over the years, we will address some of the implications of using a creative approach in midwifery education and the processes involved.

Hughes (1995) states that the current Western educational system is based primarily on knowledge that has been generated and collected through the positivist approach to learning and meaning-making. It is based on a reductionist approach and is largely aimed at delivering facts and information through cognitive lectures and content.

Most students view this educational setting as a passive way of learning. They are not actively engaged in the process. There is often little discussion, participation or engagement in the lecture by the student. Opportunities to challenge what the authority figure is saying and the freedom to propose alternative theories through personal experience are few and far between.

The pitcher metaphor is useful in relation to discussion of this didactic approach to teaching and learning (Samples 1987). The teacher acts as the pitcher who contains the knowledge. They pour knowledge into the empty vessel, which is the student. After the transaction, it is assumed that the glass is at least half full. When using creative teaching activities, the student is very much at the centre of the learning experience and some of the knowledge, at least, will have been self-generated.

You may not be able to teach someone to be creative, but you can facilitate creative thinking and, by teaching creatively, we can role model creative thinking. Teachers cannot be expected to develop the creative abilities of the students if their own creative abilities are suppressed. By teaching creatively, we can make learning more interesting, exciting and effective and fire the students' interests and motivate their learning.

In teaching for creativity, we must aim to allow for both broad and narrowly focused experimental activity but always specify and explain the purpose of the activity. The students have to feel prepared and secure enough to be willing to take risks and make mistakes in a non-threatening, non-judgemental environment that challenges but also reassures.

We perhaps should also consider that there are important links between lifelong learning and creativity. Learning and creativity are enhanced and sustained by a range of abilities, attributes and activities common to both, including intrinsic motivation, enterprise, persistence and resilience, curiosity, questioning and reflecting, assessing and testing, moving from problems to solutions and back to new problems, understanding and using failures on the road to success.

This chapter is loosely divided into six sections exploring different ideas, and we have called the chapter 'Feeling the Fear and Doing it Regardless' because it really is a question of letting go of long-held assumptions and jumping in at the deep end.

Quickies and icebreakers

Icebreakers are activities used to help groups relax and ease into a learning situation. When used effectively, they allow the group leader to foster interaction, stimulate creative thinking, challenge basic assumptions, illustrate new concepts and introduce specific material (Newstrom & Scannell 1995). However, our experience of working with student groups (especially teaching practical skills for parent education) has led us to believe that many midwives and student midwives have an almost pathological aversion to icebreakers!

It is all too easy to be sceptical about the value of icebreakers. We have frequently heard comments that suggest that they are designed to patronise and humiliate group members. In this chapter, we intend to demonstrate that icebreakers can be introduced in a non-threatening and inclusive way, that can offer the group members an opportunity to get to know one another and to learn things about themselves. We are convinced that if we get the icebreaking right, then we are 95% of the way to creating a good group dynamic.

The major clue is to use an icebreaker that is appropriate for the particular purpose that you wish it to serve. For example, if we consider the situation where people are meeting for the first time and may feel self-conscious, nervous and even defensive, what sort of icebreaker is going to be least threatening? Perhaps introducing someone other than themselves, so choose an icebreaker that does just that. If you want to recap names, then think of an icebreaker that will allow the group to briefly introduce themselves.

As facilitator, it is important that you role model for the group, who may be apprehensive. They will invariably take your lead and offer similar sort of information. This gives you some degree of control, but can also narrow the information offered. However, your finely honed facilitation skills will ensure that you are able to elicit more information with gentle probing.

There are probably 101 ways to use an icebreaker, and 1001 different icebreakers. However, the icebreaking activities listed in this chapter are an assorted selection of the ones that we have used in midwifery education, for getting-to-know-you sessions, parent education, etc.

Box 13.1

Pairs icebreaker

- Select a number of characters who come in pairs, such as those listed below.
- Ensure that you have the right number of paired characters for the numbers in your group.
- Write the names of the individual characters onto pieces of paper.
- Get the group to take a piece of paper each naming their character.
- When everyone has a character, get them to find their matching pair in the room.
- Ask them to talk for 2 minutes about their journey, their hobbies, etc.
- Reconvene and get the characters to introduce their matching pair to the group, e.g. Adam will introduce Eve and vice versa.

ADAM / EVE
LAUREL / HARDY
TOM / JERRY
ROMEO / JULIET
DASTARDLY / MUTLEY
HOLMES / WATSON
POSH / BECKS
CHARLES / CAMILLA
JEKYLL / HYDE
ABBOTT / COSTELLO
SAMSON / DELILAH
BUSH / BLAIR
ANT / DEC
ROSIE / JIM

Points to consider

- *This is a good initial icebreaker because it enables the group members to divert attention from themselves whilst they are introducing their 'other half'.*
- *However, it is quite lengthy and, depending on the size of your group, may take some time to complete.*
- *You can choose a theme, e.g. children's character, comedians, biblical characters, etc.*
- *It is possible to double the pairs activity up to fours, fives or even eights, by finding suitable groupings of people or objects. This is particularly useful when you have a larger group.*

Setting the scene

Role playing as a learning tool is a well-utilised methodology (Bolton & Heathcote 1999) and we use it as a basic tool of life without often even realising it. The 'what

---

Box 13.2

The touchstone exercise

For this icebreaker you will need enough small, attractive, coloured stones for everyone in the group, placed within a basket. Get the group to sit in a circle, close enough to each other to hand on and receive stones easily. Explain to the group that this exercise is designed to help us get in touch with three aspects of life that contribute to our overall health and well-being: a good relationship with ourselves; a good relationship with all other living beings; and a good relationship with the earth.

Get everyone to select a stone from the basket. Ask each group member to share briefly with the group:

- their full name and some mention of its possible meaning or significance (representing relationship with oneself)
- an animal that has been special in our life, as a pet, e.g., or as an object of fascination and interest (representing relationship with all other living beings)
- a place on earth that is special as a place of beauty, comfort, good memories, inspiration, relaxation (representing relationship with the earth).

When the first person has finished sharing, everyone should pass their stone to the person on their left and receive the stone from the person on their right. By the time the exercise is completed, everyone will have had their stone touched by everyone in the group and will have touched everyone else's stone, but will each end up with their own stone. Explain to the group that they may keep their stone for the rest of their life, or give it back to the universe at some point.

Points to consider
- *This is a very powerful icebreaker as it has the potential to unleash some deeply held beliefs and values. Therefore the group need to feel very safe and comfortable with one another.*
- *It is an ideal introduction to issues around spirituality in the childbearing period.*
- *It is quite time consuming and has the potential to take over the whole session, so be prepared.*

Box 13.3

Birthday and other lines

Tell the group to imagine that one end of the room is January and the opposite end, December. Get them to stand on an imaginary line in between January and December where their birthday falls. When they are all in place, get them to turn to the person beside them and talk for 2 minutes. Return to the group and ask everybody to introduce their partner.

Box 13.3 (Continued)

Points to consider
- *Similar rationale to the pairs game; a good introductory icebreaker.*
- *Additionally serves to establish common ground between group members.*
- *You could use the same principle and apply it to other 'lines', such as the geography line. One end of the room is the north of Scotland, the other the south of England. Students then decide where to stand according to where they come from – the geography obviously has to be adapted to the group!*

Box 13.4

Uncle Robert's seat game

- Sit the group in a circle and explain that you are going to give them a series of instructions (examples of these are listed below).
- If any of the group members can fulfil the requirement, they will be asked to move round the seated circle for a nominated number of places, determined by the facilitator.
- This will mean that two or more people may end up sitting on the same seat at the same time.
- The person who manages to return to their seat first is declared to be the winner.

Sample instructions
- If you watched Coronation Street on Monday night, move two places.
- If you can say the alphabet backwards, move one place.
- If you buy your undies from Marks and Spencers, move three places.
- If you can tell me the names of the members of the group All Saints, move two places.
- If you own more than three pets, move one place.
- If you have eaten an Indian takeway in the last week, move two places.

Points to consider
- *This is an example of an icebreaker where more is better. The bigger the group, the more effective the activity.*
- *Clarify with the group that no-one has any injuries that may put them at risk from the activity (bearing in mind that someone may end up with four or more people 'sitting' on them).*
- *This game can get very noisy, which is great for icebreaking but less so for the facilitator's voice – it can be really useful to have a microphone for this one!*

---

if' scenarios that we sometimes play out in our own heads allow us to project into the future and are a form of role play.

This section includes a few of the methods that we have used in order to create a mood or atmosphere. These activities can be extremely effective, giving the students

---

Box 13.5

Heraldic shield

- Have large pieces of paper and coloured pencils/crayons available as the group members arrive.
- Ask each person (as they arrive) to draw a shield on the paper which they should then divide into quarters.
- Ask them then to draw something which represents their life in each quarter.
- Get them to feed back to group.

Points to consider

- *This icebreaker is good for a first session because it gives members something to do whilst waiting for everyone to arrive.*
- *They also have something to focus on when talking about themselves which deflects immediate attention from themselves.*

---

a deeper sense of understanding by making sense of the theory by gathering together concepts into a practical experience. As Kirsten Baker identifies in Chapter 9, role play can be used to enrich and deepen the experience of the performer and the observer.

It should be remembered that if the introduction of role play is not handled well, it can become an ineffective and even a damaging exercise, as some people will almost certainly feel uncomfortable about participating. The need for a safe space cannot be overstated. Several of the exercises listed are led by the facilitator who takes on the role of 'lead' actor and takes the students into a 'virtual world' where they unwittingly become participant observers. This allows the students to engage in the immediacy of the exercise without feeling compromised or self-conscious. It may be prudent to consider using something similar as an introduction to role play.

Triggers for learning

Problem-based learning (PBL) is a facilitative educational method that challenges students to 'learn to learn', working cooperatively in groups to seek solutions to real-world problems. It prepares students to think critically and analytically, and to acquire life-long learning skills which include the ability to find and use appropriate learning resources.

Problem-based learning transfers control of the learning process from the teacher to the student. The students formulate and pursue their own learning objectives and select those learning resources which are best suited to their current information needs. Teachers contribute to PBL by providing suggestions. In problem-based learning, the traditional teacher and student roles change. The students assume increasing responsibility for their learning, giving them more motivation and more feelings of accomplishment, setting the pattern for them to become successful life-long learners. Teachers do not prescribe or dominate. The classic model consists of 6–10 students who need to resolve a phenomenon or a set of events that require explanation. There is a strong emphasis on the use of group dynamics to facilitate motivation and the elaboration of an issue.

> **Box 13.6**
>
> ## The wrong room
>
> This is a ploy to get the students to really consider the importance of the environment within parent education. The group are asked to turn up at a specific room for a session on facilitation skills. When they arrive, the room is set in traditional classroom style, with desks in rows. The teacher arrives late, making all manner of excuses for lack of punctuality.
>
> She then distributes a worksheet such as a facilitation assessment tool and asks the students to work on it. She wanders in and out of the room, makes a mobile phone call and looks out of the window.
>
> The students are then asked to feed back their findings without any clear instruction and the teacher takes little part in the ensuing feedback. At this point, ideally the teacher should have arranged to receive a telephone call. After taking it, she informs the group that they are in the wrong room and will have to move.
>
> The new room has been carefully set up. The seats are in a circle, there are refreshments available, posters and pictures decorate the room, music is playing and essential oils scent the air. The teacher has undergone a personality transplant and becomes the enabling facilitator. The group are then asked to reflect on how they felt initially and how they feel now.
>
> **Points to consider**
>
> - *This is an incredibly illuminating exercise and is worth the effort involved for the profound effect that it has on the students.*
> - *Although it is possible to discuss how to create a safe and permissive environment, actually living the reality is so very much more effective.*

> **Box 13.7**
>
> ## No place like home
>
> The students arrive for the session to be greeted by a room that looks as though it has been hit by a bomb. Dirty dishes, piles of clothes and a variety of equipment should be scattered around the room. The facilitator should be sitting or lying in the midst of this looking mildly puzzled, holding a baby doll.
>
> Once the students have taken in the tableau, they should be invited to talk to the 'woman' and find out what is going on in her life.
>
> **Points to consider**
>
> - *If you are fortunate enough to have access to a 'community/home' based midwifery practice room within your facility, and you have aspirations of a theatrical nature, then this role play carries a powerful message.*
> - *It could be used within a session on coping skills for parenting or postnatal depression.*

Box 13.8

The handover

A group of three or four volunteers are requested to act as a group receiving the handover from the charge midwife on the postnatal ward of a hospital. The 'charge' role should be played by the lecturer who will have prepared notes for the handover and will read from these. The student 'actors' are given specific roles, such as a newly qualified midwife, a student midwife and a healthcare assistant. They are informed that they can develop their characters as they wish and may ask questions or make comments at any point during the process.

The remaining students within the group are asked simply to observe and take notes and when the handover is completed, the lecturer opens up the floor for discussion.

Points to consider

* *Although the facilitator has some degree of control, this is an improvisation activity and therefore is likely to develop a life of its own.*
* *A reasonable amount of time should be allowed for both presentation and discussion, as in our experience this particular activity may run for some time.*
* *The exercise may raise some serious issues for some students within the group and debriefing may be needed for some.*

Box 13.9

Special parents, special needs

This activity is introduced as part of a theoretical session about working with parents with physical disability.

Two volunteers are identified and one is asked to role play the mother and the other the midwife. The mother is kitted out with a personal stereo, held firmly in place below a hat that covers the ears, so that the vast majority of her hearing is occluded. The second volunteer adopts the role of the midwife and, equipped with a doll, is asked to demonstrate latching on and positioning during breastfeeding for the mother.

Another volunteer is asked to don a blindfold. The room is set up with a hospital crib and a baby with a crying mechanism. When the volunteer is settled, the crib is moved to another part of the room and the crying mechanism is activated. The blindfolded student is then asked to find her way to the baby.

Points to consider

* *This is a very potent exercise, that really gives the students an understanding of some of the challenges that sensory-deprived new parents may encounter. It encourages the group to adopt a problem-solving approach in dealing with such difficulties.*
* *It often leads to lateral thinking, such as, 'wouldn't a woman with visual impairment be better giving birth at home, where everything is familiar?'.*
* *The facilitator does need to initiate the session by establishing the boundaries and explaining the sensitive aspects of the activity to the group.*
* *It should ideally be followed by a visit from mothers (or parents) with special needs, to authenticate the experiential nature of the exercise.*

During the first tutorial for the module, students are provided with a 'trigger' that acts as a catalyst for their learning. The trigger may be anything which stimulates the inquiry process.

The students explore the trigger and identify learning issues arising from it. They choose to explore individually, or as part of a coupling or small group, a specific issue that they then take away from the tutorial to research.

Boxes 13.10–13.16 show some of the triggers that we have used during our experiences with PBL.

Box 13.10

Video production

We have used 'home-made' videos on two occasions, with a relative degree of success. The first was an interview with a couple who were expecting their first baby and we questioned them very generally about the experience. The second was a recording of a 'live' trigger of a woman who encountered a whole range of problems during her pregnancy and birth. She spoke about the experience and of how it felt to have been classified as a 'high-risk patient'.

Points to consider

- *If you have a media production department, use them if you can. They have expertise in filming and will be able to produce a more professional film.*
- *Ensure that you have good sound recording equipment. We discovered that a white noise type whistle was very jarring and distracting.*
- *Informed consent is essential and any participants should be made fully aware of the purpose of the exercise and should give signed consent for its use.*
- *Recording a live event enables the student to go back and reexamine the trigger for clarification at a later date.*
- *A recording may also be used for subsequent groups where it may be impractical to attempt to reproduce the same 'live' material.*

Box 13.11

Birth videos

Commercially produced birth videos/DVDs can be useful as trigger material. We have found that comparing two very different scenarios can be a useful source of feedback.

Points to consider

- *Make sure that you check out the copyright situation. Many universities have licences to use videos for educational purposes, but it needs to be cleared with your media production department.*
- *Be aware of your own biases and remember that the video production company equally may have an agenda.*

Box 13.12

Poetry

As we were delivering a programme that contained a fairly significant PBL component, we felt that it might be a good idea to use a poem to stimulate discussion during the group interview process.

We identified a poem about a woman experiencing labour, that had been written by one of our previous students, and sent it out to the applicants with other information about the interview. During the group interview, the applicants were asked to discuss the poem and to identify what the learning issues were for them. This seemed to work very well and served to introduce the prospective students to PBL as well as give the interview team insight into their suitability.

We have also used poetry as a trigger for a postregistration module. On that occasion, we chose a Winnie the Pooh poem by A A Milne, which was found to be a little byzantine for some of the group members.

Points to consider

- *Remember that not everyone feels comfortable with poetry, so it may not be the best choice for an initial trigger.*
- *Choose poetry that is not too complex or the group may need excessive guiding to compensate for a lack of direction.*

Box 13.13

Goldfish bowl

An ambitious trigger that we attempted was to use a group of pregnant women as a 'live trigger' within a staged early pregnancy class. The women were identified by the antenatal clinic coordinator at the local hospital and were contacted by the module leader from the university who invited the women to take part.

The participants turned up at the planned time and were seated centrally within a larger circle where the student midwives sat to 'view' the session. The module leader then took on the role of facilitator and introduced a series of activities to encourage the women to raise issues relating to early pregnancy. At the end of the session, which lasted about $1\frac{1}{2}$ hours, the student midwives were invited to ask the women questions to clarify anything that they were unsure about.

Points to consider

- *Again, consent by those taking part is essential. The women need to be explicitly informed about what the exercise involves and what is expected of them.*
- *The students need to understand that whatever is discussed within the confines of the session is confidential.*
- *It may be useful to offer some sort of remuneration to the women for giving their time, travel expenses or the offer of continuing antenatal sessions for the duration of their pregnancies (minus the student audience, of course!).*

Box 13.14

Using films

We have used a number of films as triggers for learning. However, before we launch into this one, we should make clear that there are copyright implications which need to be thought through, i.e. around showing films to large groups. However, it is entirely possible to ask students to find and watch films at home in student-managed learning time, or to take groups to the cinema. We have also known of groups who have planned evenings together to watch a film that was set as a trigger.

Some of the films that we have either used or would use as potential triggers include the following.

- *Bicentennial Man* – a Robin Williams film which, although long, explores numerous issues which can be related to culture, values and society. Williams plays a robot who wants to become human and a number of really interesting issues are raised about what makes a 'person' and about human rights. There are a number of other Robin Williams films which raise poignant issues for healthcare, including *Patch Adams* and *Awakenings*.
- *How to Make an American Quilt* – is a slow-moving and sentimental film about women's lives, crafts and stories. It is one of those which raises questions about assumptions, and we recommend to students that they might like to watch it as part of a 'girl's night', along with a glass of wine and some chocolate!
- *Castaway* – is a Tom Hanks film which raises some very interesting questions about our modern, Western attitudes to time, which can be related to pregnancy and birth.
- Other films which we have not used personally but which we have thought might prove fruitful in this way include *The Village*, which raises some very deep questions about modern life, values and attitudes. There are some older films which considered topics such as male pregnancy (*Junior*) and body image (*The Nutty Professor*) in a relatively superficial way and then, of course, some deeper and more complex films such as *The Color Purple*, which raises questions about feminism, human rights and domestic violence.

Points to consider
- *Always watch the film at least once or twice yourself before using it, and make enough notes of what issues you think it raises so that you can help facilitate discussion if necessary. However, be prepared for students to find totally different things to discuss as well!*
- *Be aware that there will almost always be someone who has already seen the film with their kids or at the cinema. This is not, however, a problem, as you can ask them to watch it again and use the fact that they have seen it before to think about the deeper messages it raises, either deliberately or accidentally.*
- *Do have a plan for leading a discussion after the film, and for enabling people who didn't pick up everything you hoped they would to think about the film in different ways.*

Box 13.14 (Continued)

- *Also, do be warned that, once you have started to include films in your teaching, you will never be able to switch your brain off in the cinema in quite the same way again, as you will find yourself seeing something in almost every film that could be a useful educational trigger!*

Box 13.15

Information, quotes and controversies!

We have used a number of 'handout' triggers that began their life as articles or postings on Internet sites and discussion boards. This takes a bit of preparation time but it is relatively easy to compile a page or two of anonymised quotes, thoughts and/ or controversial statements for discussion around a particular topic. These can be used as a whole, e.g. ask students to read and think about the entire handout before discussion, or they can be discussed one at a time.

Points to consider

- *It can be quite interesting to put together a wide range of perspectives on the same topic in this way, or to bury one really controversial statement in a list of others which are relatively innocuous.*
- *It can also be useful to build up a 'library' of these, perhaps on overhead transparency, so that you always have something which will enliven a group and/or generate a few minutes of discussion.*

Box 13.16

Birth plan/hospital notes

We have used a few variations on this theme, which involves compiling a complete or partial set of midwifery/medical notes or something like a birth plan, which can be given to students to see what issues are raised for them. This kind of thing can raise literally hundreds of issues and you can obviously decide whether the notes will represent a woman experiencing normal pregnancy/birth/postnatal period, a woman who is perceived to be 'high risk' or a woman who had a completely unique set of circumstances in an area you want the students to study more closely.

Points to consider

- *While there is obviously a need to create 'fake' notes rather than contravene anyone's confidentiality, it is possible to base the notes or plan on a 'real' woman, who becomes anonymised, which can make it easier to create this kind of tool. If you want to use this to look at fairly generic issues, you could also 'book' one of your colleagues (with anonymised name, address, etc.) as if she were pregnant, so that there are no contradictions.*

- *If you are making something complex, like a complete set of notes, it is not necessary to make a copy for every student; you can make one or two and ask them to share in groups, or enable students to have access at different times, or lodge them somewhere where all students can borrow them for an hour or so if they need to go back to them, perhaps in the library or in an administration office.*
- *This idea can be adapted to look at almost anything, e.g. you could mock up a blood/ultrasound/screening report form, a partogram, a CTG readout or a letter from a midwife to another professional.*

Getting out and about

The value of taking a group of students 'on the road' to visit workplaces, galleries, or even other countries, may fill the educator with anticipation or equally with dread. The sheer logistics of organising such events may be intimidating or time consuming and at a time when educationalists are pressed for time, additional work may not hold a great deal of appeal. However, the enjoyment of the students and the value of trips and visits for them makes it a rewarding and valuable experience for all concerned.

A field trip can provide students with opportunities to develop a greater sense of themselves in relation to the world. Subjects learned in the classroom take on new meaning when students are able to connect them to people, places, occurrences and events outside the classroom. Field trips are effective as developmental or culminating activities to consolidate what has been learned in the classroom. They may provide opportunities for hands-on learning experiences where students are exposed to concrete examples rather than the abstract examples studied in the classroom. They also, very importantly, provide added social benefits, offering the group members an opportunity to get to know each other better.

There are many opportunities for field trips and educational visits available. It is chiefly a question of looking carefully and sometimes laterally in order to tap in to these opportunities. We have taken both undergraduate and postregistration groups on a wide variety of visits, including art galleries, birth centres, the theatre and The Farm Midwifery Center in Tennessee, amongst others.

In our experience, funding has never been a problem, as the students have been more than willing to pay their own transportation costs and entry fees. However, there is often funding available from a range of sources, as we will discuss in some of the specific examples in Boxes 13.17–13.21.

Rites of passage

In Western industrialised society, we seem to have lost sight of the sacred value of specific events in the lives of women that once took on considerable significance, such as menarche, childbirth and the menopause. These landmarks in a woman's life cycle have in many ways been demeaned in terms of importance and are sometimes even stigmatised.

Box 13.17

Art exhibitions

Admittedly, this is probably easier for those living near larger cities, but occasionally birth specific-related exhibitions can be found, such as Jonathan Waller's Birth exhibition in Cheltenham in 2000 (see Chapter 1). There are other less specific but equally useful opportunities. For example, the Tate Modern has a number of art works that are birth related. The Body Works Exhibition was a fascinating if somewhat gory insight into human anatomy whilst the Museum of Emotions and the Spectacular Bodies Exhibition were enjoyed by different groups of students.

Points to consider
- *It may be better to combine an art exhibition visit with another such as a theatre performance or a visit to a birth centre.*
- *Art gallery visits may be useful for modules relating to women or women's health more generally.*
- *If visiting a generic gallery, devise some sort of quiz or treasure hunt to encourage the students to identify relevant works.*

Box 13.18

Formula factory visit

As part of a breastfeeding module, we arranged to take a cohort to observe the production of artificial formula at a factory. The company actually provided transport to ferry the group to and from the factory.

This proved to be a very insightful experience and it transpired that some of the students did not even realise that formula was in fact modified cow's milk until the trip.

Points to consider
- *A useful visit to combine with a session on the politics or environmental impact of breastfeeding.*
- *The agenda for the company may be different from your own, and the students may be bombarded with 'freebies' during the visit, so you do need to address that prior to the visit and unpack it again on return.*

Box 13.19

Birth centres

There are birth centres in many parts of the country now and many of them are happy to accommodate reasonably sized groups of students. We visited a variety of birth centres as part of a module exploring practice management and the students found the visits to be a useful experience.

Box 13.19 (Continued)

Points to consider

- *Birth centre staff in our experience are generally very proud of their workplace, outcomes, etc., and consequently their input is vibrant and positive.*
- *Ensure that the students are well prepared in their understanding of what a birth centre does and how it performs.*

Box 13.20

Theatre visits

Again, you may have to wait for an appropriate production to come along but the excitement and value of the theatre visit make the planning and arranging worthwhile.

The Vagina Monologues is a production that is usually on tour and performing in many different towns and cities, and is a rich source of discussion and debate for issues around women's sexuality. It can have a profound and almost Damascene effect on some students.

We have also taken groups to see *Singing the Bones* by Canadian writer Caitlin Hicks, which is directly related to childbirth. You could also consider bringing the theatre to your own institutions. In her chapter on theatre, Kirsten Baker discusses the use of Boal's Theatre of the Oppressed methods which can be introduced with powerful effect

Points to consider

- *Allow ample time for debriefing following a theatre visit. Live theatre is a powerful medium and performances may raise personal issues for those in the audience.*
- *We have managed to secure arts grant funding for theatre visits and staged productions on several occasions, so it may be worth exploring the availability of local arts grants.*

Box 13.21

The Farm Midwifery Center

Some years ago whilst running the postregistration Advanced Diploma in Midwifery programme, we were approached by the cohort who wondered if, as their alternative placement period that was built into the programme, they could arrange a visit to the home of 'spiritual midwifery', The Farm Midwifery Center in rural Tennessee.

By pulling out all the stops, we were able to make this a reality in a relatively short period of time and on a cold morning in February, a group of 10 of us set out on what was unquestionably our most ambitious field trip to date.

Prior to leaving for the US, we were able to arrange a number of 'micro trips' which included visits to a hospital obstetric unit, a birth centre in Nashville and the home of an Amish midwife. These visits enabled the group to gain valuable insight into the spectrum of maternity care in the US. These visits were supported by a series of workshop sessions at the clinic on The Farm, which were facilitated by The Farm midwives and ourselves.

Box 13.21 (Continued)

Many of the midwives who made the trip managed to secure funding from their hospital trusts, and some student midwives who have made the trip subsequently have managed to obtain travel bursaries from their own universities, Iolanthe award, etc.

This was a seminal moment in our careers because it demonstrated that almost anything is achievable if you are prepared to have faith and put in the graft.

Box 13.22

Setting the scene

Teaching rooms within institutions of higher education are frequently sterile and functional places, offering little nourishment for the soul.

The days of dedicated teaching rooms that can be decorated and personalised may be behind us but the ambience of a teaching session can be enhanced quite simply with a relatively small amount of effort or planning.

By bringing in something as simple as a single stem flower in a vase or a small sculpture or piece of artwork, the energy of the room and within the group can be subtly altered. Something as simple as playing some relaxing music as the students arrive or burning essential oils can have an amazing effect.

Points to consider

- *Electric oil warmers are obtainable and may help to keep the health and safety officer happy!*
- *The style of the image, music and oils can be altered to suit the needs of the group. A post-lunch session may need music and oils to revitalise, whereas a session following a controversial and challenging class may need to be relaxing and soothing.*

As a result, we have also lost the sense of initiation that ritual brings to these rites of passage. In other cultures, however, rituals and celebrations of these events abound.

This section contains some of the ways in which we encourage students to consider the significance of these milestones and how their recognition may add to a holistic approach to practice. It helps them to address their own values and beliefs and to consider the cultural needs of individual client groups that they may work with. For further ideas and inspiration, you may find it useful to read Chapter 14, on creativity, spirituality and birth, by Jenny Hall.

Fun and games

'We don't stop playing because we grow old; we grow old because we stop playing.'

(George Bernard Shaw)

Box 13.23

Poem for the baby

As part of the examination of the newborn programme, the students are read a poem relating to the early neonatal experience. They are then asked to write a poem about a baby that they have encountered in practice or about the memory of meeting their own baby, if they prefer.

Points to consider

- *This activity resulted from recognising that the students were addressing the baby very much as a series of systems. It seems to help them to focus on the baby and its parents more holistically.*
- *There may be some reticence initially but in our experience, once the students overcome their shyness, they have some amazing talent.*

Box 13.24

Mother's birth story

The students are given several weeks' notice and asked, if it is at all possible, to see if they can get the story of their own birth from their mother. If that is not possible, then they can use their own account of giving birth or share the story of a special birth that they have been privileged to attend.

The group then gather and, if they feel able, they share the stories that they have brought, and relevant issues are raised for discussion.

Points to consider

- *This activity will only work with a small group of students who feel very safe with each other and within the environment created.*
- *An opt-out clause should be available for any group members who do not wish to attend.*
- *It may come as a surprise how many students have not really ever talked to their own mothers about their births. This activity almost seems to legitimise the discussion for many.*
- *This can be a very emotional session and it is probably a good idea to have a box of tissues on standby.*
- *Debriefing of this activity is essential. The stories relating to their own birth give the students a link with their past and help them to gain a further understanding of who they are and where they come from. During pregnancy, women often experience a need to know more about their place in the universe.*

This final section lists a number of games and activities that we have used within our teaching. Some of these we have designed ourselves; with others, we have borrowed the idea and adapted it (usually beyond recognition); and some have been designed by students.

Box 13.25

Birthing bundle

Pam England introduced us to the idea of preparing a 'birthing bundle' for the baby. Couples are encouraged to bring along a number of items for their baby which they have wrapped in a bundle and, if they are comfortable, share this with the group.
   The items must include:

- something that symbolises the life of one of the grandparents (the past)
- something from the parents that represents who they (singly or jointly) are (the present)
- something that represents the soul of the baby (the future).

We never cease to be moved at the offerings that group members have made when this activity is used. Items include such things as poetry, pressed flowers, family bibles and patchwork quilts.
   The birthing bundle makes the group members consider connections with the past and the future and in doing so, gives them a sense of their own place in the world. It also highlights the changing relationship with their own parents at this significant time and lastly, it makes them consider the relationship that they want to have with their new baby, often beyond a material level.

In our busy and serious lives, we need to learn to play a bit more. The mention of games may have the effect of 'ruffling the feathers' of some people, leading them to mutter about being treated in a patronising manner. However, there is sound evidence to suggest that games can be used for a number of beneficial purposes (Schaefer 2002). They can offer an opportunity to revitalise as a break in a more conventional teaching and learning session. With careful handling, they may offer a safe environment in which to practise social and life skills and, as a result, may improve group cohesiveness. The games involve all group members which means that there is less chance of anyone falling asleep in the back row. They encourage the group to take responsibility, allow for flexibility and increase relevance. Finally, they allow a framework and structure within which the group can experiment and experience. Happy playtime!

Conclusion

Teaching for creativity is not an easy option but it can be deeply fulfilling. It may involve more time and planning to generate and develop ideas, but the results will pay dividends by producing students who demonstrate skills such as self-awareness, reflection, critical analysis, problem solving, team-building skills and evaluation. These are higher-order transferable skills, which could help to improve both the quality of service to mothers, their babies and families, and the development of midwifery.
   There is debate around so-called 'progressive' pedagogical methods and the effectiveness of using methods that encourage exploratory and experiential learning activities. It is possible that some of the activities listed within this chapter will ask the participants,

---

Box 13.26

Pub-style quiz

This can be a way of teaching, of checking learning or of breaking up an otherwise 'heavy' day by adding some fun. Divide participants into teams of between three and six people each. (If you wanted to get people to join with people they don't usually sit with, you could do this by means of the 'pairs' icebreaker in Box 13.1, but use threes or fours instead.) Make sure each team has a table to sit around or a space to sit in together, and invite each team to come up with their own name, and write a list of these somewhere. Distribute paper and pens to each team.

You will need to have previously compiled a list (or several lists, if you are going to have more than one 'round') of questions, which you can then read out loud. Allow time for the teams to think of their answer and get the teams to swap papers at the end of each round, to mark each others'. They can then give you the total scores and you can keep a record.

This can either be competitive, where the highest scoring team wins a prize, or friendly, where the scoring is 'played down'. The best kind of prizes are big bags of sweets; they are inexpensive and can easily be shared.

Points to consider

- *This activity lends itself well to topics where answers can be easily quantified, e.g. anatomy and physiology, rather than topics where there is often room for debate on what the 'correct' answer is.*
- *The questions can be enhanced by the use of audio-visual aids, e.g. an acetate with a picture of the bony pelvis and an arrow pointing to the bone you want them to name.*
- *It is worth clarifying the rules at the outset, and telling people how many times you will repeat the questions; otherwise, you can end up having to read out each question several times for one group, while another wants to move on!*
- *To make it more fun, you can throw in the odd popular culture or general knowledge question, but it is worth trying to cater for a range of age groups with this, e.g. ask questions about the Beatles as well as Dido or Eminem!*
- *This kind of activity can get competitive, so it is up to you to set the tone and decide whether you are happy to encourage that or whether you want to play the 'competition' aspect down.*
- *As with Uncle Robert's seat game, a microphone can be really useful as you may otherwise find yourself shouting over discussions!*

both teachers and students, to step outside their comfort zone because we are breaking away from the traditional approach of addressing specific skills and content. We believe that there is room for both traditional and progressive methods within midwifery education. A healthy balance of formal instruction of content and skills countered with activities that offer the students the freedom to inquire, question, experiment and express their own ideas is, in our opinion, the key to effective learning. We feel that

---

Box 13.27

A bloody mess!

Students enter a room to find the remnants of several births: sheets, inco (chux) pads, sanitary towels and perhaps even, in one case, a big bloody mess that might cause you to think a postpartum haemorrhage has occurred! Their job is to estimate the blood loss in each case and write it down either on scrap paper or on pre-prepared sheets. Following the guesstimation, you can reveal what the actual blood loss is in each case, and talk about how hard it is to estimate blood loss and the implications of this.

This exercise takes a fair amount of preparation, both beforehand and on the day itself. You need to decide what kinds of blood loss you want to represent, and thus how many 'stations' you will need. It can be fun to try to make 250 ml look like a lot of blood and 1500 ml look like less than it is – which is, of course, part of the point! If you think you might do this, it is worth asking hospital-based colleagues if they can make you a stockpile of any items from delivery packs which would have been thrown away but which are actually clean; you can pick up old sheets and towels very cheaply from charity shops and you may be able to enhance some of your 'birth stations' with things like placenta dishes and bedpans. It is much more fun to do this with a friend and experiment with making 'blood'! We have found that damson jam makes good blood clots and you can make very realistic blood from a mixture of water, flour and food colouring!

Points to consider

- *Compared to the time that the students will spend carrying out the exercise, this does take a lot of preparation, and it may be worth creating the mess in one room which is not otherwise being used, so that more than one group of students can access it on the same day.*
- *Try to create stations which are as realistic as possible. It can help to have scenarios in your head, i.e. a normal physiological birth on the floor with a couple of incos and a few sanitary pads; a forceps birth on the bed with an episiotomy and significant blood loss; a PPH. However, we would recommend against adding too many visual clues which will lead students in one direction or the other; it might add to the effect to leave a pair of bloody forceps on the floor but it will add information which will influence the student's estimates.*
- *Allow time for the students to revisit the stations after they have learned how much 'blood' is actually there, so they can consolidate this information and learn from it.*
- *Do take lots of big binbags, both to put under your 'messes' to save the carpet and to put everything in to take home and dispose of afterwards!*

---

it also makes the job of the teacher far less arduous and much more satisfying! However, we must remember that teaching with and for creativity includes all the individual characteristics of good teaching, such as strong motivation, high expectations, the ability to communicate and listen, and to interest and inspire. It is not a cop-out.

May you have as much fun as we have had introducing some of the ideas outlined into your teaching sessions.

Box 13.28

Designing a super drug

During a session on pain, the group are given flipchart paper and coloured board markers (there is no reason why paints, pastels, etc. could not be used, time permitting). The group are divided into groups of four or five and asked to spend 10–15 minutes designing a super drug that gives them everything that they could possibly desire from a pain-relieving medication.

They then reconvene and describe their wonder medication and some rationale as to why they require such qualities in a medication, e.g. 'we don't want anything that will make the baby drowsy'.

They then compare their fantasy drug with what is currently available for use in labour.

Points to consider

- *This is a great way of getting the students to really take on board the potent effects of medication in labour.*
- *It works to make the students consider non-pharmacological methods of pain relief as a first-line approach in labour.*

Box 13.29

Take a stand

Using three sheets of flipchart paper, write 'AGREE' on the first, 'DISAGREE' on the second and 'ON THE FENCE' on the third. Place these in different areas of the room.

Think of a controversial statement that relates to an issue within midwifery, such as:

- women should be free to make a choice of mode of birth, including the freedom to choose caesarean section for whatever reason
- co-sleeping is a negative practice and should not be actively encouraged
- a woman with a previous history of stillbirth should be advised that hospital is the best place to give birth.

The group are then asked to take a stand and move to the standpoint where they feel most comfortable. Once everyone has settled, the groups on the standpoint should reach a consensus about why they are there in order to produce a cogent argument. Each group then feeds back their collective reasoning and the floor is open to debate. If at any point in the procedure, a group member feels that they have changed their mind, they are free to move to a new standpoint and support the argument of that group. When the facilitator feels that the issue has been adequately addressed, the next statement is announced and the group move on.

Box 13.29 (Continued)

Points to consider

- *This is a useful activity to raise awareness of difficult subject areas, including ethical dilemmas.*
- *It demonstrates that there are rarely black and white answers and often shades of grey relating to practice-related issues.*
- *It does have the potential to become raucous and needs careful monitoring, so it is useful if the facilitator can circulate within the groups to maintain a sense of order.*
- *It is possible to ask the group members to contribute to the statements themselves.*
- *This can be easily adapted to use in parent education sessions.*

Box 13.30

Is she in labour?

Use the template below to create cards which each hold a statement from the table. Distribute the cards equally amongst a group of student midwives.

Ask the group to imagine that they are a midwife on a labour ward who receives a telephone call from an anxious woman, saying that whatever is printed on the card is happening to her at that time.

Each group member should decide what they would advise a woman to do in the event of the scenario on their particular card. You should explain that they may advise the woman to:

- stay at home
- call the midwife/hospital
- come straight to hospital
- or take another course of action if they so wish.

Baby moving less than usual	Irrational urge to carry out cleaning duties	Membranes rupture with a gush of clear amniotic fluid
Membranes rupture, amniotic fluid greeny/brown in appearance	Overwhelming contractions every 2 minutes lasting for 1 minute, with hardly time to catch breath	Moderate strong contractions, one every 10 minutes lasting 30 seconds
Urge to push at the height of a contraction	Heavy, mucoid, bloodstained 'show'	Baby's head feels very low in the pelvis. Feels very uncomfortable
Membranes may have broken, trickle of amniotic fluid noticeable	Fair contractions: one in every 15 minutes, variable in strength and length	Strong contractions: one every 5 minutes lasting 40 seconds
	Upset tummy with diarrhoea	

Box 13.30 (Continued)

Points to consider

- *This is a useful way to introduce what is happening physiologically at onset of labour to a group of students at an early stage in their programme.*
- *It also helps in the development of communication skills and by asking them what they might say to the woman and how they would document the call, you are addressing broader professional issues.*
- *If you have more students than cards, you could make extra sets of cards and split the cohort into smaller groups for the purposes of the exercise.*
- *It can be adapted to use in parent education sessions.*

Box 13.31

Designing a birthing environment

Create a template that represents the layout of a simple rectangular room. Have a selection of coloured pencils, crayons, pastels, etc. available. Simply ask the students to create what they would consider to be the ideal birthing environment. Then feedback to the whole group to initiate discussion about the points raised during the exercise.

Points to consider

- *This activity will raise awareness of many aspects relating to an optimal environment for birth.*
- *Colour schemes, architecture and actual location (i.e. hospital, birth centre and home) will invariably arise.*

Box 13.32

The crying baby

This is a good exercise to use during a parenting session on coping with a newborn baby. It is particularly effective when utilised as the surprise element of a theoretical session. Either use one of the sophisticated baby dolls that has a crying programme or a audio recording of a baby crying. When least expected, activate the doll or switch on the recording of the baby crying. Allow the 'crying' to continue for several minutes. After turning the programme/recording off, ask the students how they feel in response to the crying. Open up a discussion with the group about how they feel about the crying.

Points to consider

- *A pre-recorded crying baby CD may be purchased from the BBC Archives series. Or you may wish to make your own recording.*
- *You need to run the programme/recording for long enough to provoke a distressed reaction from the group. They need to feel what it is like to be subjected to a lengthy period of unabated crying in order to imagine how new parents may feel and react.*

Box 13.33

Equipment cards

Cut out a selection of pictures of merchandise from baby catalogues and stick them to postcard-sized pieces of card. Add a few others such as a picture of a mother holding a new baby and a breastfeeding mother.

Label each of the items on the cards, including 'a loving carer' and 'breastmilk'.

Write each of the following statements separately on three pieces of A4 paper:

- essential
- important but not essential
- waste of money.

Distribute the cards equally between the students and ask them to individually place their cards on the statement that reflects their views about the equipment, etc. and to explain why they made that decision.

When all the cards have been laid, get the group to identify what items are really considered to be essential and which are really only cosmetic. When they are asked what is really essential, the only two cards that usually remain on the 'essential' pile are 'a loving carer' and 'nutrition'.

Points to consider
This activity has many different advantages.

- *It addresses parenting issues for the students. Any number of discussion points may spin off, such as co-sleeping (is a cot really necessary?), reusable nappies, etc.*
- *By focusing on consumerism, it effectively demonstrates the pressures that new parents are under to purchase more and more often unnecessary equipment.*
- *It can be modified to use in parent education sessions.*
- *It may take some time to carry out because it will raise so many discussion points.*

Box 13.34

The isoimmunisation dance!

This is a way of getting students to participate in a 'walking dance' where they will play various people, cells and reactions in order to enact isoimmunisation and explore the role of anti-D. It is best explained in a step-by-step process and the only introduction needed is that I have large, pre-prepared cards which people can hold so that they and everyone else will know what role they are playing.

I always play the rhesus-negative mother and direct the dance, but someone else could do this if you want to direct from the sidelines. I invite someone to play my partner (they don't have to move!) and give them two cards which say 'rhesus positive' and 'rhesus negative' so that we can explore the different possible combinations and the implications of these. (I have also used cards for 'homozygous' and 'heterozygous' in order to talk about this aspect, but this is best left for students who have enough knowledge of genetics to not need a full explanation at this point.)

Box 13.34 (Continued)

I also ask someone to play my first rhesus-positive baby, and invite this person to sit on the floor about 10 feet from me. I have a very long scarf (actually a series of scarves tied together!), which represents the umbilical cord, and my baby and I tie one end of this around our waists.

Three or four students then become fetal red blood cells and they dance around the baby and up and down the cord, but not around me at first. I talk about how fetal cells do not usually enter the maternal circulation but, if there is a sensitising episode, they can. We then create a birth scenario where there is a sensitising episode, release the baby (who is well and gets to sit down and enjoy the rest of the show) and the red blood cells dance around me.

I then need some antibodies to come along and mop up the red blood cells (who get to sit down temporarily!) and who remain in my blood and dance around me until I become 'pregnant' again with another rhesus-positive baby. Once this baby is tied to me and the red blood cells have returned to dance around her and the cord, the antibodies can dance up and down the 'cord' and enter her bloodstream, haemolysing the red blood cells, which is often the best bit, as I explain what happens during haemolysis and the students get to enact this! The baby is asked to respond as well, and we have created a depiction of isoimmunisation.

We then reenact the dance, but with additional students playing the part of synthetic anti-D. They mop up the red blood cells as they enter my bloodstream, and the second baby's red blood cells do not become haemolysed. We also look at scenarios in which we have a rhesus-negative baby, who is not affected by the antibodies, and at different combinations of women and partners.

Points to consider

- *This works best in a group of around 20 students, where almost everyone (excluding the people who seriously hate this kind of thing!) can play a part. It will still work in a bigger group, especially if they know each other and will remember one of their friends haemolysing another!*
- *Depending on how well I know the group and how enthusiastic they are, I might give out all the cards before we start the dance, or I might hang onto some and hand them out as we go along. If I choose people from a group I know well, I always pick the extraverts to be the red blood cells and the rhesus antibodies!*
- *In order to make this exercise work, you need a really good understanding of the process, and it is probably worth practising with colleagues, friends or stuffed animals before unleashing it on students!*
- *This idea can also be adapted for other physiological processes – imagination is the only limit!*

'I may safely predict that the education of the future will be inventive minded. It will believe so profoundly in the high value of the inventive or creative spirit that it will set itself to develop that spirit by all means within its power.'

(Overstreet 1949)

(Burkhardt & Nagai-Jacobson 2002, p.174). It could be through everyday tasks, where people are 'naturally visually creative' as in choosing the clothes we wear, how we decorate the place we live or plan out gardens (Campbell 1993, p.3). The suggestion is that even if consciously people have lost the exploratory creative nature they had as a child, it is still there in their unconscious behaviour. Further, the aesthetic responses to our everyday world can move us into a 'spiritual journey' (Pike 2002, p.10). Labun (1988) writes: 'Meaningful purposeful work or creative expression is often an expression of spirituality'. The emphasis here is the 'meaning' and 'purpose' of the activity as being key to the spiritual aspect. What is not clear is whether the meaning and purpose are solely personal to the one undertaking it or also in the understanding of others. Edassery & Kuttierath (1998) indicate the importance of the 'rediscovery of self-worth' and suggest that the use of creative arts may help this process.

Creative activity for the spirit

It appears that it does not particularly matter which type of creative activity a person undertakes, for it to be regarded as 'spiritual'. Demonstration of spirituality may occur through painting, story telling, sculpture, poetry, music, ritual or gardening.

Guare (2001) discusses the spiritual potential of poetry and states that 'every person has a kind of poet living within the soul' (p.86). She describes the prophetic nature of poetry and the desire of poets to 'try to make us feel the truth'. She states that 'the prophet calls people to be faithful to their vocation of becoming fully human subjects' (p.79). Her standpoint is more about poetry being the message of the spirit rather than poetry acting as a spiritual voice for the writer. A concern with poetry is that it depends so much on the language used to express it. If the reader is unable to read the language or to understand the message that is being portrayed then the spiritual message may be lost. If poetry is to be prophetic it must speak in the language and metaphor of that generation and that culture. Others have indicated the spiritual value of the person writing themselves (Harrison 1993, Labun 1988). Writing may be used to release intuition (Rew 1989) or creative potential (Cameron 1993). The spiritual nature of words could be appreciated, therefore, in the reading and receiving of others' words or in writing them ourselves.

Words may also be used within story telling. The suggestion has been made that this is a specific aspect of women's spiritual expression (Burkhardt 1994). However, many of the stories and messages passed down through religions were told by men (Hall 2001, p.25). Also, Stanworth (1997) has shown that story telling is not limited to women, through a study that explored the use of language and metaphor as indicators of spirituality. There may also be differences in the spiritual expressions of story telling: some may be created stories that lead the listeners to personal growth (Pinkola Estés 1992) while others may be the telling of personal story (Burkhardt 1998, Taylor 1997).

Music is suggested to have a particular spiritual effect (Wynn 2004). It is thought to invoke intense feelings through the meanings put on particular pieces by the listener (Updike 1994, p.292, Wynn 2004). Music touches and expands the imagination (Palmer 1995, p.96) in a deeply intimate way (Wynn 2004, p.42) and has powerful properties for healing (Updike 1994, p.299). It is not surprising that these properties have been incorporated into therapeutic methods (Evans 2002). However, it could be encouraged more as a method of healing and restoration.

The selection of music is important. What is soul music for one could be unpleasant for another. One piece of music will calm us while another will provide stimulation

(Cameron 1993, p.22). The effects of the tempo, rhythm and harmony may be positive or negative (Updike 1994, p.297). There is also the question of whether the powerful effects are in the listening or at the point of making the music or a combination of both (Cameron 1993, pp.110–111). It has been noted that it is beneficial for a person in therapy to have the therapist playing along, accompanying 'the patient on their journey' (Robinson et al 2003, p.205).

Creativity and women

Carl Jung (1966, p.103) wrote of the 'creative process as having a feminine quality'. Winnicott (1971, p.72) explores play and writes from the psychological view that creativity is 'one of the common denominators of men and women'. This indicates that although it may be viewed as a 'feminine' trait, it does not exclude men. Spirituality research relating specifically to women has been sparse and there remains the question of the appropriateness of making a division between the characteristics of men and women in this way (Hall 2001, pp.13, 17).

Burkhardt's (1994) study exploring women's understanding of spirituality in South America demonstrated the way women use stories to express spirituality. The study participants' stories were grounded in the everyday aspects of life, including ritual, care for children and parents, and caring for gardens. The research indicated that the creative nature of the story telling may be a specific aspect of spirituality for women. The study also demonstrated women's understanding of the changes on their journey. The process of change could also be regarded as an element of creativity.

Women in an art therapy group demonstrated that their willingness to express themselves through art was enhanced through the connections and relationships within the group (Levine 1989). The act of sharing gave an opportunity for the others to receive from it. Connecting relationships formed by women have been shown to be an element of spiritual nature (Burkhardt 1994, Hall 2001). The expression of women through group art efforts or through meeting together but preparing individual creations may be a demonstration of the need for women to connect together. The art that is produced may be an add-on benefit to these relationships or it may be potentially a vehicle for self-development.

Creativity and birth

Perhaps the most significant process of change and creativity a person can go through is the experience of giving birth to a child. Some women may experience the sense of being 'co-creator' (O'shea 1998). Others may experience the desire to explore aspects of nature and the environment as demonstration of their creative self. Richards (1992, p.27) emphasises that 'Birth is the most consuming of passions, an intensely spiritual act. It is one of the most powerful forces on earth and certainly the most powerful force that can occupy a human body'. This powerful force leads to an immense change within the nature and life of the woman giving birth. Creativity is not only in the making but in the 'seeing' of things in a different way. Pregnancy brings an internal 'knowing', an expansion of the 'self'. The wonder that some women experience in their internal and external changes can be viewed as beauty (Wallas LaChance 2002, p.31).

Giving life to a new person has the potential for a major shift in a woman's concept of her 'self'. In one study of women's self-development (Belenky et al 1996), some talked of childbirth as the most important learning experience in their lives and linked the creative nature of birth with an increased depth of understanding of women's creative abilities. Rubin's (1984) study of the development of maternal identity states that: '...childbearing requires an exchange of a known self in a known world for an unknown self in an unknown world'. The process of the experience then has the potential to be life-changing and creative. Marck (1994), in her study of women who have an unexpected pregnancy, identifies that women try to see their 'way to motherhood' and that ' we seek, in looking for a way, a safe passage from what we know and are to what we do not yet know and might or might not be' (p.120). She goes on to say: 'Whatever way we find, we are never as we once were. Even in trying to find a way, something in us has changed. We have a new way of being and things are not the same way...'. The challenge for any woman is to find the safe way through the process of becoming a mother. 'To mother a child is to know pain, and the pain can never be safe' (Marck 1994, p.121). The effect of this can be enhanced or suppressed through the nature of becoming pregnant, the nature of the pregnancy itself, the type of birth and the relationship with the caregivers. This places a responsibility on those caregivers to acknowledge the power of this transformational process and to establish better ways of facilitating women's safe passage through it.

The creative nature of pregnancy may lead women to become more fascinated with nature itself and to want to spend more time outside or 'in touch' with nature (Hall 2001, p.33). It has been suggested that women want to spend more time near the sea or develop a greater interest in the moon or the cyclical function of being a woman. The links with nature may also arise through becoming aware of her own bodily functions and the changes taking place. Being able to feed her baby by the breast links a woman with the mammals and is a powerful creative force.

Images of birth itself have been linked to nature through the metaphor of a flower opening and birth art often has a theme related to nature. Some midwives use this image of the flower to help a woman who is finding giving birth difficult, to enable her to open her body. A woman's pregnant abdomen no longer has to be covered up; young women today celebrate by allowing the body to be exposed and may adorn the shape with paints and jewels. The woman's pregnant form is therefore seen as beautiful and to be valued as creation is taking place.

The power of pregnancy also opens a woman's mind to different aspects of herself in her search for meaning in the event. Expression of this change to woman as nurturer may be through artistic elements, such as the creative activity of 'nesting' – providing a place for her new baby in her life. Making 'things' for the baby may be another expression of this. The nature of 'nesting', the process of preparation for the new baby, often involves creative artistic acts: decorating rooms, spending many hours making bedding or needlecrafts to enhance the baby's 'new space' or making new clothes. Family and friends (often women) also participate in this way by providing new objects for the baby and for the home.

Preparation may also involve listening, often over and over again, to particular pieces of music that enhance their feelings of well-being, or they may be drawn to playing music themselves. Others may take up art or writing to express their feelings and emotions during the pregnancy. This need to be 'creative' may arise simply through having more time, as they are 'ladies-in-waiting', and not be specifically related to the pregnancy itself. However, the child and the birth may become a focus for the creativity, which may therefore be a process through which women find meaning for the experience. Further, the use of drawing in pregnant women has shown the potential of the use of art as a diagnostic tool (Swan-Foster et al 2003). The knowledge that art could have this ability needs further exploration. The possibility may be that this information could be used by midwives to assess women's development over pregnancy or to recognise when there are potential concerns.

Some antenatal educators already encourage the use of art to enable couples to explore their feelings about the pregnancy and the forthcoming birth and to aid them in their journey towards being parents. One view is that using art to express 'secret hopes and dark fears' is vital in preparing for the birth of the child (England & Horowitz 1998, p.xi). Encouraging 'intuitive responses' in couples or discussing dreams may be beneficial (Davies 2002). Within one church-based group, use of creative materials is encouraged to give parents a focus to remind them of their beliefs during labour. Figure 14.1 shows what one father made in this group. What is made is obviously dependent on the materials provided. The fact that some of the parents have kept these pieces may indicate a certain value and meaning that they place on them as a significant reminder of the experience.

The 'art' of professional healthcare practice

The word 'art' has been used in relation to professional midwifery practice, with the suggestion that it is both an art and a science, since the days of Florence Nightingale (Whitman & Rose 2003). It is the 'art/act of the experience-in-the-moment' (Chinn 1994, p.24). The move of healthcare toward a more scientific model through the use of 'evidence' (Charles 2001) has raised concerns. Nurses' recognition of the 'unity of the mind and body' may be in 'direct conflict' with scientific approaches (Chinn 1994,

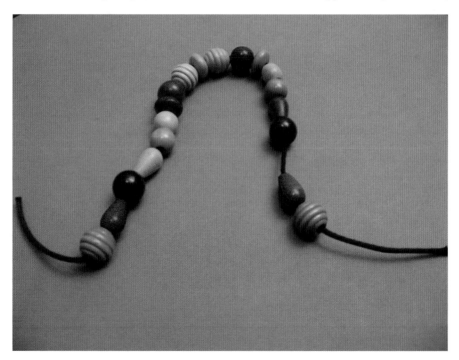

Figure 14.1 Article made by a father in a church based pregnancy group

p.23). Knowledge of the art of nursing and midwifery is required in order to develop practice appropriately. Appleton (1994) researched the experience of the art of nursing and extricated the following themes:

- being there
- being-with each other in understanding
- creating opportunities for fullness of being
- a transcendent togetherness
- a context of caring.

These themes have also been thought of as demonstrating spiritual care (Hall 2001). This indicates that the spiritual nature of caring may be more linked to what is described as the art of caring.

Titchen & Higgs (2001, p.281) suggest an understanding of professional practice through a model. In this, various issues intertwine:

- the perceived or stated needs of the client
- the client's interpreted needs
- the practitioner's technical competency
- the practitioner's ethical competency.

These authors suggest that artistry in professional practice is generated through improvisation between these issues and intuition, imagination and the unconscious. They add as a central aspect the issue of spirituality: the Muse, the Greater Self or soulfulness (p.289). They suggest that this is the place of transformation and transcendence.

The knowledge that is required to carry out this kind of care may be described as 'aesthetic knowing' (Leight 2002, p.109), which involves 'integration of the total knowledge spectrum in practice' and this then leads to transformation. Chinn (1994, p.37) writes of 'aesthetic knowing' as involving 'embodied grasp of situations and intimate experiences with the deepest and most significant life events that have been traditionally and cross-culturally associated with women's experience – birth, death, sorrow, joy, pain, life transitions'. Carers then have the ability to take what is known and to turn it into something meaningful to the person who is on the receiving end.

Professional practice in this way is also viewed as a combination of four dimensions of 'doing', knowing', 'being' and 'becoming' (Higgs & Titchen 2001, p.viii). The ability of each caregiver to integrate these dimensions successfully at any one time is affected by many external and internal forces and directly related to their personal ability to cope with change (Mullavey-O'Byrne & West 2001). Recognising that there is never total certainty in decision making appears to be an important step forward (Charles 2001) and health carers 'should consciously adopt a therapeutic position of uncertainty' when caring for patients and recognise the 'complexity of each person's life' (p.68). In order for health carers to be effective in caring, there must be wisdom, which is shown by an ability to be open-minded, 'to keep the processes of knowing in a receptive and open state of creative chaos out of which the emergence of new insights can be facilitated' (Dimitrov 2004, p.6).

Midwives and creativity

In recognising the nature of caring as art, there is evidence that exploration of the use of creative arts in the care of patients is of benefit (Evans 2002, Hunter 2002, Michael et al 2002). The role of midwives throughout history has had a creative aspect. The ability of midwives to be flexible in their behaviour demonstrates a link to creativity. The nature of midwifery knowledge is complex with the understanding that is required to care individually for each person and situation they are in contact with. Wickham (2004, p.163–164) discusses how knowledge may be gained through the use of narrative, experiential learning, intuition and female bodily wisdom. Midwifery and nursing are viewed as having paradigms of both art and science in combination. The interplay between these different ways of approaching care is complicated and presents practical challenges on an individual basis. The fact that most midwives are female suggests that they may be specifically creative by nature, which means that they may have a natural ability to approach care from a wide basis. The understanding that birth is a spiritual event adds to the depth and intensity that is required in order to facilitate the care.

In traditional societies the midwife's role is often viewed as spiritual, and her activities may include rituals that enable 'spiritual transition' for the woman becoming a mother (Kitzinger 2000, p.85–88). The vision of women giving birth is said to have great beauty and it has been suggested that midwives should explore this in greater depth (Anderson & Davies 2004).

Over time midwives have developed creative ways of caring for and supporting women. This has led to innovative designs of equipment or use of household equipment to enhance care. In simple terms, midwives have also been pictured as sitting in the corner knitting, as waiting women along with the women in labour – sometimes making bootees or little coats for the newborn (Wickham 1999).

Creativity and education

In recent years the development of more creative approaches in higher education has been increasing. The transfer of healthcare education from college to university initially meant that staff took on many of the teaching methods that were already in place within universities (Hall & Mitchell 2005). With a greater understanding of the way that different people absorb knowledge, challenges are being made to whether these are the best methods of teaching. Exploration of learning through different methods, such as art, poetry, drama and dance, is taking place. Within healthcare settings, this is also transferred to the patient and meeting their needs through art therapies and music therapies. The use of an aesthetic approach to caring has been acknowledged in respect of chronic illness (Michael et al 2002) and within nursing (Chinn & Watson 1994, Darbyshire 1994, Wikstrom 2003), health promotion (Green & Tones 2000) and midwifery courses (Anderson & Davies 2004, Jackson & Sullivan 1999). The former paper describes innovative methods of teaching in an Australian context. Evaluation of the course demonstrated the benefits the students perceive from this method of learning. However, clarity is also required as to whether there are any problems or limitations related to this method of learning for the students or teachers involved.

A philosophy of holistic care for women and their families, as indicated at the start of this chapter, means that education programmes leading to midwifery qualification should include an understanding of the nature of spirituality and the impact of this on people's lives. However, it appears that this is an area which has been lacking within most midwifery curricula, even though women and midwives recognise this to be an important part of birth (Hall 2001). Spiritually based care is recognised within nursing, especially in the context of the end of life (e.g. Cobb & Robshaw 1998, McSherry 2000a,

Robinson et al 2003). It is a strange contradiction that there is so little appreciation of the value of recognising the spiritual potential of life at its beginnings. How issues relating to spirituality are facilitated in an effective way is challenging (McSherry 2000b).

It could also be argued that, currently, the ways in which midwifery is put across to students are not as effective as they could be. Little research has taken place into the methods that are used. The transfer of midwifery training into higher education institutions may have encouraged and expanded the factual knowledge underpinning practice. However, the philosophy of woman-centred, holistic care, as described above, may need different methods of teaching in order to facilitate deeper learning and development to enable students to become midwives (Wickham 1999).

Fasnacht (2003) has suggested that the current method of educating nurses may actually 'suppress creative potential'. If we are to enable nurses and midwives to provide spiritual care then the use of teaching methods that develop this creativity will be beneficial (Cameron 1993).

In recent years I have been involved in developing facilitative sessions where students use creative art as a medium in order to learn about spiritual issues. The belief is that spirituality is an integral part of normal midwifery practice and that the students also have a spiritual aspect to their nature. To give them an opportunity to explore their feelings about their spiritual selves and as potential midwives was felt to be necessary. There was also a belief that students undertaking any course are not just 'intellectual' and that giving them opportunity to explore the more creative and artistic aspects of themselves will open their minds and beings to a more holistic approach to care.

Studies have demonstrated that the two hemispheres of the brain have different roles and functions and it is suggested that both can be trained through the use of artistic exploration (Quinn Patton 1987, p.155). Further, it is recognised that individuals have different psychological systems for understanding the world (Gardner 1985, Quinn Patton 1987, p.154) and that we all learn through different forms and methods (Cassidy 2004). Those who have developed art as a form of therapy recognise that this more 'rounded' way of approaching issues is of value (e.g. Robbins 1994). Others propose that using different methods of teaching 'emphasise creative awareness and reasoning' (Koithan 1996 in Wikstrom 2003). Also it is suggested that strengthening imagination in a person will help in developing 'adaptive behaviour' as it enables the person to 'improvise when faced with a changing set of circumstances' (Palmer 1995). This means that enabling the students to use their imagination may help them to be more open in how they respond to those they encounter on a day-to-day basis in practice, as they will then recognise others in a more complete way. Steiner (2002, p.101) wrote: 'The more we strengthen our creative tendencies, the sooner we will find ourselves capable of the right attitude'. His implication is that creativity encourages self-growth and consequently a desire for wholeness and good. Though we cannot teach or force someone to have 'right attitudes', there is potential that appropriate use of more creative methods in education may encourage the development of positive attitudes.

Creativity research

Practitioners of the arts and humanities have consistently explored art in research as part of their profession. Whether dance, music, words or visual art, researchers have explored and tried to understand meanings created. Social scientists have also used visual images to explore society from different standpoints, albeit with some limited acceptance (Pink 2001, p.7). However, the current explosion of technology is enabling new developments in the realms of research (Banks 2001, Pink 2001, Rose 2001). Digital video is creating a new media for social researchers and dance practitioners and technology is bringing progress in the research of music.

The choice of methodology for art research will be dependent on the nature of the research. The use of quantitative research is not impossible; for example, in research I have undertaken, students' creative pieces were quantified through frequency of the use of a particular symbol or type of material (Hall & Mitchell 2005). However, qualitative methodology is generally used as the researcher is applying principles of interpretation to another's work and usually making value judgements. Quinn Patton (2002, pp.172–173) writes of a 'connoisseurship approach' to evaluation.

The process of the research could take many forms. The visual, for example, could be researched from the basis of history, from the basis of the symbols in the piece or from a technological perspective. The visual could also be used as part of the method of the research, providing the participants with art to view and react to or by providing them with the means with which to create their own visual representation. In this situation the participants can also be co-researchers and their views can be incorporated as part of the research findings. Video research is opening up new avenues with participant co-research or with the researcher as controller of the video. The nature of this type of research requires extensive reflexivity and the researcher is embedded in the social arena in which he or she is placed (Pink 2001, p.80).

Within music research, the process may involve investigation of music that has already been created as well as the creation and exploration of new works. The same processes may be used with dance. Ylonen (2003, p.565) states that the research of dance utilises the researcher's use of the body and observations of what happens. It is also seen as a 'form of inquiry into the research process' (Cancienne & Snowber 2003, p.237).

As the arts are beginning to be used in the care of patients, research is beginning to emerge. Some is establishing the worth of particular forms of interventions while others use the intervention to understand a particular aspect of the person or the condition.

The use of art as research exposes a different type of truth which is dependent on the aesthetic understanding of the viewers as well as the 'seeing' of the individual. As technology becomes more advanced, there arises the potential of 'doctoring' the data so that the viewer or listener will not know what has been erased from the research, in the same way as selective use of data may occur in other forms of research.

The use of artistic expression as a type of data may provide a different 'truth' for that individual at that moment in time. The indication is that the issue of truth in relation to methodology appears to be important, as the researcher needs to know what truth they are trying to elicit in order to make the right choice of direction. However, Charmaz (2004, p.983) states that our personal standpoint affects how we look at things and will affect our view of truth. This means that the researcher also needs to address their own values and personal bias and those of the researched to establish the total place of truth for them and for the reader/observer.

My journey of development of a teaching programme relating to spirituality, which enables students' creative expression, lead to investigation of the products of those sessions (Fig. 14.2). The different knowledges explored within this study meant that the analysis of any data required an approach that would reflect this investigation. It was based on a 'critical visual methodology' (Rose 2001). Rose (p.3) states that this is 'an approach that thinks about the visual in terms of the cultural significance, social practices and power relations in which it is embedded'. She also recognises that perceptive criticism of visual

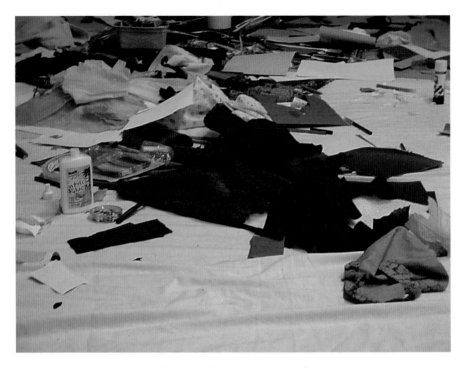

Figure 14.2 Creative materials

images also 'depends on the pleasure, thrills, fascination, wonder, fear or revulsion of the person looking at the images and then writing about them' (p.4). She encourages success through 'passionate engagement' of the researcher with what is observed. The choice of this methodology was related to the need to explore the creative pieces in the context of the whole experience of the student in the teaching session and within their experience as student midwives and in their life outside the course. This reflects the principle of holism and recognising that the students do not experience or create anything that is not affected by and does not impact on all aspects of their personality and being.

In order to analyse images, Rose (2001, p.188) indicates that there needs to be understanding of:

- the site of production – how an image is made
- the site of the image itself – what it looks like
- the site of its audiencing – how the image is seen.

Within the context of the study, the focus was mostly on the construction of the image and the image itself as the researchers would be the only 'audience'. However, analysis can also be made of the impact of the image on ourselves as the viewer.

Rose (2001) describes different methods of analysis of visual images. She describes content analysis, where the images are coded according to descriptive labels; semiology, which enables analysis of signs from within images; psychoanalytic criticism, which explores subjectivity, sexuality and the unconscious; and discourse analysis, which places the image in the context in the world in which it is being created. These methods are specifically for photographs. The difference with this study is that the images were created pieces using many different media, with abstract forms as well as recognisable shapes and symbols. Therefore analysis involved using a series of questions about the pieces based on those suggested by Rose (2001, pp.188–190).

The process involved two researchers examining the pieces individually, extracting data on the images that had been created. This was further examined in light of the explanation the students had given and in combination with a short questionnaire to establish how the students felt about the teaching session and the use of art to explore the meaning of birth (Hall & Mitchell 2005). The study has shown that these students felt that the use of art was a valuable way to explore these issues (Hall & Mitchell 2005) (Fig. 14.3).They also indicated the value of exploring the nature of meaning in relation to birth and their future role as midwives.

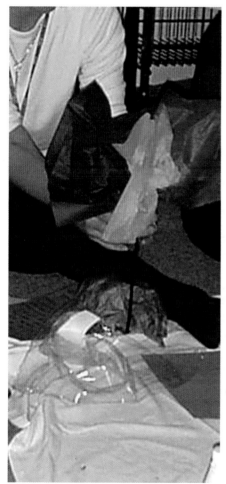

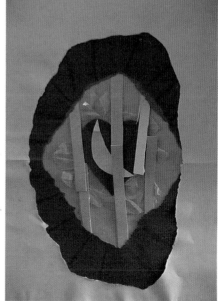

Figure 14.3 Examples of art made relating to spirituality

It has yet to be shown whether the personal development that these sessions facilitate in some students will have an effect on their future selves as people or in their role as midwives. Similar approaches have been used in brief sessions with midwife educationalists and with educators from other healthcare professions and verbal feedback indicated this was personally beneficial. Use of art as a group activity in a research group revealed some interesting insights as there was a concern about being led by a 'title' and some felt more comfortable in an approach where they could 'do their own thing'.

Conclusion

Artistic expression is a demonstration of spirituality. For women and their partners in pregnancy, encouragement of the use of art may enable them to explore some of the difficult and challenging issues of the changing state they are experiencing. Enabling them to address their fears and anxieties prior to birth may have long-term benefits as these will have been reduced prior to going through labour. The use of art to facilitate learning in midwives may also be beneficial as they may develop greater openness toward being flexible and creative in the care that they give. In understanding the rich potential of birth as having a powerful effect on future generations, seeking new strategies to enable women and midwives to share in this knowledge must be a priority.

> 'In nursing in the twentieth century spirituality was separated from art and art was separated from science. Nursing must be radically reimagined if it is to restore its caring-healing fine art and the view of body/mind/spirit unity that is the basis of its practice. In this revision, nursing art and spirituality – the sacred – need to be seen again as one.'
>
> (Chinn & Watson 1994, p.xvi)

References

Anderson T, Davies L 2004 Celebrating the 'art' of midwifery. Practising Midwife 7(6): 22–25

Appleton C 1994 The gift of self: a paradigm for originating nursing as art. In: Chinn P, Watson J (eds) Art and aesthetics in nursing. National League for Nursing, New York

Banks M 2001 Visual methods in social research. Sage, London

Belenky M, Clinchy B, Goldberger M, Mattuck Tarule J 1996 Women's ways of knowing: the development of self, voice and mind. Basic Books, New York

Burkhardt M A 1994 Becoming and connecting: elements of spirituality for women. Holistic Nursing Practice 8(4): 12–21

Burkhardt M A 1998 Reintegrating spirituality into healthcare. Alternative Therapies 4(2): 127–128

Burkhardt M A, Nagai-Jacobson M G 2002 Spirituality: living our connectedness. Delmar, New York

Burnard P 1988 Searching for meaning. Nursing Times 84(37): 34–36

Cameron J 1993 The artist's way: a course in discovering and recovering your creative self. Pan Macmillan, London

Campbell J 1993 Creative art in group work. Wilmslow Press, Oxford

Cancienne M B, Snowber C N 2003 Writing rhythm: movement as method. Qualitative Inquiry 9(2): 237–253

Cassidy S 2004 Learning styles: an overview of theories, models, and measures. Educational Psychology 24(4): 420–444

Cawley N 1997 An exploration of the concept of spirituality. International Journal of Palliative Nursing 2(1): 31–36

Charles C 2001 Uncertainty in treatment decision-making. In: Higgs J, Titchen A (eds) Professional practice in health education and the creative arts. Blackwell Science, Oxford, pp.62–71

Charmaz K 2004 Premises, principles and practices in qualitative research: revisiting the foundations. Qualitative Health Research 14(7): 976–993

Chinn P L 1994 Developing a method for aesthetic knowing in nursing. In: Chinn P, Watson J (eds) Art and aesthetics in nursing. National League for Nursing, New York

Chinn P L, Watson J (eds) 1994 Art and aesthetics in nursing. National League for Nursing, New York

Cobb M, Robshaw V (eds) 1998 The spiritual challenge of healthcare. Churchill Livingstone, London

Craft A 2001 An analysis of research and literature on creativity in education: report prepared for the Qualifications and Curriculum Authority. Available online at: www.ncaction.org. uk/creativity/creativity_report.pdf#search='anna%20craft%20creativity%20in%20education'

Darbyshire P 1994 Understanding caring through arts and humanities: a medical/nursing humanities approach to promoting alternative experiences of thinking and learning. Journal of Advanced Nursing 19: 856–863

Davies L 2002 Antenatal classes and spirituality. Practising Midwife 5(11): 19–21

Dimitrov V 2004 Complexity, chaos and creativity: a journey beyond system thinking. Available online at: www.zulenet.com/VladimirDimitorv/pages/complexthink.html

Dyson J, Cobb M, Forman D 1997 The meaning of spirituality: a literature review. Journal of Advanced Nursing 26: 1183–1188

Edassery D, Kuttierath S K 1998 Spirituality in the secular sense. European Journal of Palliative Care 5(5): 165–167

England P, Horowitz R 1998 Birthing from within. Partera Press, Albuquerque, NM

Evans D 2002 The effectiveness of music as an intervention for hospital patients: a systematic review. Journal of Advanced Nursing 37(1): 8–18

Fasnacht P H 2003 Creativity: a refinement of the concept for nursing practice. Journal of Advanced Nursing 41(2): 195–202

Gardner H 1985 Frames of mind: the theory of multiple intelligences. Basic Books, New York

Goddard N C 1995 Spirituality as integrative energy: a philosophical analysis as requisite precursor to holistic nursing practice. Journal of Advanced Nursing 22: 808–815

Green J, Tones K 2000 The health promoting school, general practice and the creative arts: an example of inter-sectoral collaboration. Health Education 100(3): 124–130

Guare R E 2001 Educating in the ways of the spirit: teaching and leading poetically, prophetically, powerfully. Religious Education 96(1): 65–87

Hall J 2001 Midwifery mind and spirit: emerging issues of care. Books for Midwives, Oxford

Hall J, Mitchell M 2005 Creativity and spirituality: student midwives' creative expression of the meaning of birth. University of the West of England, Bristol

Hall J, Taylor M 2004 Birth and spirituality. In: Downe S (ed) Normal childbirth: debate and the evidence. Churchill Livingstone, Edinburgh

Harrison J 1993 Spirituality and nursing practice. Journal of Clinical Nursing 2: 211–217

Helson R, Srivastava S 2002 Creative and wise people: similarities, differences and how they develop. Personality and Social Psychology Bulletin 28: 1430–1440

Higgs J, Titchen A (eds) Professional practice in health education and the creative arts. Blackwell Science, Oxford

Hunter L P 2002 Poetry as an aesthetic expression for nursing: a review. Journal of Advanced Nursing 40(2): 141–148

Jackson D, Sullivan J R 1999 Integrating the creative arts into a midwifery curriculum: a teaching innovation report. Nurse Education Today 19: 527–532

Jung C G 1966 The collected works, vol 15. Princeton University Press, Princeton, NJ

Kitzinger S 2000 Rediscovering birth. Little, Brown, London

Labun E 1988 Spiritual care: an element in nursing care planning. Journal of Advanced Nursing 13: 314–320

Leight S B 2002 Starry night: using story to inform aesthetic knowing in women's health nursing. Journal of Advanced Nursing 37(1): 108–114

Levine C G 1989 Women and creativity: art-in relationship. Arts in Psychotherapy 16: 309–325

Long A 1997 Nursing: a spiritual perspective. Nursing Ethics 4(6): 496–510

Marck P B 1994 Unexpected pregnancy. In: Field P A, Marck P B (eds) Uncertain motherhood. Sage, London

McSherrry W 2000a Making sense of spirituality in nursing practice. Churchill Livingstone, London

McSherrry W 2000b Education issues surrounding the teaching of spirituality. Nursing Standard 14(42): 40–43

Meraviglia M G 1999 Critical analysis of spirituality and its empirical indicators: prayer and meaning in life. Journal of Holistic Nursing 17(1): 18–33

Michael S R, Candela L, Mitchell S 2002 Aesthetic knowing: understanding the experience of chronic illness. Nurse Educator 27(1): 25–27

Mullavey-O'Byrne C, West S 2001 Practising without certainty: providing healthcare in an uncertain world. In: Higgs J, Titchen A (eds) Professional practice in health education and the creative arts. Blackwell Science, Oxford

National Advisory Committee on Creative and Cultural Education 1999 All our futures: creativity, culture and education. DFES, London

O'shea M 1998 An exploratory study of women's experience of childbirth specifically identifying the spiritual dimension. Dissertation for BSc Midwifery Studies. Nightingale Institute, King's College, London

Palmer A J 1995 Music education and spirituality: a philosophical exploration. Philosophy of Music Education Review 3(2): 91–106

Pike M A 2002 Aesthetic distance and the spiritual journey: educating for spirituality and morally significant experiences across the arts curriculum. International Journal of Children's Spirituality 7(1): 9–21

Pink S 2001 Doing visual ethnography. Sage, London

Pinkola Estés C 1992 Women who run with the wolves. Rider, London

Price J L, Stevens H O, La Barre M C 1995 Spiritual caregiving in nursing practice. Journal of Psychosocial Nursing 33(12): 5–9

Quinn Patton M 2002 Qualitative research and evaluation methods. Sage, London

Rew L 1989 Intuitions: nursing knowledge and the spiritual dimension of persons. Holistic Nursing Practice 3(3): 56–68

Richards H 1992 Cultural messages of childbirth. International Journal of Childbirth Education 7(3): 27–29

Robbins A 1994 A multi-modal approach to creative art therapy. Jessica Kingsley, London

Robinson S, Kendrick K, Brown A 2003 Spirituality and the practice of healthcare. Palgrave Macmillan, Basingstoke

Rose G 2001 Visual methodologies. Sage, London

Rubin R 1984 Maternal identity and maternal experience. Springer, New York

Stanworth R 1997 Spirituality, language and depth of reality, International Journal of Palliative Nursing 3(1): 19–22

Steiner R 2002 How to know higher worlds. Anthroposophic Press, Great Barrington

Swan-Foster N, Foster S, Dorsey A 2003 The use of human figure drawing with pregnant women. Journal of Reproductive and Infant Psychology 21(4): 293–307

Swinton J 2001 Spirituality and mental healthcare. Jessica Kingsley, London

Tanyi R A 2002 Towards clarification of the meaning of spirituality. Journal of Advanced Nursing 39(5): 500–509

Taylor E J 1997 The story behind the story: the use of story telling in spiritual caregiving. Seminars in Oncology Nursing 13(4): 252–254

Titchen A, Higgs J 2001 Professional artistry and creativity. In: Higgs J, Titchen A (eds) Professional practice in health education and the creative arts. Blackwell Science, Oxford

Updike P A 1994 Aesthetic spiritual healing dimensions in music. In: Chinn P, Watson J (eds) Art and aesthetics in nursing. National League for Nursing, New York

Vaughan F 2002 What is spiritual intelligence? Journal of Humanistic Psychology 42: 16–33

Wallas LaChance C 2002 The way of the mother: journey of the lost feminine. Chrysalis, London

Waugh L A 1992 Spiritual aspects of nursing: a descriptive study of nurses' perceptions. PhD thesis, Queen Margaret College, Edinburgh

Whitman B L, Rose W J 2003 Using art to express a personal philosophy of nursing. Nurse Educator 28(4): 166–169

Wickham S 1999 Reclaiming the art in birth. Midwifery Matters 83: 6–7

Wickham S 2004 Feminism and ways of knowing. In: Stewart M (ed) Pregnancy, birth and maternity care: feminist persepectives. Books for Midwives, Oxford

Wikstrom B-M 2003 A picture of a work of art as an empathy teaching strategy in nurse education complementary to theoretical knowledge. Journal of Professional Nursing 19(1): 49–54

Winnicott D W 1971 Playing and reality. Tavistock, London

Wynn M 2004 Musical affects and the life of faith: some reflections on the religious potency of music. Faith and Philosophy 21(1): 25–44

Ylonen M E 2003 Bodily flashes of dancing women. Qualitative Inquiry 9(4): 554–568

INDEX

A

'Aesthetic knowing,' 224
'Agitprop' (agitational propaganda), 131
Alienation, professional, 131
Antenatal care, music and *see* Music/music
    therapy
Antenatal education, 106
  birth poetry use, 88–89
ARMS (Association of Radical Midwives),
    121–122
'Arrival' exhibition, 58
Art
  birth art *see* Birth art
  childbirth, representation of *see* Artistic
    representation (of childbirth)
  delivery in maternity hospitals *see* Maternity
    hospitals, arts delivery/curatorship
  exhibitions, midwifery education, field trips,
    204
  research, 227
  therapy, 221, 226
Artemis, 16
Artistic representation (of childbirth), 9–29
  ancient history, 13–16
  Christianity, influences, 16–18
  early 20th century
    male perspectives, 20–21
    social realism, 21–24
  feminism and, 24–26
  future of, 26–27
  see also Birth art
'A Shared Experience' exhibition, 55
The Association for Poetry Therapy, 90
Association of Radical Midwives (ARMS),
    121–122

B

*Baby Catcher: Chronicles of a Modern
  Midwife,* 103

Becker, Paula Modersohn, 21
Belly dancing, 164
Berger, John, 24
'Bibliotherapy,' 90
Birth (process of) *see* Childbirth
Birth art
  process in holistic care, parental involvement,
    31–48
    assignments, 37–38
    drawing, 34–35
    LabOrinth project *see* LabOrinth project
    materials needed, 34–37
    painting, 35
    sculpture, 35–36, 38
    time requirements, 36–37
  social context, 18–19
  see also Artistic representation (of
    childbirth); *specific forms*
Birth centres, midwifery education field trips,
    204–205
Birth choreography *see* Dance
Birthday lines (icebreaker) activity, midwifery
    education, *194–195*
Birthing bundles, midwifery education, *208*
Birthing from Within, 15, 151
Birthing stools, 15–16
Birth mythology, 15, 65
Birth narratives *see* Birth stories
'The Birth of Mary,' 18–19
Birthplace significance, 51
Birth plans, midwifery education use,
    202–203
Birth poetry, 5, 75–94
  antenatal education and, 88–89
  ethical aspects, 80, 91–92
  feminism and, 78
  history, 76–79
  midwifery education, 80–86, *200, 207*
  midwifery research, 88
  professional development, 87
  therapeutic application, 89–92

Birth Project, 24–25
Birth Reborn, 162
Birth stories, 31, 103–107
  healing and, 118–120
  midwifery education, *207*
  traumatic, 119
  see also Childbirth; Literature; Story
    telling
'Birth Tear,' 25
Birth videos, *199*
  see also Video production
Boal, Augusto, 127, 128, 130
Brain synchrony, 41
Brain, thinking styles, 175–176
  whole-brain, 2–3, 187, *189*
Brain waves, 41, 44
Breastfeeding
  creativity and, 222
  music and, 152
  neonatal intensive care, 159
Brecht, Bertold, 128
Breech birth, 124

C

Caesarean sections, 148, *211*
Call the Midwife, 103
Cervical dilatation, 32, 44–45, 46
Chadwick, Helen, 25–26
Chanting, antenatal music therapy,
    146–147, 151
Chicago, Judy, 24–25
Childbirth
  artistic representation *see* Artistic
    representation (of childbirth)
  breech, 124
  caesarian sections, 148, *211*
  crafts, expression through *see* Crafts
  creativity and, 221–223
    see also Creativity
  dance and *see* Dance
  environment/settings
    clinical, 33–34
    design, midwifery education, *213*
  forceps delivery, 86
  holistic preparation *see* Holistic care
  imagery, feminism and, 24–26
  induced, 32, 162
  literary portrayal *see* Literature

Childbirth—*cont'd*
  medical imagery, 33
  medicalisation *see* Medicalisation of
    childbirth
  metaphor and *see* Metaphor
  music and *see* Music/music therapy
  mythology, 15, 65
  pain associated, 149–150, *211*
  poetry and *see* Birth poetry
  sexuality of, 13
  social context, 18–19
  technological intervention, 26–27, 162
  theatre and *see* Theatre
  universality, 27
  women's narratives *see* Birth stories
  see also Labour
Childbirth websites, 79
Childbirth Without Fear, 149
Child loss
  emotions triggered, arts delivery/curatorship
    and, 57–58
  poetry associated, 82–83, 88
  see also Grief
Choreography *see* Dance
'The Christening Feast,' 19, *19*
Christianity, 16–18
Clay (as medium), 36, 38
Clinical settings, 33–34
Coda, Áine Nic Giolla, 50
  '100 Names and Dates' project, 50–51, *51,*
    52, 53, 54, 60
Cold Comfort Farm, 98
Community midwives, 117–118
Contact improvisation, 163–164
Contextual art practice, maternity hospitals
    see Maternity hospitals, arts delivery/
    curatorship
Coyote Circle, 151–152, 154
Crafts, 5, 63–74
  definition, 63–64
  goddess-related imagery, 65
  history, 64–66
  needlework, 24–25, 222
  'nesting' and, 222
  therapeutic potential, 68–70
  workshops, 71–74
  see also *individual crafts*
Creative materials, *228*
Creative writing groups, 78

Creativity
  breastfeeding and, 222
  definitions, 1–2, 170, 218–219
  in midwifery education *see* Midwifery
      education
  potential, 219–220
  research, 226–230
  spirituality and *see* Spirituality
  stifling of, 2
Crisis facing profession, 27, 121–124, 131
'Critical visual methodology,' 227
Crying babies, midwifery education, *213*
Cultural issues, 135
Curatorship in maternity hospitals *see*
      Maternity hospitals, arts delivery/
      curatorship
Cusk, Rachel, 105
'Cyborg' mother, 26–27

D

Dance
  of childbirth, 6, 157–165
      'belly dancing' and, 164
      contact improvisation, 163–164
  midwifery education as, 187–188
  research, 227
The Diary of a Mad Mother to Be, 102
Die Kraft in Mir (Inner Strength), 151
'Dinner Party' exhibition, 25
Dix, Otto, 21
Down's syndrome, 91
Drabble, Margaret, 99–100
Drawing
  as diagnostic tool, 222–223
  materials required, 34–35
  see also Artistic representation (of
      childbirth); Birth art

E

Early Childhood Education curriculum,
      New Zealand, 160
Education
  antenatal, 106
      birth poetry use, 88–89
  children's early learning, 160
  learning styles, whole-person, 81
  midwifery *see* Midwifery education

Empathy, 136
Empowerment (of women), 12
  crafts as catalyst, 71
Enright, Ann, 105
Epidural anaesthesia, 162
Episiotomy, 86, 162
Epistemic discrimination, 112
Epstein, Jacob, 9
  'Genesis' sculpture, 9, *10*
Ethical issues, birth poetry and, 80,
      91–92
Expressionist movement, 21

F

The Farm Midwifery Center, 153
  midwifery education field trips, *205–206*
Fathers-to-be, poetry participation, 89
The Fat Ladies Club, 106
Feminism
  birth poetry and, 78
  childbirth imagery and, 24–26
Fertility goddess, 15
Fetal Attraction, 101
Fetal hearing, music and, 142–144
Fiction *see* Literature
Field trips, midwifery education, 203,
      204–206
Films
  birth videos, *199*
  midwifery education use, *201–202*
  research, 227
Forceps delivery, 86
Friedman's (labour) graph, 38–41
Frontier School of Midwifery and Family
      Nursing, 124

G

Games for Actors and Non Actors, 127
Gender, 13
'Genesis' sculpture, 9, *10*
Giving Birth, 84–85
Goddess-related imagery, 15, 65
'God Giving Birth,' 24
Grief
  following miscarriage, 79
      see also Child loss
  poetry expressing, 88–89

H

Halliday, Caroline, 78
Handcrafts *see* Crafts
The Handmaid's Tale, 100
The handover (activity), midwifery education, *198*
Healing, birth stories and, 118–120
Healthcare, arts therapies role, 3–4
  see also specific therapies
Heraldic shield (icebreaker activity), midwifery education, *196*
History/historical aspects, 13–16
  birth poetry, 76–79
  crafts, 64–66
  early 20th century imagery, male perspectives, 20–21
  medicalisation of childbirth, 19
Holistic care, 4, 6, 225
  birth art role *see* Birth art
  midwifery education and, 180–183, 184–188
  see also Mind-body connection
Howard, Ghislaine, 55, 59
Humane Neonatal Care Initiative, 158
'100 Names and Dates' project, 50–51, *51, 52, 53, 54,* 60

I

Icebreaker activities, midwifery education, 192, *193, 194–195, 196*
Inanna, 15, *15,* 16
In Celebration of my Uterus, 77
Induction, 32, 162
Inner Strength *(Die Kraft in Mir),* 151
Intelligences, multiple, 2–3
'Introspection,' 26
Isis, 16
Isoimmunisation dance, *214–215*

J

Jane Eyre, 97

K

Kahlo, Frida, 22–23
Kangaroo Mother Care (KMC), 159–160
Kelly, Mary, 24

Kitzinger, Sheila, 162
Knitting *see* Crafts
Knowledge base (of midwifery), storytelling and, 111–113, 123–124
Kollwitz, Kathe, 21

L

Laban movement philosophy, 163
LabOrinth project, 38–45, *39*
  materials needed, 41–42
  metaphor and, 40, 43–45
  template, *42*
Labour, *212–213*
  brain waves in, 41
  graphical representation (partogram), 38–41
  induced, 32, 162
  music during, 145, 148–152
    see also Music/music therapy
  see also Childbirth
Labour graph (partogram), 38–41
Learning styles, whole-person, 81
Leicestershire Maternity Services Liaison Committee, 120
Lessing, Doris, 99
Levin, Adik, 158
Liebowitz, Annie, 9
Life Isn't All Ha Ha Hee Hee, 101
A Life's Work, 105
Literature, 6, 95–110
  childbirth portrayal, 96–107
    20th and 21st century, 106–107
    American authors, 101–102
    non-fictional, 103–105
    romantic comedy novels, 101
  midwives' portrayal, 95–107
    fictional, 102–103
    non-fictional, 103
  see also Poetry; Story telling; *specific titles*
Loss of child *see* Child loss
Lullabies, 147, 148, 152, 154

M

'Madonna and Child,' *17,* 17–18, *18,* 25–26
Male perspectives, early 20th century imagery, 20–21
The Mastery of Movement, 162–163
Maternal-child relationship, 142, 158–160

Maternity, 103
Maternity care *see* Midwifery
Maternity hospitals, arts delivery/curatorship, 49–61
'100 Names and Dates' project, 50–51, *51, 52, 53, 54*, 60
child loss, emotions triggered, 57–58
staff involvement, 58
'Viewer' project, 51–53, 60
Maternity Leave, 102
Medical imagery, 33
Medicalisation of childbirth, 4–5, 26
history, 19
midwifery education, socialisation process, 115–116, 168
as topic of birth stories, 107
Medical notes, midwifery education use, *202–203*
Meningitis, 91
Menstruation at Forty, 77
Metaphor, 81, 112
of childbirth, 222
LabOrinth project and, 40, 43–45
creative midwifery education, 176–180, *178, 179*, 184, 191
see also Birth poetry
Metis, 112
Midwifery
arts therapies role, 4–5
see also specific therapies
crisis facing profession, 27, 121–124, 131
education in *see* Midwifery education
holistic *see* Holistic care
knowledge base, storytelling and, 111–113, 123–124
mindful, 123–124
political issues, crisis and identity, 121–123, 131
professional alienation, 131
professional development, birth poetry use, 87
professional socialisation, 115–116, 168
spirituality and *see* Spirituality
theory, gulf with practice, 168
see also specific topics
Midwifery education
birth environment design, *213*
birth poetry use, 80–86, *200, 207*
birth stories, *207*

Midwifery education—*cont'd*
creativity in, 167–216, 225–226
expressions, 171, 184
factors affecting, *172*, 172–176, *188–189*
field trips, 203, *204–206*
holistic care and, 180–183, 184–188
icebreaker activities, 192, *193, 194–195, 196*
metaphor and, 176–180, *178, 179*, 184, 191
perceptions, 170, 171–172, 176–180, *178*
problem-based learning methods, 196–199, *197–203*
role play, 193–196
student activities, 206–208, *209, 210–215*
video production use, *199*
crying babies, *213*
socialisation process, 115–116, 168
spirituality and, 225–226
student midwives' experiences, story telling, 113–118
Midwifery Matters, 122
Midwifery professional development, birth poetry use, 87
Midwifery research
birth poetry use, 88
creativity and, 226–230
video production use, 227
spirituality and, 221
The Midwife's Apprentice, 97
Mind-body connection, 32, 134–135, 146, 188, 223
see also Holistic care
'Mind Where You Look' exhibition, 59
Miscarriage, grief associated, 79
see also Child loss
Misogynism (in imagery), 17
The Moment the Two Worlds Meet, 88
Moore, Demi, 9
Mother-baby bond, 142, 158–160
'Motherese,' 152
Motherhood myth, 34
'Mother No.44,' Jonathan Waller, *11*
Multiple intelligences, 2–3
Music and Therapy in Healthcare, 141
Music/music therapy, 6, 139–156
antenatal, 142–152, 222
chanting, 146–147, 151

Music/music therapy—*cont'd*
  antenatal—*cont'd*
    fetal hearing, 142–144
    relaxation through, 144–146
    singing, 147–148, 154
    toning, 150–152, 154
    use in labour, 145, 148–152
  benefits
    metaphysical, 140–141
    physiological, 139–140
  midwives and, 153–154
  as origin of speech, 141–142
  postnatal, 152–153
    neonatal intensive care units, 153
  research, 227
  spirituality and, 220–221
'Mutter mit Kind,' 21, 23
'My Birth,' 22–23
'My Nurse and I,' 22, 23
Mythology, 15, 65

N

National Advisory Committee on Creative and
    Cultural Education, 219
National Association for Poetry Therapy
    (NAPT), 90
National Childbirth Trust (NCT), 106
National Maternity Hospital (NMH), Dublin,
    50
National Network for Arts in Health, 3–4
Natural Birth, 77
NCT (National Childbirth Trust), 106
Needlework, 24–25, 222
Neel, Alice, 23–24
Neonatal intensive care units (NICUs)
  breastfeeding, 159
  Humane Neonatal Care Initiative, 158
  music value, 153
'Nesting,' 67–68, 222
'Newborn Baby on Hands,' 21
NICUs *see* Neonatal intensive care units
    (NICUs)
No place like home (activity), midwifery
    education, *197*
Novels *see* Literature
Nurse education
  arts and health modules, 4
  midwifery *see* Midwifery education

O

Occupational therapy, 68
Odent, Michel, 13, 147, 162
'One Flesh,' 25
'One Mother, One Midwife' campaign, 121
Oxytocin, 88

P

Pain, 149–150, *211*
Painting
  birth art, materials required, 35–36
  holistic care role, 35
  see also Artistic representation (of childbirth);
      Birth art
Paintings in Hospitals, 56
Pairs icebreaker exercise, midwifery education,
    193
Partogram, 38–41
Partograph, *40*
Parturition, 77
Perineal wound repair, 67
Phantom pregnancy, 21
Photography, 9
Placenta, 26
Plath, Sylvia, 78
'Poems for the Waiting Rooms' project, 90
Poetry, 5
  birth and *see* Birth poetry
  child loss and, 82–83, 88
  definition, 79
  grief expression, 88–89
  spirituality and, 220
'Poets-in-residence' scheme, 90
Political issues, crisis and identity, 121–123, 131
Pollock, Griselda, 24
Postnatal period, music and, 152–153
'Post Partum Document,' 24
Pregnancy
  high-risk, music as therapy, 148
  phantom, 21
  unexpected, 222
'Pregnant Woman and Death,' 20, *20*
Premature babies, 52, 159
  see also Neonatal intensive care units
      (NICUs)
Problem-based learning (PBL), midwifery
    education, 196–199, *197–203*

Professional alienation, 131
Professional development, birth poetry use, 87
Professionalisation, 135
Professional socialisation, 115–116, 168
Progress Theatre, 127–134
A Proper Marriage, 99
'Psychopoetry,' 90
    see also Birth poetry
Puffball, 100
The Pursuit of Love, 98–99

R

Reddjedet, 15
Reflective techniques, theatre and, 134–135
Relaxation
    antenatal music therapy, 144–146
    brain waves in, 41
Relaxation Through movement (RTM),
    145–146
Religious aspects, 16–18
Research *see* Midwifery research
Rhesus positive babies, *214–215*
Role play, 135–137
    midwifery education, 193–196
    see also Theatre

S

Sancisi, Gabriella, 54–55
Schiele, Egon, 20
Sculpture
    birth art
        assignments in clay, 38
        materials required, 35–36
    representation of childbearing/childbirth,
        9, 27
Seven-circuit labyrinth, 41–42, *42*
    see also LabOrinth project
Sewing *see* Crafts
Sexton, Anne, 77–78, 90
Sexual abuse survivors, 130
Sexuality (of childbirth), 13
Singing, antenatal music therapy, 147–148,
    154
Small Changes, 101–102
Social context of birth art, 18–19
Social realism, artistic representation of
    childbirth, 21–24

Special care baby units *see* Neonatal intensive
    care units (NICUs)
'Special parents, special needs' (activity),
    midwifery education, *198*
'The Spirit of Birth: Nature, Nurture and the
    Evidence,' 162
Spirituality, 217–233
    creative potential and, 219–220
    creativity research, 226–230
    definitions, 217–218, *218*
    midwifery education and, 225–226
    midwifery practice and, 224–225
    midwifery research and, 221
    music and, 220–221
    poetry and, 220
    story telling and, 220
The Squire, 98
Stanislavski, Konstantin, 136
Stillbirth, *211*
Story telling, 5, 111–125
    midwifery knowledge base and, 111–113,
        123–124
    political issues and, 121–123
    spirituality and, 220
    student midwives' experiences, 113–118
    theatre and, 132–134
    see also Birth stories; Literature
Student midwives, 113–118, 206–208, *209,*
    210–215
    see also Midwifery education
Summers, Llew, 27
    sculpture, *28*
'Swimming in Concrete,' 129–130, 131
Synectics, 81

T

Tao of Birthing, 44
Technological intervention, 26–27, 162
Terra Mater, 16
Te Whariki, 160
Theatre, 5–6, 127–138
    midwifery education, field trips, *205*
    political issues and, 131
    Progress Theatre group, 127–134
    reflective techniques, 134–135
    role play, 135–137
    story telling and, 132–134
Theatre of the Oppressed, 130, 131

Thinking styles, 175–176
  whole-brain, 2–3, 187, *189*
  'zig-zag,' 175
'Third entity,' 163
Three Women, 78
Threshold Stone, 42, 43
Time will Tell, 100
Tlazolteotl, 16
Toning, antenatal music therapy, 150–152, 154
Touchstone (icebreaker) exercise, midwifery
      education, *194*
Traditional societies, midwife's role, 225
Tristram Shandy, 96

U

Ulrich, Laurel Thatcher, 97
Ulrich, Roger, 57, 59
Uncle Robert's seat game (icebreaker activity),
      midwifery education, *195*

V

Venus of Willendorf, 13–14, *14*
Video production
  midwifery education, *199*
  research, 227
'Viewer' project, 51–53, 60
Virgin birth, 16

W

Waller, Jonathan, 9–13, *11, 12*
Waterbirth, 11, *12,* 147
Waterbirth (Mother No.5), Jonathan
      Waller, *12*
The Waterfall, 100
Waterford Healing Arts Trust, 58
Weaving *see* Crafts
Weldon, Fay, 100
The Westcar Papyrus, 15
Whole-brain thinking, 2–3, 187, *189*
Whole-person learning, 81
'The Widow,' 21, *22*
The Wives of Bath, 101
'Woman waiting, Antenatal Unit,' *56*
Women, 104
The wrong room (activity), midwifery
      education, *197*

Y

Yantra, *44*

Z

Zen training, 43
'Zig zag thinking,' 175

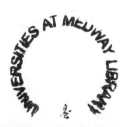